Veterinary Medicine: A Practical Approach

Veterinary Medicine: A Practical Approach

Edited by Kevin McLeod

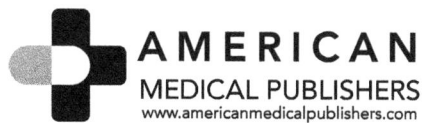

AMERICAN
MEDICAL PUBLISHERS
www.americanmedicalpublishers.com

American Medical Publishers,
41 Flatbush Avenue,
1st Floor, New York,
NY 11217, USA

Visit us on the World Wide Web at:
www.americanmedicalpublishers.com

ISBN: 978-1-63927-528-1

Cataloging-in-Publication Data

Veterinary medicine : a practical approach / edited by Kevin McLeod.
    p. cm.
Includes bibliographical references and index.
ISBN 978-1-63927-528-1
1. Veterinary medicine. 2. Animals--Diseases. 3. Animal health. I. McLeod, Kevin.
SF745 .V48 2022
636.089--dc23

Table of Contents

Preface

The branch of medicine which deals with the diagnosis, prevention and treatment of diseases, injury and disorders in animals is known as veterinary medicine. It covers all the species of animals including wild and domestic animals. It is involved in preventing the transmission of diseases from animals to humans. Veterinary medicine also deals with the welfare and basic biology of animals. Specialization in veterinary medicine could be in a particular category of animals such as companion animals or farm animals. It can also be in a particular area of medicine like anesthesiology or dentistry. This book provides comprehensive insights into the field of veterinary medicine. It strives to provide a fair idea about this discipline and to help develop a better understanding of the latest advances within this field. The book aims to equip students and experts with the advanced topics and upcoming concepts in this area.

The information contained in this book is the result of intensive hard work done by researchers in this field. All due efforts have been made to make this book serve as a complete guiding source for students and researchers. The topics in this book have been comprehensively explained to help readers understand the growing trends in the field.

I would like to thank the entire group of writers who made sincere efforts in this book and my family who supported me in my efforts of working on this book. I take this opportunity to thank all those who have been a guiding force throughout my life.

Editor

Correlation of post-operative pain and levels of creatin phosphokinase enzyme following ovariohysterectomy in cats

Tavakoli, A.*, Shafiee, B.

Department of Clinical Sciences, Faculty of Veterinary Medicine, Islamic Azad Univeristy, Garmsar Branch, Garmsar, Iran

Key words:
cortisol, creatin phosphokinase enzyme, feline, post-operative pain

Correspondence
Tavakoli, A.
Department of Clinical Sciences, Faculty of Veterinary Medicine, Islamic Azad Univeristy, Garmsar Branch, Garmsar, Iran

Email: azin.tavakoli@gamil.com

Abstract:

BACKGROUND: Recognition of pain is challenging in veterinary medicine due to lack of verbal communication and universal pain assessment system. Increase in biochemical parameters have been shown to have direct correlation with level of postoperative pain. **OBJECTIVES:** The purpose of the present study is to evaluate the serum levels of CPK and investigate any correlation in serum levels of CPK and postoperative pain following ovariohysterectomy in feline. **METHODS:** Conventional midline ovariohysterectomy was performed in 24 healthy female queens. Serum levels of cortisol, CPK and glucose were measured prior to surgery and at 1 and 3 and 24 hours after the surgery. Also, VAS was used to assess level of post-operative pain. Data was analyzed using repeated measure ANOVA. Spearman's rank correlation coefficient was used to identify any correlation between level of pain and CPK after the surgery. **RESULTS:** The score of pain significantly increased at 1 and 3 hours after the surgery in all of the cats (p=0.001). The concentration of cortisol and CPK significantly increased after the surgery in comparison to the values prior to surgery (p<0.001). Also, the concentrations increased significantly at 3 hours after the surgery compared to the values at 1 hour after the surgery (p<0.001). In 24 hours after the surgery results revealed that serum level of cortisol returned to its normal values but CPK was still higher compared to the values prior to surgery. Significant correlation was detected between the level of pain and CPK after surgery (p<0.05). **CONCLUSIONS:** It is concluded that there is a correlation with VAS score of pain and serum levels of Cortisol and CPK at early hours after the surgery. CPK might be used as an indicator of pain in early hours after the surgery in feline. However, the assessment of pain in cats is not possible based on its values alone.

Introduction

Pain is a result of tissue damage following surgery that is associated with decreased gastrointestional motility, tachycardia, respiratory depression, decreased food intake, and even delayed wound healing. Therefore, recognition of pain in patients is very valuable in pain management in veterinary medicine since it results in earlier recovery of the patient and, consequently, earlier return to normal conditions (Minto et al., 2013; Johnson, 1991; Taylor, 2000). Because of the lack of verbal communication, pain assessment in small animals seems challenging. Many pain scales and indicators of pain like visual analogue scale, numerical rating scale, simple descriptive scale, and behavioral and physiological response rating scales have been introduced in veterinary medicine but there is no universal or self-sufficient pain assessment system (Firth and Haldane, 1999; Holton, 1998; Mathews, 2000; Mich and Helleyr, 2008). Most of the developed scales are subjective and rely on many external factors. Due to the lack of a certain subjective assessment of pain in animals, a multimodal approach is considered accurate and appropriate (Maticic et al., 2010; Mich and Hellyer, 2008). Therefore, if there is a measurable quantitative indicator of pain to be proved to have a correlation with the level of pain, assessment of pain will be very precise, easy, and reliable.

The visual analogue scale is proved to be a sensitive and reliable behavioral scale to assess pain and has been successfully applied in many studies (Pascoe, 2000; Conzemius et al., 1996; Budsburg et al., 2002). However, the subjectivity of the scale and the difference among observers is still an issue (Grant, 2006; Maticic et al., 2010). In addition, biochemical parameters have been shown to be indicators of pain and stress in veterinary medicine. Serum levels of cortisol and blood glucose were used as a marker to interpret post-operative pain (Smith, 1996). Serum cortisol concentration is recognized as one of the most objective criteria for pain assessment in animals and found to have a direct relation with post-operative pain in dogs (Grisneaux et al., 1999; Feldsien et al., 2010). Also, another marker of muscle injury is Creatin phosphokinase enzyme (CPK) that has been used in the assessment of pain in veterinary medicine (Hancock et al., 2005). It is shown that the serum level of the enzyme in-

creases after the surgery and there is a correlation with its activity and the histologic changes of the back muscles (Kawaguchi et al., 1997; Arts et al., 2011). Since pain makes the animal reluctant to move and also the severity of pain is related to the invasiveness of the surgery, inflammation, and muscle injury (Maticic et al., 2010; Hancock et al., 2005), we hypothesized that if CPK has a correlation with scores of post-operative pain, it might be used as a biochemical indicator of pain. Therefore, this study was conducted to evaluate the serum levels of CPK and investigate any correlation in serum levels of CPK and post-operative pain following ovariohysterectomy in cats.

Materials and Methods

After approval was received from the University Research Committee, 24 healthy DSH queens were selected for the study. Their body weights ranged from 3.1 to 4.4 kg, and they were aged 6 months to 3.4 years with a mean of 1.1 ± 0.6 years. The cats were maintained at the same place and lighting conditions a few days prior to surgery. A control blood sample was taken from all the cats to measure the biochemical parameters including serum levels of glucose, cortisol, and CPK prior to surgery. The blood samples for the biochemical parameters analysis were collected from the cephalic vein at the same time. General anesthesia was performed with the administration of a combination of ketamin (Ketalar®, 10%, Alfasan, Woerden, Holland) 6.5 mg/kg and diazepam (Valium®, 10mg/2mL, Razi, Iran) 0.27 mg/kg, intravenously and continued by 1.5-2.2% isoflurane (Forane, Abbott Laboratories Ltd, UK) in oxygen following the intubation of the cats. A single dose of cefazolin (Ancef; Kefzol®, 1gr, Razi, Iran) 20 mg/kg/IV was administered as prophylaxis immediately prior to surgery. Also, all the cats received 0.5 mg/kg/ IV meloxicam (Metacam®, 7.5 mg/ml, Boehringer- Ingelheim, Germany) at the time of induction of anesthesia. Aseptic preparation of the patients' abdomen was performed in dorsal recumbency similarly. A midline skin incision was started from the umbilicus and extended 3-4 cm caudally. Following the identification of the more accessible ovary, the suspensory ligament and mesovarium were transected. Then, two simple ligatures using 3-0 polygalactin 910 were placed around the ovarian pedicle, and the ovary was transected and removed. The uterine artery and vein were ligated and severed 0.5 cm above the cervix. The stump was checked for hemorrhage and released to the abdomen. Finally, the incision was closed in a routine three-layer manner. The same surgeon performed all the surgeries.

Serum level of cortisol, CPK, and glucose were measured prior to surgery and at 1, 3, and 24 hours after the surgery. For cortisol, the blood samples were taken in the EDTA tubes and the samples were analyzed by a Dia Plus Immunoanlayser kit and using Roche Cobas e 411. For CPK and glucose, blood was taken in 1.5 mL microvettes and tested on an Idexx VetLab. In order to assess the level of pain, a trained observer recorded the score of pain in all the cats just before the surgery and at 1, 3, and 24 hours after the surgery using the Visual analogue scale (VAS) used by Conzemius et al. (1997) and Slingsby et al. (2000). The scale used subjective criteria including behavior, movements, mental status, temper, etc. An analysis of repeated measures with 95% Confidence Interval was carried out by the General Linear Model (GLM) procedure of the SPSS version 16.0. A p-value of less than 0.05 was statistically considered significant. A spearman's rank correlation coefficient was used to relate VAS scores to serum Cortisol, CPK, and glucose. Data were presented as Mean±SEM. A value of $p<0.05$ was considered significant.

Results

Mean pain score measured by Visual Analogue Scale was 2.3±0.22 and 2.8±0.29 and at 1 and 3 hours following the surgery respectively. The score of pain significantly increased at 1 and 3 hours after the surgery in all of the cats (p=0.001). Although 3 hours after the surgery Mean±SEM of pain score was higher compared to 1 hour after the surgery, the difference was insignificant ($p>0.05$). The cats did not seem to have any pains 24 hours after the surgery. The concentration of blood glucose was significantly increased one hour after the surgery (p=0.0013). However, the increase was insignificant in cats at 3 hours following the surgery ($p>0.05$). Results regarding serum levels of cortisol and CPK indicated that the concentration of cortisol and CPK significantly increased after the surgery in all the cats comparing to the values prior to the surgery ($p<0.001$). Moreover, the concentrations increased significantly at 3 hours after the surgery compared to the values at 1 hour after the surgery ($p<0.001$). 24 hours after the surgery, the results revealed that serum level of cortisol returned to its normal values but CPK still was higher compared to the values prior to surgery. Values of blood concentration of glucose, cortisol, and CPK are illustrated in Table 1. There was a strong correlation between the VAS pain scores and serum cortisol. Also, a significant correlation was detected between the VAS pain scores and CPK at 1 and 3 hours

Table 1. Serum levels of glucose (mg/dl), cortisol (µg/dl), CPK (IU/l), and score of pain (Mean±SEM) prior, 1, and 3 hours following ovariohysterectomy in cats. [abc] Values within rows with different superscripts differ (p<0.05).

	Prior to surgery	1 hr after the surgery	3 hr after the surgery	24 hr after the surgery
Glucose (mg/dl)	129±21.21[a]	323.2±47.05[b]	256±74.9 [a]	198±48.3 [a]
Cortisol (µg/dl)	3.21±0.32 [a]	6.93±0.76 [b]	9.00±0.96 [c]	4.33±0.83 [a]
CPK (IU/l)	670.18±130.33 [a]	2752.18±358.27 [b]	3332.27±481.88 [c]	3248.23±544.33 [c]

after the surgery (p<0.05; Table 1).

Discussion

Successful pain management requires a valid and reliable assessment of the degree of pain. Because of the inability of animals to describe the level of pain they suffer, it is believed that the accurate recognition of pain needs a multimodal approach and the application of multiple parameters (Maticic et al., 2010). Thus, in this research we used VAS that has been successfully used to evaluate pain in dogs and cats to evaluate post-operative pain (Conzemius et al., 1997; Slingsby et al., 2000). In addition, because biochemical parameters have been used as markers of pain in veterinary medicine (Maticic et al., 2010), the alteration of serum concentration of cortisol, CPK, and glucose were assessed to investigate any correlation with pain.

Ovariohysterectomy produces mild to moderate post-operative pain and is used as a standard surgery to assess pain in animals (Genta and Fee, 1992). The score of pain significantly increased at the early hours after the surgery and decreased a day following the surgery. The concentration of cortisol significantly increased at 1 and 3 hours after the surgery and was very close to its normal values 24 hours after the surgery. The dynamic of changes of serum cortisol was very similar to VAS pain scores and a significant correlation was identified between these two parameters (p<0.05). Serum cortisol concentration is recognized as one of the most objective criteria for pain assessment in animals and found to have a direct relation with post-operative pain (Smith et al., 1996; Feldsien et al., 2010). Secretion of cortisol together with glucose typically increase during stress, so they are not specific indicators of pain (Maticic et al., 2010). Both the duration and extent of trauma during the surgery will result in an increase in the serum levels of cortisol. However, because the condition,

duration, and type of the surgery were similar to the patients, the increase in cortisol was mainly due to pain in this study. The changes in blood glucose did not correlate to the VAS score of pain. Therefore, the blood level of glucose was not a reliable marker of pain in the present study because it decreased at three hours after the surgery, the time that cats had the highest pain score and were greatly suffering. Glucose has been used as an indicator of pain in newborns and animals (Smith et al., 1996). Similar results were obtained in cranial cruciate rupture surgery in dogs by Maticic et al. (2010).

In the present study, CPK increased significantly at early hours following the surgery and remained high a day after the surgery. It was during the time VAS scores of pain indicated that the cats did not suffer from pain generally. The highest reported pain score was between 3 to 6 hours after ovariohysterectomy, and the use of analgesic medications is not essential after 24 hours following the procedure (Slingsby et al., 2000, Carpenter et al., 2004). There was a correlation between VAS scores of pain and CPK changes at 1 and 3 hours after the surgery. The values of CPK stayed above the normal values, while VAS scores and cortisol indicated that the cats did not experience pain 24 hours after the operation. Different results have been reported in the literature in this regard. Kawaguchi et al. in 1997 reported that the serum level of CPK reaches a maximal value 1 day after the surgery. However, Shin et al. indicated that no significant difference in the serum levels of CPK occurred 24 hours after the surgery compared with the pre-operative condition (Shin et al., 2008) .

Creatin phosphokinase has been reported to be an indicator of muscle damage and operative trauma (Hancock et al., 2005). The increase in creatinine phosphokinase has been shown to occur in response to anesthesia with halothane and propofol, as well as with intramuscular injections (Aktas et al., 1997; Maticic et al., 2010). None of the injections prior and during the procedure were intramuscular, so other sources of pain were eliminated for interpreting CPK values. Pain causes the animal to be reluctant to move after the operation. The recumbency following the surgery in addition to intra-operative trauma leads to muscle injury. This might lead to an increase in the values of CPK. Although CPK increases with skeletal muscle injury and recumbency, it has not been reported as a reliable indicator for pain in dogs (Austin et al., 2003; Hancock et al. 2005).

Conclusion: The results of our study indicated the concordance of the dynamics of pain measured by the VAS with cortisol and CPK at the early hours after the surgery. These findings demonstrated that CPK is a good indicator of pain in cats a few hours after the operation when the highest score of pain is expected. However, it is not recommended for assessing pain in cats based on its values alone. In addition, glucose was not a reliable indicator of pain.

Acknowledgments

The authors would like to acknowledge Dr. Mahmoodi Ashtiani and Dr. Akbarein for their sincere collaboration in collecting and statistical analysis of this study data.

References

1. Aktas, B.M., Vinclair, P., Autefage, A., Lefebvre, H.P., Toutain, P.L., Braun, J.P. (1997) In vivo quantification of muscle damage in dogs after general anaesthesia with halothane and propofol. J Small Anim Pract. 38: 565-569.

2. Arts, M., Brand, R., der Kallen, B.V., Nijeholt, G.L., Peul, W. (2011) Does minimally invasive lumbar disc surgery result in less muscle injury than conventional surgery? A randomized controlled trial. Eur Spine J. 20: 51-57.

3. Austin, B., Lanz, O., Hamilton, S.M., Broadstone, R.V., Martin, R.A. (2003) Laparoscopic ovariohysterectomy in nine dogs. J Am Anim Hosp Assoc. 39: 391-396.

4. Budsberg, S.C., Cross, A.R., Quandt, L., Pablo, L.S., Runk, A.R. (2002) Evaluation of intravenous administration of meloxicam for perioperative pain management following stifle joint surgery in dogs. Am J Vet Res. 63: 1557-1563.

5. Carpenter, R.E., Wilson, D.V., Evans, A.T. (2004) Evaluation of intraperitoneal and incisional lidocaine or bupivacaine for analgesia following ovariohysterectomy in the dog. Vet Anaesth Analg. 31: 46-52.

6. Conzemius, M.G., Hill, C.M., Sammarco, J.L., Perkowski, S.Z. (1997) Correlation between subjective and objective measurements used to determine severity of postoperative pain in dogs. J Am Vet Med Assoc. 210: 1619-1622.

7. Feldsien, J.D., Wilke, V.L., Evans, B.R., Conzemius, M.G. (2010) Serum cortisol concentration and force plate analysis in the assessment of pain associated with sodium urate-induced acute synovitis in dogs. Am J Vet Res. 71: 940-945.

8. Firth, A.M., Haldane, S.M. (1999) Development of a scale to evaluate postoperative pain in dogs. J Am Vet Med Assoc. 214: 651-659.

9. Genta, R., Fee, J.P.H. (1992) Pain on injection of propofol: comparison of lidocaine with metoclopramide. Br J Anaesth. 69: 316-7.

10. Grant, D. (2006) Pain Management in Small Animals: A Manual for Veterinary Nurses and Technicians. Butterworth-Heinemann. Edinburgh, London, New York, Oxford, Philadelphia, St. Louis, Sydney, Toronto. p. 74-75.

11. Grisneaux, E., Pibarot, P., Dupuis, J., Blais, D. (1999) Comparison of ketoprofen and carprofen administered prior to orthopedic surgery for control of postoperative pain in dogs. J Am Vet Med Assoc. 215: 1105-10.

12. Hancock, R.B., Lanz, O.I., Warldon, D.R., Duncan, R.B., Broadstone, R.V., Hendrix, P.K. (2005) Comparison of postoperative pain following ovariohysterectomy via harmonic scalpel assisted laparoscopy versus traditional celiotomy in dogs. Vet Surg. 34: 273-282.

13. Holton, L.L., Scott, E.M., Nolan, A.M., Reid, J.,

Welsh, E., Flaherty, D. (1998) Comparison of three methods used for assessment of pain in dogs. J Am Vet Med Assoc. 212: 61-66.

14. Johnson, J.M. (1991) The Veterinarians responsibility: assessing acute pain in dogs and cats part1. Compend Contin Educ Prac Vet. 13: 804-7.

15. Kawaguchi, Y., Matsui, H., Tsuji, H. (1997) Changes in serum creatine phosphokinase MM isoenzyme after lumbar spine surgery. Spine J. 22: 1018-1023.

16. Mathews, K.A. (2000) Pain assessment and general approach to management. Vet Clin North Am Sm Anim Prac. 30: 729-755.

17. Maticic, D., Stejskal, M., Pecin, M., Kreszinger, M., Pirkic, B., Vnuk, D., Smolec, O., Rumenjak, V. (2010) Correlation of pain assessment parameters in dogs with cranial cruciate surgery Vet Arhiv. 80: 597-609.

18. Mich, P.M., Hellyer, P.M. (2008) Objective, Categoric Methods for Assessing Pain and Analgesia. In: Handbook of Veterinary Pain Management. Gaynor, J.S., Muir, W.W. III, (eds.). (2nd ed.) Mosby, St. Louis, USA. p. 78-109.

19. Minto, B.W., Rodrigues, L.C., Steagall, P.V.M., Monteiro, E.R., Brandão, C.V.S. (2013) Assessment of postoperative pain after unilateral mastectomy using two different surgical techniques in dogs. Acta Vet Scand. 55: 60-69.

20. Pascoe, P.J. (2000) Perioperative pain management. Vet Clin North Am Small Anim Pract. 30: 917-932.

21. Shin, D.A., Kim, K.N., Shin, H.C., Yoon, H. (2008) The efficacy of microendoscopic discectomy in reducing iatrogenic muscle injury. J Neurosurg Spine. 8: 39-43.

22. Slingsby, L.S., Water-Pearson, A.E. (2000) Postoperative analgesia in the cat after ovariohysterectomy by the use of carprofen, ketoprofen, meloxicam or tolfenamic acid. J Small Anim Pract. 41: 447-450.

23. Smith, J.D., Allen, S.W., Quandt, J.E., Tackett, R.L.(1996) Indicators of postoperative pain in cats and correlation with clinical criteria. Am J Vet Res. 57:1674-1678.

24. Taylor, P.M., Houlton, J.E.F. (1984) Post-operative analgesia in the dog: A comparison of morphine, buprenorphine, and pentazocine. J Small Anim Pract. 25: 437-451.

Effect of subacute exposure of nano Zinc particles on oxidative stress parameters in rats

Hejazy, M.[1], Koohi, M.K.[2*]

[1]*Department of Basic Sciences, Faculty of Veterinary Medicine, University of Tabriz, Tabriz, Iran*

[2]*Department of Basic Sciences, Faculty of Veterinary Medicine, University of Tehran, Tehran, Iran*

Key words:

FRAP, GPx, nano Zinc, oxidative stress, rat

Correspondence

Koohi, M.K.

Department of Basic Sciences,
Faculty of Veterinary Medicine,
University of Tehran, Tehran,
Iran

Email: mkkoohi@ut.ac.ir

Abstract:

BACKGROUND: Zinc (Zn) is one of the most important essential elements in the body of animals and plants. Zinc plays a significant role in the structure of more than 300 different proteins and in many life supporting biochemical and metabolic processes such as cellular respiration and protection against free radicals. Nanoparticles of zinc are the new form of Zinc used in cosmetic and personal care products and also in livestock feed and food packaging. **OBJECTIVES:** The aim of this study was to evaluate the effects of several sizes and doses of zinc nanoparticles on antioxidant defense system in rat compared to controls. **METHODS:** Zinc nanoparticles (10, 20 and 30 nm) at 3 doses (3, 10 and 100 mg/kg bw) were administrated orally for 28 days among 9 experimental groups (n=5). One experimental group was treated orally with ZnCl2 (100 mg/kg bw) for 28 days and control group received normal saline (n=5). After 28 days, the rat was decapitated and serum was separated from the blood samples. The ferric reducing ability of Plasma (FRAP), thiobarbituric acid reactive substances (TBARS) and activity of glutathione peroxidase (GPx), and superoxide dismutase (SOD) enzymes in serum samples were measured as biomarkers of oxidative stress and compared with control group. **RESULTS:** This survey showed that zinc nanoparticles cause induction of GPx and SOD activity (p<0.05) and also increased the level of TBARS (p<0.05). This assay also showed zinc nanoparticles cause significant decrease in total antioxidant activity of plasma (FRAP) (p<0.001). **CONCLUSIONS:** Nano zinc induced oxidative stress in a dose dependent manner in large sizes, while their effects depend on the level of ionization in small sizes.

Introduction

Zinc (Zn) is one of the most important essential elements in the body of animals and plants. Zinc plays a significant role in the structure of more than 300 different proteins, metalloenzymes and transcription factors. Zinc is involved in many life supporting biochemical and metabolic processes such as the metabolism of protein, lipid, and carbohydrates, cellular respiration, detoxification of free radicals, and protection against lipid peroxidation (Hendy et al., 2001; Yousef et al., 2002; Carlson et al., 2004; Prasad, 2009; Frassinetti, 2006).

Zinc deficiency and the increase in the

production of reactive oxygen species lead to the generation of free radicals and lipid peroxidation in the tissues. A wide range of physiologic defects including disorders of the skin, growth retardation, and impaired neurologic, reproductive and immune systems are associated with zinc deficiency. Zinc deficiency alters the activities of some enzymes such as copper/zinc superoxide dismutase (Cu-Zn SOD). As an antioxidant, zinc inhibits the induction of oxidative stress through protecting sulfhydryl groups of proteins against free radicals, reducing the formation of free radicals by protective mechanisms (Jomova and Valko, 2011; Valko and Morris, 2005; Prasad, 2008).

Zinc nanoparticles (zinc NPs) are particles between 1 and 100 nanometers in size. Increasing the surface area of the particles changes the pressure and surface properties, viscosity and magnetic properties of the particles, leading to a change in the distance between the particles or their atoms, an increase in the ionization potentiality as well as a change in chemical reactions of the matter. Numerous applications of zinc NPs paved the way for oral, dermal and respiratory contacts with them. Oral contact with zinc nanoparticles happens through zinc supplements in the livestock food and food packaging. Dermal contact occurs through sunscreen, cosmetics, paint, paper and plastics. Respiratory contact happens in working environments (paint and nanoparticle producing factories). Despite the commercial production and widespread applications of zinc nanoparticles the safety of zinc NPs for humans, animals and other biological systems is still a controversial problem (Vandebriel and De Jong, 2012).

Some previous studies suggested that zinc nanoparticles are safe and revealed protective effects of zinc NPs against oxidative injuries (Afifi et al. 2015; Dawei et al., 2009; Malekshahinia et al., 2012). However, some other studies showed that exposure to zinc NPs resulted in oxidative stress and other adverse effects on animal and human health as well as cell cultures (Yousef, 2015; Xiong et al., 2011; Xia et al., 2008; Li et al., 2012). Some other studies showed that dissolved zinc ions induced metallothionein synthesis, and enhanced cellular resistance to oxidative stress. However, at higher doses zinc ions induced oxidative stress injuries. This suggested that different oxidative response mainly depend on the effect of size, dose, duration and route of exposure of zinc NPs (Zhang et al., 2012; Hejazy et al., 2012)

The present study aims to investigate the effects of subacute oral exposure to different sizes and doses of zinc NPs in comparison to bulk zinc on the oxidative stress parameters in rats.

Materials and Methods

Characterization of Zinc nanoparticles: Zinc NPs powder with 99.9 % purity, grey color, approximate concentration 0.2-0.4 g/m3 and specific surface area of 0.2-0.4 g/m3 was bought from Nanoshel Company. This powder is provided from zinc metal with high purity via the process of vaporization. The process of vaporization produces zinc with high purity, very small, very reactive and very reactant particles. The size and shape of the particles were determined by transmission electron microscopy (TEM). The particles were in three sizes of 10, 20 and 30 nm and they were mostly spherical.

Preparation of particle suspension: Prior to use, the particles were suspended in 1 % sodium carboxy methyl cellulose. The particles were dispersed by ultrasonic vibration for 15 min, and some glass beads were added to avoid aggregation of the particles in the suspension (Wang et al., 2006).

Animals and treatment: 60 adult (10-week-old) male Wistar rats, weighing 253±25 g, were used in the study. During the whole experiment, animals were housed in controlled conventional conditions (temperature, 22±2 °C; relative humidity, 50-70 %; 12- h light-dark cycle). They were given free access to water and a conventional rodent pellet (2,390 kcal kg−1 metabolic energy and 10,320 kcal kg−1 digestible energy; crude protein, 19.5 %; crude fiber, 10 %; phosphor, 0.69 %; and calcium, 0.76 %).The design of experiments was approved by the local ethics committee. After a period of 2 weeks of acclimation, the rats were randomly divided into 9 experimental and control groups containing five animals each. The administrable zinc nanoparticles in each size (10, 20 and 30 nm) with 3, 10 and 100 mg/kg doses were mixed in 1% carboxy methyl cellulose solution by ultrasonic machine for 15 minutes. To prevent the aggregation of nanoparticles, glass globes were added to the suspension and it was subjected to vortex before every application (Wang et al., 2006). The administration of nanoparticles was done orally by gavage for 28 days.

. The control group received clean water without zinc plus carboxy methyl cellulose.

. Group 1-3: 3, 10 and 100 mg/kg doses of 10 nm Zinc NPs.

. Group 4-6: 3, 10 and 100 mg/kg doses of 20 nm Zinc NPs.

. Group 7-9: 3, 10 and 100 mg/kg doses of 30 nm Zinc NPs.

. Group 10: 100 mg/kg dose of bulk Zinc chloride.

At the end of the administration period the rats were anesthetized by chloroform and decapitated and blood sample was collected in the citrate-containing tubes. Blood serum was separated after centrifugation and kept at -80 oC until testing time.

Measurement of Oxidative Stress Biomarkers (Measurement of Plasma Total Antioxidant Capacity): Ferric Reducing Ability of Plasma (FRAP) method was used to assess plasma total antioxidant capacity. This method evaluates the ability of plasma in reducing ferric ions to ferrous. The basis of this assay is the formation of colorful complex of ferrous tripyridyltriazine [Fe (II)-TPTZ]. The amount of FRAP (micromol/liter) is achieved by comparing the absorption changes in 593 nm in the sample with solutions containing distinct concentrations of ferrous ion (Benzie and Strain, 1996).

Measurement of TBARS (ThiobarbituricAcid Reactive Substances): Plasma levels of MDA were estimated by the thiobarbituric acid reaction according to the method of Ledwoz et al. (1986). Briefly, 1 ml of plasma was mixed with 2 ml of freshly prepared thiobarbituric acid-trichloric acid-hydrochloric acid (TCA-TBA-HCl) reagent (30 g trichloroacetic acid, 0.75 g thiobarbituric acid and 4.2 ml concentrated HCl were mixed and diluted to 200 ml with distilled water) and 1.5 µl butylhydroxytoluene (0.05%). This mixture was boiled for 30 min. in a boiling water bath, and cooled to room temperature. n-Butanol extractable layer was centrifuged at 3000 ×g for 10 min., supernatant layer was removed and its absorbance was read at 535 nm. Concentrations of TBARS (nmol/mL) were determined from the standard curve using malondialdehyde bis (S4258497 537,

Table 1. FRAP, TBARS, SOD and Glutathione peroxidase levels in zinc and nano zinc treated groups. [a] Significant decrease (p<0.05) compared to control group. [b] Significant increase (p<0.05) compared to control group.

Treatment groups	FRAP (micromol/liter) (Mean±SD)	TBARS (nanomol/ mL) (Mean±SD)	Superoxide dismutase(U/L) (Mean±SD)	Glutathione peroxidase (U/L) (Mean±SD)
Control group	1.761±0.0377	2.714±0.286	0.017±0.001	422.3±69.15
Zinc	1.855±0.1081	2.425±1.156	0.016±0.002	440.1±56.7
Nano Zn 10 nm (3mg/kg)	1.263±0.0915[a]	4.033±1.06[b]	0.019±0.005	175.4±48.8[a]
Nano Zn 10 nm (10mg/kg)	1.281±0.01513[a]	4.933±1.343[b]	0.017±0.001	246±35.44[a]
Nano Zn 10 nm (100mg/kg)	1.311±0.0118[a]	5.467±1.286[b]	0.022±0.003[b]	281.8±36.42[a]
Nano Zn 20 nm (3mg/kg)	1.08±0.1324[a]	3.393±1.097	0.012±0.001[a]	672±12.84[b]
Nano Zn 20 nm (10mg/kg)	1.307±0.445[a]	5.928±0.444[b]	0.015±0.002[a]	722.5±33.69[b]
Nano Zn 20 nm (100mg/kg)	1.395±0.4160	7.095±0.837[b]	0.026±0.001[b]	906.1±78.78[b]
Nano Zn 30 nm (3mg/kg)	1.579±0.0252[a]	4.333±0.650[b]	0.017±0.004	513±145
Nano Zn 30 nm (10mg/kg)	1.66±0.0816	4.367±0.611[b]	0.022±0.002[b]	618.5±183
Nano Zn 30 nm (100mg/kg)	1.644±0.346	7.933±0.404[b]	0.020±0.004[b]	870.2±93.21[b]

Merck Company, Tehran, Iran).

Measurement of Superoxide Dismutase (SOD): Superoxide Dismutase is involved in the detoxification of O2 toxic radical. In this method, Xanthine and Xanthine oxidase are used to produce superoxide radicals. They react with 2-(4-iodophenyl)-3-(4-nitrophenyl)-5-phenyl-tetrazolium chloride (INT) and red color of formazan is produced which is measured at 505nm wavelength. If SOD enzyme exists in the superoxide radicals sample, it is turned into hydrogen peroxide and O2, inhibiting the production of red color of formazan. The activity of SOD enzyme is determined by the degree of its inhibition of this reaction. One unit of SOD restrains the INT reduction speed up to 50% or restrains nicotinamide adenine dinucleotide phosphate (NADPH) oxidation up to 50% under the measurement concentrations. SOD was done by using the commercial kit of Ransod (Randox) on the basis of colorimetric method with some modifications.

Measurement of Glutathione Peroxidase: This method is based on the method introduced by Valentine and Paglia (1967). Glutathione peroxidase enzyme catalyses glutathione oxidation reaction (GSH) by Cumenehydroperoxide. In the presence of glutathione reductase and NADPH, oxidized glutathione (GSSG) turns into reduced glutathione again and this reduction is simultaneous with oxidation of NADPH into NADP+. In this reaction, light absorption reduction is measured at 340 nm wavelength. Glutathione peroxidase measurement was done by using the commercial kit of Ransod (Randox) on the basis of enzymatic method with some modifications.

Statistical analysis: Statistical analysis was done using Graph Pad InStat, version 3.06 (Graph Pad Software, Inc). The measures were expressed according to Means ± SD. T test analysis was performed to show significance between control and others groups. p<0.05 was considered statistically significant.

Results

In nano zinc (10 nm) treated groups, the amount of FRAP significantly decreased compared to the control group (p<0.05), it seems that the amount of FRAP has increased by increasing the doses and sizes of zinc nanoparticles (Table 1). As shown in

Table 1, it seems that the amount of malondialdehyde has increased by increasing the administered dose of zinc nanoparticles. The administration of 10 nm zinc nanoparticles significantly decreased ($p<0.0001$) the amount of GPx compared to controls. The administration of 20 and 30 nm zinc nanoparticles in all doses increased the amount of GPx ($p<0.0001$) in a dose-dependent manner (Table 1).

Discussion

Previous studies showed the antioxidative effects of bulk zinc (Powell and Saul 2000; Bray et al., 1990; Prasad and Anada, 2004; Rostan and Elizabeth, 2002; Zago et al., 2001; Sun et al., 2006). As shown in our study, in contrast to the bulk zinc, nano zinc remarkably decreased plasma total antioxidant capacity, especially in lower sizes. It can be due to the fast release of the high amount of Zn^{2+} ion from the administered zinc nanoparticles (Reed, 2012). Previous studies have shown that fast solubility of Zn^{2+} ion of nano zinc in the cell and other biological systems leads to the fast access of the cells and the biological systems to zinc ions (Deng, 2009; Ma et al., 2012). Zn^{2+} seems to be responsible for inducing oxidative stress.

In groups which received the smallest sizes of nanoparticles (10 nm), the amount of MDA increased whereas the amount of GPx and FRAP decreased. The lower levels of GPx along with the decrease of FRAP could cause more oxidative stress effects and raise the amount of MDA. In higher doses and sizes SOD and GPx levels increased. These observations give rise to the hypothesis that nanoparticles of smaller sizes can induce more potent oxidative stress damages as

other studies reported that the high toxicity of nanoparticles in cells increases with the reduction of size (Hanley et al., 2009; Wang et al., 2008; Cho et al., 2011). However, Guo et al. (2008) showed that the toxic effects of zinc nanoparticles in leukemia cells are related to their surface structure and dose-dependent effects are insignificant.

Compared with Wang et al.'s (2006) and (2008) studies, it seems that smaller sizes of nanoparticles with lower doses and larger size nanoparticles with higher doses produce more toxic effects. It seems release of Zn^{+2} ions in biological solutions is more convenient at lower sizes and doses of nanoparticles, while in higher doses and sizes of nano zinc, aggregation of nanoparticles decrease the release of Zn^{+2} ions and toxic effects.

Some other studies on the laboratory animals and cell culture mediums showed time dependent toxicity of zinc NPs. The duration of exposure to nano zinc plays an influential role in oxidative stress induction and also defensive responses (Bakhshiani and Fazilati, 2014; Trevisan, 2014; Valdiglesias et al., 2013). It seems that antioxidant defense system is induced gradually during the time of exposure to adapt animals against the nanoparticles adverse effects of oxidative injury (Bakhshiani and Fazilati, 2014; Trevisan, 2014). Some studies reported induction and activation of SOD and metallothioneins after nano zinc administration, while significant expressions of metallothioneins by larger sizes and higher doses of nano sized zinc were observed in our complementary studies (Xiao-bo et al., 2009; Hejazy et al., 2014). However, Zhang et al. (2012) reported that at low concentration of nano zinc, dissolved zinc ions induced metallothionein synthesis, enhanced cellular resistance to oxidative stress. At higher doses, excessive zinc destroyed mitochondrial function and cell membrane and caused cell necrosis of mouse alveolar macrophages (MH-S).

Similar to our study, some in vitro and in vivo studies showed that oxidative stress has a principle role in nano zinc induced cytotoxicity (Ahamed et al., 2011; Lenz et al., 2009; Huang et al., 2010; Kim et al., 2010; Osmond and McCall, 2010; Kao et al., 2012; Cho et al., 2011). Yousef and Mohamed (2015) reported increase in malondialdehyde (MDA), decrease in glutathione peroxidase (GPx) of rat liver tissue in response to oral administration of 500mg/kg nano zinc particles for 10 days. Zhao et al. (2013) showed acute ZnO nanoparticles exposure induces developmental toxicity, oxidative stress and DNA damage in embryo-larval zebra fish. Surekha et al. (2012) showed a significant decrease in collagen content and oxidative stress with an inverse dose relationship in nano zinc oxide-treated rats. Sharma et al. (2012) reported induction of oxidative stress, DNA damage and apoptosis in mouse liver after sub-acute oral exposure to zinc oxide nanoparticles. Wong et al. (2010) reported significant up-regulation of SOD, MT and HSP70 and oxidative stress in nano zinc oxide treated marine organisms.

Lina et al. (2009) reported that supplemental zinc oxide in broilers chicken significantly increased the activity of glutathione peroxidase and serum antioxidant and decreased MDA content in serum and liver of chickens. They also reported decrease in serum Nitric oxide and Hydroxyl radicals and increase in the activity of resisting superoxide anion free radical in liver. Decrease of SOD, catalase and GSH levels and increase in MDA content in the kidney,

spleen and heart of mice treated with the zinc oxide nanoparticles was reported by Fang et al. (2010).

However, some studies concluded protective effects of nano zinc against oxidative stress. Malekshahinia et al. (2012) reported that endurance exercise induced oxidative stress in the male reproductive system and can be protected by nano zinc oxide supplementation. Afifi et al. (2015) showed significant decrease in the MDA levels and significant increase in the activity and mRNA expression of SOD, CAT, GPx, GRD, and GST, in testicular tissue of diabetic rats treated with Zinc oxide NPs. Dawei et al. (2010) revealed protective effects of nano zinc on the primary culture mice intestinal epithelial cells against oxidative injury.

Nano zinc particles are expected to be more toxic than their bulk ones because of their greater surface reactivity and their capacity to penetrate into cells and organisms (Ispas et al., 2009; Mironava et al., 2010). Dissolved Zinc ions increase in the cells, leading to increase of intracellular ROS generation, membrane damage, Ca2+flux and mitochondrial activity impairment, apoptosis, inhibition of mitochondrial respiratory chain. ROS generation leads to oxidative stress and in consequence, lipid peroxidation and oxidative DNA damage (Xiong et al., 2011; Vandebriel & De Jong, 2012).

As reported in different studies, our study showed change of oxidative stress parameters in treated animals. However, different results in various studies may relate to different physicochemical properties of the nanoparticles such as size, surface shape, agglomeration property, liberation and solubility. Moreover, exposure duration, animal species, administration route may have some effects on oxidative stress parameters.

Dose response relationship of Zinc nanoparticles must be investigated in more detail. In some cases inverse dose dependency effects were reported. Therefore, more experiments are required to understand the dose -response and size-response relationship of nano Zinc. New concept of dose metric that was introduced in nanotoxicology should be further investigated.

References

Afifi, M., Almaghrabi, O.A., Kadasa, N.M. (2015) Ameliorative effect of zinc oxide nanoparticles on antioxidants and sperm characteristics in streptozotocin-induced diabetic rat testes. Biol Med Res Int. dx.doi.org/10.1155/2015/153573.

Ahamed, M., Akhtar, M.J., Raja, M., Ahmad, I., Siddiqui, M.K.J., AlSalhi, M.S., Alrokayan, S.A. (2011) ZnO nanorod-induced apoptosis in human alveolar adenocarcinoma cells via p53, survivin and bax/bcl-2 pathways: role of oxidative stress. Nanomedicine: Nanotech, Biol Med. 7: 904-913.

Bakhshiani, S., Fazilati, M. (2014) Vitamin C can reduce toxic effects of nano zinc oxide. Int Res J Biol Sci. 3: 65-70.

Benzie, I.F., Strain J.J. (1996) The ferric reducing ability of plasma (FRAP) as a measure of "antioxidant power": the FRAP assay. Anal Biochem. 239: 70-6.

Bray, T.M., Bettger, W.J. (1990) "The physiological role of zinc as an antioxidant." Free Radical Biol Med. 8.3: 281-291.

Carlson, D., Poulsen, H.D., Sehested, J. (2004) Influence of weaning and effect of post weaning dietary zinc and copper on electrophysiological response to glucose, theophylline and 5-HT in piglet small intestinal mucosa. Biochem Physiol A. 137: 757-65.

Cho, S., Sayes, C.M., Reed, K.L. (2011) Nanoscale and fine zinc oxide particles: can in vitro assays accurately forecast lung hazards following inhalation exposures. Environ Sci Technol. 43: 7939-7945.

Dawei, A., Zhisheng, W., Anuo, Z. (2009) Protective effect of nano-ZnO on primary culture mice intestinal epithelial cell in in vitro against oxidative stress. Int J Nanotech Appl. 3: 1-6.

Deng, X., Luan, Q., Chen, W., Wang, Y., Wu, M., Zhang, H., Jiao, Z. (2009) Nanosized zinc oxide particles induce neural stem cell apoptosis. Nanotecholgt. 20: 115101.

Fang, H., Li, M., Cui, Y.B. (2010) Impact of Nano-ZnO Particles on the antioxidant system of mice. J Environ Health. 1: 010.

Frassinetti, S., Bronzetti, G.L., Caltavuturo, L., Cini, M., Della Croce, C. (2006) The role of zinc in life: a review. J Environ Path Toxicol Oncol. 25: 3.

Guo, D., Wu, C., Jiang, H., Li, Q., Wang, X., Chen, B. (2008) Synergistic cytotoxic effect of different sized ZnO nanoparticles and daunorubicin against leukemia cancer cells under UV irradiation. J Photochem Photobiol B: Biol. 93: 119-126.

Hanley, C., Thurber, A., Hanna, C., Punnoose, A., Zhang, J., Wingett, D.G. (2009) The influences of cell type and ZnO nanoparticle size on immune cell cytotoxicity and cytokine induction. Nanoscale Res Lett. 4: 1409-1420.

Hejazy, M., Koohi, M.K., Asadi, F., Behrouz, H.J. (2014) Induction of renal metallothionein expression by nano-zinc in cadmium-treated rats. Comp Clin Pathol. 23: 1477-1483.

Hendy, H.A., Yousef, M.I., Naga, N.I. (2001) Effect of dietary zinc deficiency on hematological and biochemical parameters and concentrations of zinc, copper, and iron in growing rats. Toxicology. 167: 163-70.

Huang, C.C., Aronstam, R.S., Chen D.R., Huang, Y.W. (2010) Oxidative stress, calcium homeostasis, and altered gene expression in human lung epithelial cells exposed to ZnO nanoparticles. Toxicol In Vitro. 24: 45-55.

Ispas, C., Andreescu, D., Patel, A., Goia, D.V., Andreescu, S., Wallace, K.N (2009). Toxicity and developmental defects of different sizes and shape nickel nano particles in Zebra fish. Environ Sci Technol. 43: 6349-6356.

Jomova, K., Valko, M. (2011) Advances in metal-induced oxidative stress and human disease. Toxicology. 283: 65-87.

Kao, Y.Y, Chen, Y.C., Cheng, T.J., Chiung, Y.M., Liu, P.S. (2012) Zinc oxide nanoparticles interfere with zinc ion homeostasis to cause cytotoxicity. Toxicol Sci. 125: 462-472.

Kim, Y.H., Fazlollahi, F., Kennedy, I.M., Yacobi, N.R., Hamm-Alvarez, S.F., Borok, Z., Crandall, E.D. (2010) Alveolar epithelial cell injury due to zinc oxide nanoparticle exposure. Am J Respir Crit Care Med. 182: 1398-1409.

Ledwoż, A., Michalak, J., Stpień, A., Kadziołka, A. The relationship between plasma triglycerides, cholesterol, total lipids and lipid peroxidation products during human atherosclerosis. Clinica Chimica Acta. 155: 275-283.

Lenz, A.G., Karg, E., Lentner, B., Dittrich, V., Brandenberger, C., Rothen-Rutishauser, B., Schmid, O. (2009) A dose-controlled system for air-liquid interface cell exposure and application to zinc oxide nanoparticles. Part Fibre Toxicol. 6: b16.

Li, J.H., Liu, X.R., Zhang, Y., Tian, F.F., Zhao, G.Y., Jiang, F.L., Liu, Y. (2012) Toxicity of nano zinc oxide to mitochondria. Toxicol Res. 1: 137-144.

Lina, T., FengHua, Z., HuiYing, R., JianYang, J., WenLi, L. (2009) Effects of nano-zinc oxide on antioxidant function in broilers. Chin J Anim Nutr. 21: 534-539.

Ma, H., Williams, P.L., Diamond, S.A. Ecotoxicity of manufactured ZnO nanoparticles - A review (2012) Environ Pollut. 17: 76-85.

Malekshahinia, H., TeymuriZamaneh, H., Dorostghola, M., Kesmati M., NajafzadehVarzi, H. (2012) Effect of nano zinc oxide supplementation on testicular oxidative stress in adult male rats exposed to endurance exercise. Int J Fertil Steril. 6: 63.

Mironava, T., Hadjiargyrou, M., Simon, M., Jurukovski, V., Rafailovich, M.H. (2010) Gold nanoparticles cellular toxicity and recovery: Effect of size, concentration and exposure time. Nanotoxicology. 4: 120-37.

Osmond, M.J., McCall, M.J. (2010) Zinc oxide nanoparticles in modern sunscreens: an analysis of potential exposure and hazard. Nanotoxicoogy. 4: 15-41.

Paglia, D.E., Valentine, W.N. (1967) Studies on the quantitative and qualitative characterization of erythrocyte glutathione peroxidase. J Lab Clin Med. 70: 158-169.

Powell Saul, R. (2000) The antioxidant properties of zinc. J Nutr. 130.5: 1447-1454.

31.Prasad, A.S. (2009) Zinc: role in immunity, oxidative stress and chronic inflammation. Curr Opin Clin Nutr Metab Care. 12: 646-652.

Prasad, A.S. (2008) Clinical, immunological, anti-inflammatory and antioxidant roles of zinc. Exp Gerontol. 43: 370-377.

Prasad, A.S., Bao, B., Beck, F.W., Kucuk, O., Sarkar, F.H. (2004) Antioxidant effect of zinc in humans. Free Radical Biol Med. 37: 1182-1190.

Reed, R.B., Ladner, D.A., Higgins, C.P., Westerhoff, P., Ranville, J.F. (2012) Solubility of nano-zinc oxide in environmentally and biologically important matrices. Environ Toxicol Chem. 31: 93-99.

Rostan, E.F., DeBuys, H.V., Madey, D.L., Pinnell, S.R. (2002) Evidence supporting zinc as an important antioxidant for skin. Int J Dermatol. 41: 606-611.

Sharma, V., Singh, P., Pandey, A.K., Dhawan,

A. (2012) Induction of oxidative stress, DNA damage and apoptosis in mouse liver after sub-acute oral exposure to zinc oxide nanoparticles. Mutat Res/Genetic Toxicol Environ Mutagen. 745: 84-91.

Sun, J.Y., Jing, M.Y., Wang, J.F., Zi, N.T., Fu, L.J., Lu, M.Q., Pan, L. (2006) Effect of zinc on biochemical parameters and changes in related gene expression assessed by cDNA microarrays in pituitary of growing rats. Nutrition. 22: 187-196.

Surekha, P., Kishore, A.S., Srinivas, A., Selvam, G., Goparaju, A., Reddy, P.N., Murthy, P.B. (2012) Repeated dose dermal toxicity study of nano zinc oxide with Sprague-Dawley rats. Cutaneous Ocular Toxicol. 31: 26-32.

Trevisan, R., Bouzon Andrew, S., Fisher David, L. (2014) Gills are an initial target of zinc oxide nanoparticles in oysters Crassostreagigas, leading to mitochondrial disruption and oxidative stresss. Aquat Toxicol. 153: 27-38.

Vallee, B.L., Falchuk, K.H. (2013) The biochemical basis of zinc physiology. Physiol Rev. 1993: 79-118.

Valdiglesias, V., Costa, C., Kiliç, G., Costa, S., Pásaro, E., Laffon, B., Teixeira, J. P. (2013) Neuronal cytotoxicity and genotoxicity induced by zinc oxide nanoparticles. Environ Int. 55: 92-100.

Vandebriel, R.J., De Jong, W.H. (2012) A review of mammalian toxicity of ZnO nanoparticles Nanotech Sci Appl. 34: 284-87.

Wang, B., Feng, W.Y., Wang, M., Wang, T.C., Gu, Y.Q., Zhu, M.T. (2008) Acute toxicological impact of nano-and submicro-scaled zinc oxide powder on healthy adult mice. J Nanopart Res. 10: 263-276.

Wang, B., Feng, W.Y., Wang, T.C., Jia, G., Wang, M., Shi, J.W. (2006) Acute toxicity of nano-and micro-scale zinc powder in healthy adult mice. Toxicol Lett. 161: 115-123.

Wong, S.W.Y., Leung, P.T.Y., Djurišić, A.B.,

Leung, K.M.Y. (2010) Toxicities of nano zinc oxide to five marine organisms: influences of aggregate size and ion solubility. Anal Bioanal Chem. 396: 609-618.

Xia, T., Kovochich, M., Liong, M., Mädler, L., Gilbert, B., Shi, H., Nel, A.E. (2008) Comparison of the mechanism of toxicity of zinc oxide and cerium oxide nanoparticles based on dissolution and oxidative stress properties. ACS nano. 2: 2121-2134.

Xiao-bo, D., Li-xin, W., Hui, Y. (2009) Effect of nano-zinc oxide on liver metallothionein of AA chicken. Chin J Vet Sci. 2: 31.

Xiong, D., Fang, T., Yu, L., Sima, X., Zhu, W. (2011) Effects of nano-scale TiO 2, ZnO and their bulk counterparts on zebrafish: acute toxicity, oxidative stress and oxidative damage. Sci Total Environ. 409: 1444-1452.

Yousef, J.M., Mohamed, A.M. (2015) Prophylactic role of B vitamins against bulk and zinc oxide nano-particles toxicity induced oxidative DNA damage and apoptosis in rat livers. Pak J Pharm Sci. 28: 175-184.

Yousef, M.I., Hendy, H.A., Demerdash, F.M., Elagamy, E.I. (2002) Dietary zincdeficiency induced-changes in the activity of enzymes and levels offree radicals, lipids and protein electrophoretic behavior in growingrats. Toxicology. 175: 223-34.

Zago, M.P., Oteiza, P.I. (2001) The antioxidant properties of zinc: interactions with iron and antioxidants. Free Radical Biol Med. 31: 266-274.

Zhang, J., Song, W., Guo, J., Zhang, J., Sun, Z., Ding, F., Gao, M. (2012) Toxic effect of different ZnO particles on mouse alveolar macrophages. J Hazar Mater. 219: 148-155.

Zhao, X., Wang, S., Wu, Y., You, H., &Lv, L. (2013) Acute ZnO nanoparticles exposure induces developmental toxicity, oxidative stress and DNA damage in embryo-larval zebrafish. Aquat Toxicol. 136: 49-59.

3

Anatomical study of the Iranian brown bear's skull (*Ursus arctos*)

Yousefi, M.H.*

Department of Anatomy, Faculty of Veterinary Medicine, Semnan University, Semnan, Iran

Key words:
anatomy, brown bear, skull

Correspondence
Yousefi, M.H.
Department of Anatomy, Faculty
of Veterinary Medicine, Semnan
University, Semnan, Iran

Email: myousefi@semnan.ac.ir

Abstract:

The Brown bear (*Ursus arctos*) is a species at risk of extinction. It is considered the largest carnivore and lives in northern Iran. Several studies on the structure of skull have been accomplished in different animals. The aim of this study was the inscription of gross anatomical characteristics of skulls of three Iranian adult male brown bears that were transferred to the Anatomical Department of the Faculty of Veterinary Medicine of Semnan University. After processing, that included cleaning, degreasing and bleaching, skulls were studied from the dorsal or frontal, ventral, lateral, rostral, caudal and medial views. The facial part of the brown bear's skull from dorsal view was small and the cranium was seen quadrilateral and larger than the dogs. The facial part of lacrimal bone and also the optic groove of presphenoid were absent. There was not articulation between maxillary and nasal bones. The interincisive canal was present and situated inter palatine processes of incisive bones. The orbital cavity was small in brown bear. Lacrimal canal was formed by lacrimal and maxillary bones. The interparietal bone and external sagittal crest in brown bear were seen as being shorter than the dogs. Tympanic bulla was very small and jugular foramen rounded. The external acoustic meatus was formed by squamous and tympanic part of temporal bone. In conclusion, the brown bear's skull has different important macroscopic characteristics compared to other carnivores.

Case History

Many carnivores that live in Iran such as brown bears are at risk of extinction (Mclellan et al., 2008). In recent years the Iranian wildlife has been exposed to various risks such as illegal hunting and road kill (Qashqaei et al., 2012). Ecological study was accomplished about the Iranian brown bear (Ataei et al., 2012). The Iranian Brown bear (Ursus arctos) is considered the largest carnivore living in the north of Iran and parts of Lorestan and Khuzestan (Ebrahimi et al., 2011). There are several present studies about osteology of carnivorous animals (Evans and Christensen, 1964, Getty, 1975, Tomar et al., 2014). Several studies on the structure of skull have been conducted in different animals (Atalar et al., 2009., He et al., 2002., Jurgelenas et al., 2007., Petrov et al., 1992., Sarma et al., 2001., Singh, 1997).

The morphometrical skull of brown bear was studied in Golestan province of Iran (Movahedi et al., 2014). The length of brown bear's skull was reported 368mm and width 205mm. In another report about the skull of brown bear in Iran it was concluded that different parts of the skull in males is stronger, whereas female skulls have been reported to have more length, and are narrower and weaker (Nezami and Eagdari, 2014). The length of Bulgarian brown bear's skull was clarified, 370mm and width 223/8mm (Mihaylov et al., 2013). To the best of the author's knowledge, there is no macroscopic study about Iranian brown bear's skull, therefore, this investigation, for the first time, was focused on the macroscopic skull features in Iranian brown bear in order to extend the knowledge in this field. Results were compared with the data available for other carnivores.

The specimens including the three skulls were obtained from the carcasses of brown bears in Golestan forest in Iran. These skulls were provided by the Department of Environment (DoE), Semnan, Iran and transmitted to the dissection part of the Faculty of Veterinary Medicine of Semnan University. The macroscopic features of skulls were studied from dorsal or frontal, ventral, lateral, medial and caudal views. Seventeen craniometrical indices of the brown bear's skull were measured in this study (Figures 1, 2, 3). Linear values of the head skeleton parameters were measured using a caliper (Petrov et al., 1990, Yamaguchi et al., 2009).

Clinical Presentation

Morphometrical findings were shown in Tables one, two and three. The mean of the condylobasal length or distance between the incisive and occipital condyle was 260.44mm. The mean of the rostral width of hard palate was 50.97 mm. The mean of greatest length of the skull and the mean of the dorsal length of the cranium were 289.31mm and 177.87 mm respectively. The mean of the zygomatic width was 165.55 mm. The mean of the width of the cranium of the brown bear's skull was 100.54 mm. The mean of the length of the mandible and the mean of the high of the ramus of the mandible were 192.27 mm and 83.26 mm re-

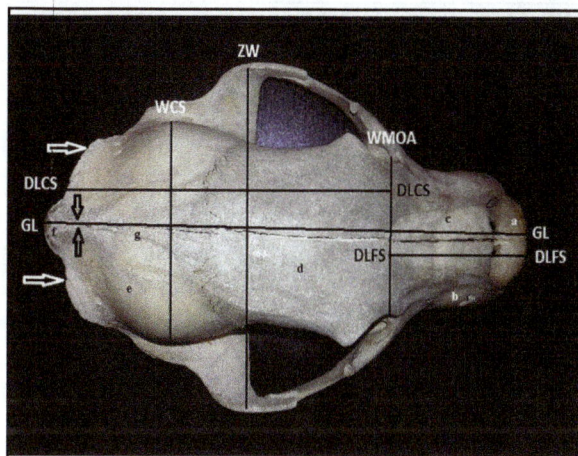

Figure 1. Dorsal view and craniometrical parameters of brown bear's skull showing: a. Incisive bone. b. Maxilla. c. Nasal bone. d. Frontal bone. e. Parietal bone. f. Interparietal bone. g. Temporal line. Black arrow: External sagittal crest. White arrow: Nuchal crest. (GL): Greatest length of the head skeleton. (WCS): Width of the Cranium of the Skull. (ZW): Zygomatic Width. (DLFS): Dorsal Length of the Face of the Skull. (DLCS): Dorsal Length of the Cranium of the Skull. (WMOA): Width between the Medial eye Angles.

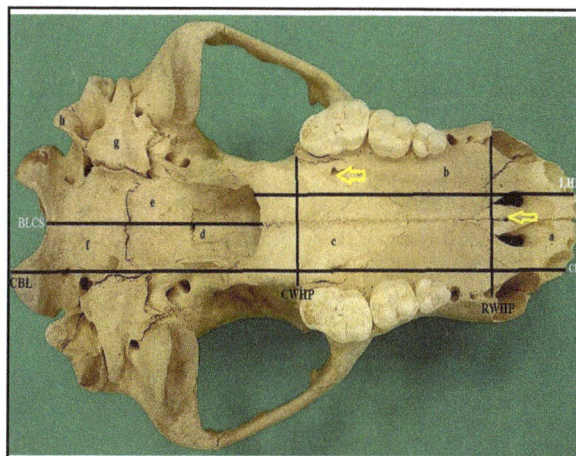

Figure 2. Craniometrical parameters of brown bear's skull (Ventral view): (RWHP): Rostral Width of the Hard Palate. (CWHP): Caudal Width of the Hard Palate. (LHP): Length of the Hard Palate. (CBL): Condylobasal Length of the head skeleton. (BLCS): Basal Length of the Cranium of the Skull. a. Incisive bone b. Palatine process of maxillary bone c. Horizontal plate of palatine bone. d. Presphenoid bone e. Basisphenoid bone. f. Basilar part of occipital bone. g. Tympanic bulla. h. Jugular process. Rostral arrow: Interincisive canal. Caudal arrow: Major and Minor palatine foramen.

spectively.

Macroscopically important specifications of the skull were explained from different views:

The skull of brown bear, like other animals, was divided into two portions. The rostral and

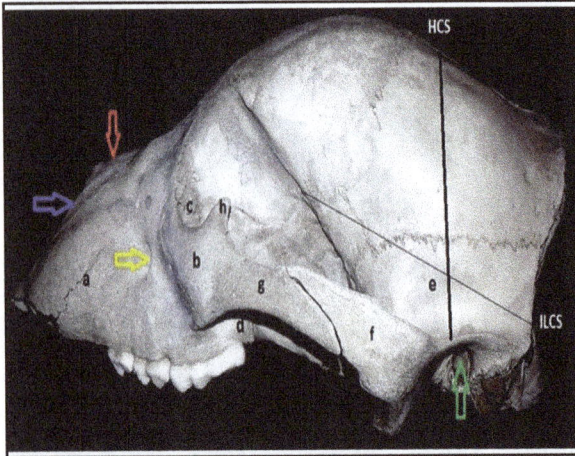

Figure 3. Craniometrical parameters of brown bear's skull (Lateral view): (HCS): Height of the Cranium of the Skull. (ILCS): Internal Length of the Cranium of the Skull. a. Maxilla. b. Zygomatic bone. c. Lacrimal bone. d. Maxillary tubercle. e. Squamous temporal bone. f. Zygomatic process of temporal bone. g. Temporal process of zygomatic bone. h. Frontal process of zygomatic bone. Red arrow: Nasal bone. Blue arrow: Nasal process of incisive bone. Yellow arrow: Infraorbital foramen. Green arrow: External acoustic meatus.

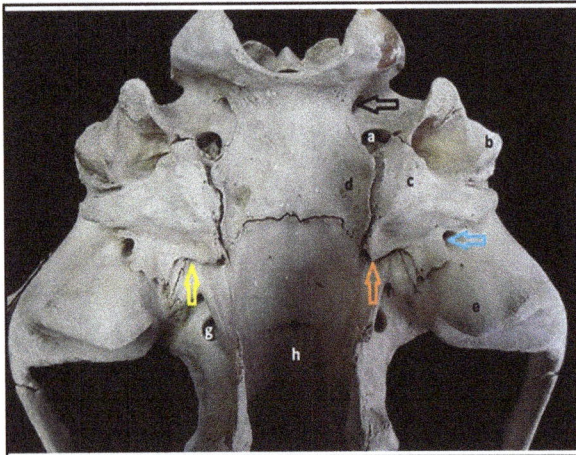

Figure 4. Cranium of brown bear's skull (Ventral view): a. Jugular foramen. b. Mastoid process. c. Tympanic bulla. d. Muscular tubercle. e. Retroarticular process. f. Oval foramen. g. Caudal alar foramen. h. Presphenoid bone. Black arrow: Hypoglossal foramen in condyloid fossa. Blue arrow: Retroarticular foramen. Yellow arrow: Carotid foramen. Orange arrow: Auditory opening.

small part was the face and the caudal part was the cranium. The cranium was observed quadrilateral shape from dorsal view. Frontal, nasal, parietal and interparietal bones were seen from this view (Fig. 1).

Frontal bone covered half of the cranium's roof approximately. External surface of frontal bone was crossed by temporal line, which extends in a curve from external sagittal crest to short zygomatic process. Temporal line was not prominent (Fig. 1). The nasal part of frontal bone was long, which fits between nasal bone and maxilla. This part was rostrally joined with the nasal process of incisive bone (Fig. 6). External sagittal crest was short and less prominent. This crest was formed by two parietal bones (Fig. 1). The rostral end of interparietal bone was narrower than the caudal end. The caudal ends of two nasal bones were convex and form the semicircular border, which was caudolaterally joined with the nasal part of frontal bone and the nasal process of incisive bone, rostrolaterally (Fig. 1, 3, 6).

The nuchal crest at the dorsal part of the squamous occipital was high and the external occipital protuberance was formed by the occipital and interparietal bones. The median occipital crest was sharp and extended to foramen magnum. The jugular process was short and hypoglossal canal present in condyloid fossa.

The ventral surface of basioccipital was concave and the lateral border of basioccipital at the tympanic bulla reflected ventrally. The muscular tubercle was not prominent. Jugular foramen was seen round and formed by basioccipital, lateral part of occipital and tympanic part of temporal bones (Fig. 4). The body of basisphenoid was seen wide and concave ventrally. Infratemporal fossa was small and presents oval and caudal alar foramens in this region. The groove was seen between the body and wing of the basisphenoid. This groove continued to the auditory opening of tympanic bulla caudally and choanal opening rostrally, which transmits the auditory tube (Fig. 4). The small body of presphenoid was present in the ventral wall or floor of cranium, rostral to the basisphenoid (Fig. 4). There were four foramens, including ethmoidal, optic, orbital and rostral alar, on the wing of presphenoid, at the caudal part of the orbit. These fo-

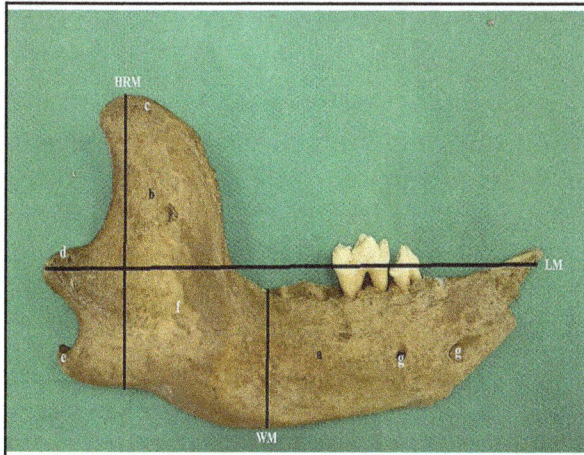

Figure 5. Lateral view of brown bear's mandible: (LM): Length of the Mandible. (WM): Width of the Mandible. (HRM): High of the Ramus of Mandible. a. Body of mandible. b. Ramus of mandible. c. Coronoid process. d. Condylar process. e. Angular process. f. Masseteric fossa. g. Mental foramen.

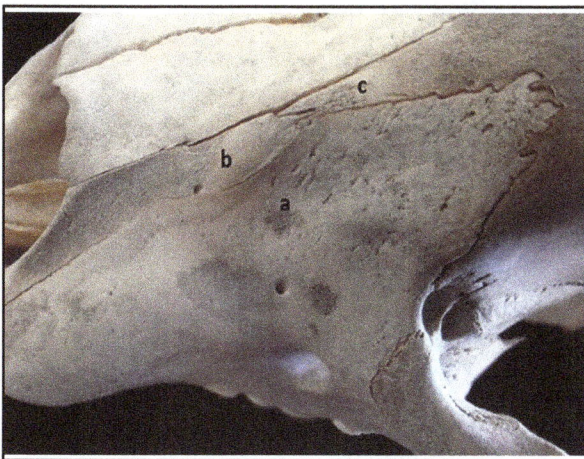

Figure 6. Face of brown bear's skull (Dorsolateral view): a. Maxilla. b. Nasal process of incisive bone. c. Nasal part of frontal bone.

ramens were situated respectively from dorsal to ventral and approximately the same distance from each other. The round foramen opened to the rostral alar foramen.

The palatine bone was situated in the caudal portion of the hard palate. The horizontal plate was approximately large. On the oral surface of horizontal plate, caudal part of palatine groove was present, extending to the major palatine foramen. The minor palatine foramen presents in each side, but was not separated from the major palatine foramen (Fig. 2). The caudal part of perpendicular plate was thick and joined medially with pterygoid bone and laterally with pterygoid process of basisphenoid. The Hamulus or muscular process of pterygoid bone was thick and large. The ramus of mandible was short and wide. The wider coronoid process, condylar and angular process were present in the ramus. The masseteric fossa was not depressed. The ventral border of the mandible was direct and not convex. There were two mental foramen rostralaterally of the body of mandible (Fig. 5). Interincisive canal was observed between the right and left palatine process of the incisive bones. The nasal process of incisive bone was extended to the rostral part of the nasal bone laterally and joined with the nasal part of the frontal bone. The nasoincisive notch was not clear or absent (Fig. 1, 3, 6).

The lateral surface was smooth and depression rostrally to the infraorbital foramen. Maxilla formed the rostral portion of the orbital cavity, dorsal to the zygomatic bone. The lacrimal canal in the orbital cavity was formed by maxilla and lacrimal bone (Fig. 3, 6, 7). Zygomatic process of maxillary bone was attached to the ventromedial aspect of the rostral part of zygomatic arch. This process was articulated with lacrimal bone under the maxillary foramen. The maxillary tubercle was prominent, sharp and clear. The caudal palatine foramen had formed between the maxillary tubercle and pterygopalatine fossa. The sphenopalatine foramen was situated in pterygopalatine fossa next to the caudal palatine foramen (Fig. 7). The facial surface of lacrimal bone was absent (Fig. 6, 7). The maxillary foramen was situated medial to the zygomatic bone and formed by the lacrimal bone. The zygomatic bone had two processes including the high frontal process and long temporal process (Fig. 3).

The external acoustic meatus was formed between squamous and tympanic part of temporal bone. The tympanic bulla was small and indicates short muscular process. The prominent mastoid process was situated between the squamous temporal and lateral part of occipital

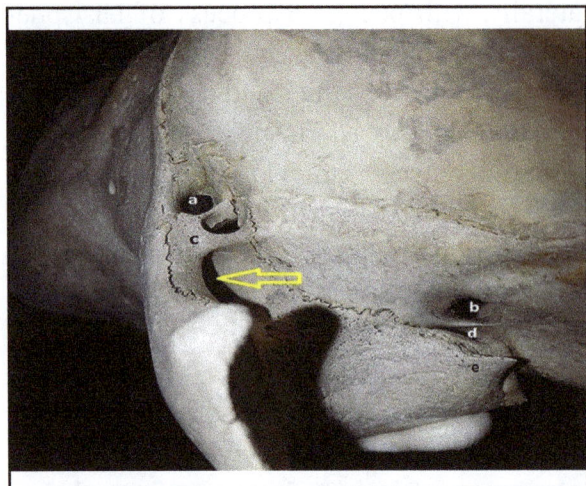

Figure 7. Rostral part of orbit of brown bear's skull: a. Lacrimal canal. b. Sphenopalatine foramen. c. Lacrimal bone. d. Caudal palatine foramen. e. Maxillary tuber. Yellow arrow: Maxillary foramen.

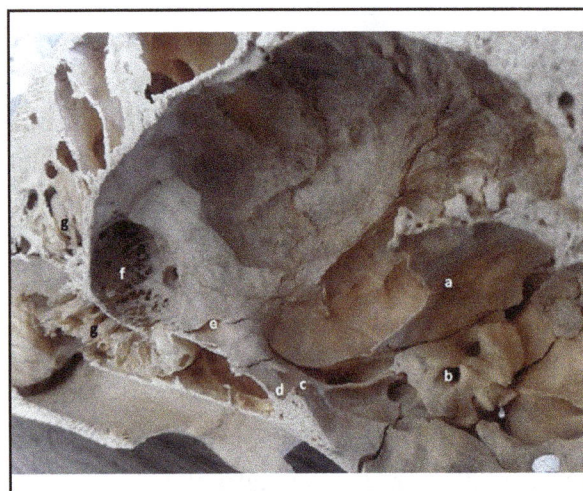

Figure 8. Cranium of brown bear's skull (Medial view): a. Septum between cerebellum and right cerebral hemisphere. b. Internal acoustic meatus. c. Dorsum sellae. d. Hypophyseal fossa. e. Optic canal. f. Cribriform plate of ethmoid. g. Ethmoidal turbinate.

bone (Fig. 3, 4).

The dorsum sellae was present and prominent on the dorsal surface of basisphenoid. The optic groove was absent in brown bear's skull and entrance of the optic canals was separated from them (Fig. 8).

Discussion

This study shows that the skull of the brown bear is the same as the skull of the other carnivores but there were different points between them. The skull of brown bear was wide and the facial part, small, like the tiger (Singh, 1997) and ferret (He et al., 2002). The results of this study show a groove is present between the body and the wing of basisphenoid. This groove continues to the auditory opening of tympanic bulla caudally and choanal opening rostrally, which transmits the auditory tube. To the best of the author's knowledge there is not a report about this groove in other carnivores.

This research showed that optic groove is absent in the brown bear's skull and optic canals are separated from each other. The optic groove was present on the dorsal surface of presphenoid in the dogs and cats (Dyce et al., 2010).

The results of this study revealed that the facial part of lacrimal bone is not present in the brown bear, but the orbital part of lacrimal bone is greater than that of the dog (Getty, 1975) and composed the maxillary foramen medially to the rostral part of zygomatic arch. This study showed that maxillary bone is not articulated with the nasal bone and composed the dorsal part of rostral border of orbit and partially to the lacrimal canal. The maxillary bone in felis bengalencis built the rostral part of orbit (Sarma et al., 2001).

The external surface of frontal bone was smooth and slightly convex like that of the dog (Evans and Christensen, 1964). This surface is more convex in the felis bengalencis (Sarma et al., 2001) and tiger (Singh, 1997), but in the wolf it is slightly concave (Atalar et al., 2009). The zygomatic process of the frontal bone in the brown bear's skull, like the most carnivores, was short, while this process is longer in cats (Evans and Christensen, 1964) and the felis bengalencis (Sarma et al., 2001). The results of this study shows the external sagittal crest and temporal line are present, but not prominent like the felis bengalencis (Sarma et al., 2001) and fox (Atalar et al., 2009). The orbital cavity in the brown bear was small against the greater skull and resembles the

Table 1. Values of the investigated ventral of cranium indices. **T.S**: This study. **I.S.M**: Iranian study by Movahhedi. **B.S.M**: Bulgarian study by Mihaylov.

Parameters	T.S	I.S.M	B. S.M
LHP- Length of hard palate (mm)	149/47	-	152/75
CBL- Condylobasal length (mm)	260/44	266/8	292/83
BLCS- Basal length of cranium of skull (mm)	103/83	-	145/23
RWHP- Rostral width of hard palate (mm)	50/97	66	71/27
CWHP- Caudal width of hard palate (mm)	56/87	-	82/22

Table 2. Values of the investigated dorsal of cranium indices. **T.S**: This study. **I.S.M**: Iranian study by Movahhedi. **B.S.M**: Bulgarian study by Mihaylov.

Parameters	T. S.	I.S.M	B.S.M
GL- Greatest length of the skull (mm)	289/31	290	319/05
DLFS- Dorsal length of face of skull (mm)	111/55	-	112/75
DLCS- Dorsal length of cranium of skull (mm)	177/87	-	207
WMOA- Width between of medial ocular angles (mm)	71/08	66/7	78/45
ZW- Zygomatic width (mm)	165/55	171	189/5
WCS- Width of cranium of skull (mm)	100/54	101	107/23
ILCS- Internal length of cranium of skull (mm)	106/79	-	138/73
VCS- Volume of cranium of skull (cm3)	320		343
HCS- High of cranium of skull (mm)	90/34	-	91/23

Table 3. Values of the investigated of mandible. **T. S**: This study. **I.S.M**: Iranian study by Movahhedi.

Parameters	T.S.	I.S.M
LM- Length of mandible (mm)	192/27	189/5
WM- Width of mandible (mm)	38/35	-
HRM- High of ramus of mandible (mm)	83/26	-

dogs' near to the median line. It was a distant median line in cats (Miller et al., 1964). The infraorbital foramen, the same as the tiger (Singh, 1997), felis bengalencis (Sarma et al., 2001) and ferret (He et al., 2002), was situated rostroventrally near the orbital cavity. The maxillary tubercle in the skull of brown bear was raised and sharp, but it is small in the dogs (Miller et al., 1964). The frontal process of the zygomatic bone in brown bear was longer than the dogs. The nuchal crest was shorter in brown bear than the dogs. The external occipital protuberance was distinguished and median occipital crest present and sharp, similar to the fox (Atalar et al., 2009). The median occipital crest is not present or not prominent in other carnivorous animals (Dyce et al., 2010, Evans and Christensen, 1964, Getty, 1975). In this study the interincisive canal present between the right and left palatine process of incisive bones was observed, but this canal exists in the interbody of incisive bones in dogs (Nickel et al., 1986). The minor palatine foramen in the brown bear is present in each side, but not separated from the major palatine foramen, while the minor palatine foramen is independently present in tiger (Singh, 1997), and absent in felis bengalencis (Sarma et al., 2001).

The jugular process was short in the skull of brown bear. The jugular process was reported short and sharp in felis bengalencis (Sarma et al., 2001). Atalar et al., (2009) observed the long jugular process in fox and wolf. The hypoglossal foramen was seen in condyloid fossa, while it was observed rostrally to the condyloid fossa in the dogs (Miller et al., 1964).

This study showed the external acoustic meatus in brown bear, formed by the squamous and tympanic part of temporal bone, while in dogs, this meatus is formed by the tympanic part of temporal bone (Miller et al., 1964). This study revealed that the tympanic bulla in brown bear was small and short like the equids (Nickel et al., 1986). The tympanic bulla is large in dogs and muscular process is long (Miller et al., 1964). The large tympanic bulla is present in tiger (Singh, 1997), felis bengalencis (Sarma et al., 2001) and ferret (He et al., 2002). This research showed that the prominent and clear mastoid process is present in brown bear as the same as equine (Nickel et al., 1986). The mastoid process was reported large in the wild cat (Atalar et al., 2009).

The mandible is described in dogs (Evans and Christensen, 1964) and in tiger (Tiwari et al., 2011). The mandible of brown bear closely resembled that of other carnivores.

The masseteric fossa of the mandible of the brown bear's skull was not depressed and the ventral border of the body of this bone was approximately direct, the same as the mandible of tiger (Tiwari et al., 2011), while it was convex in dogs and cats (Getty, 1975).

Acknowledgements

The author would like to thank Dr. Salimi-Bejestani, for reviewing this manuscript and the following individuals for different roles that they played, Dr. Mirbehbehani, and Dr. Rasouli from the Department of Anatomy, Mr. Rostami and Mr. Pourafshar the senior technologist of Faculty of Veterinary Medicine, Semnan, Iran, Dr. Behnam and Mr. Adiby from the Department of Environment, Semnan, Iran.

References

1. Atalar, O., Ustundag, Y., Yaman, M., Ozdemir, D. (2009) Comparative anatomy of the neurocranium in some wild carnivore. J Anim Vet Adv. 8: 1542-1544.
2. Dyce, K.M., Sack, W.O., Wensing, C.J.G., (2010) Text Book of Veterinary Anatomy. (4th ed.) W. B. Saunders Co., Philadelphia, London, Toronto, Montreal, Sydney, Tokyo.
3. Ebrahimi, M., Hosseinizavarei, F., Rajabzadeh, M., Ghafari, H., Ghelichpour, M., Mobaraki, A., Nezami, B. (2011) Iranian wildlife encychopedia. (3rd ed.) Tehran Golden Publisher. Tehran, Iran.
4. Evans, H.E., Christensen, G.C. (1964) Miller's Anatomy of the Dog. Publ., W. B. Saunders Co., Philadelphia, USA.
5. Getty, R. (1977) Sisson and Grossmans. The Anatomy of the Domestic Animals. (5th ed.) W.B. Saunders. Philadelphia, London, Toronto.
6. He, T., Friede, H., Kiliaridis S. (2002) Macroscopic and roentgenographic anatomy of the skull of the ferret (*Mustela putorius furo*), Laboratory Animals Ltd. Laboratory Animals. 3: 86-96.
7. Mihaylov, R., Dimitrov, R., Raichev, E., Kostov, D., Stamatova-Yiovcheva, K., Zlatanova, D., Bivolarski, B. (2013) Morphometrical Features Of the head Skeleton In Brown (*Ursus arctos*) in Bulgaria. Bulgarian J Agric Sci. 19: 331-337.
8. Miller, M.S., Christensen, G.C., Evans, H.E., (1964) The skeletal system, skull. In Anatomy of Dog. W.B. Saunders Co., Philadelphia, USA. p. 6-49.
9. Movahhedi, N., Kemi, H., Shajiei, H. (2014) The study of skull of mammal carnivorous in Golestan state of Iran. Iran J Anim Biol. 6: 81-89.
10. Nezami, B., Eagdari, S. (2014) Allometric Growth Pattern of Skull on Brown Bear (*Ursus arctos*) of the Alborz Mountain. J Appl Biol Sci. 8: 52-58.
11. Nickel, R., Schummer, A., Seiferle, E. (1986) The Anatomy of the Domestic Animals. Vol. 1: The Locomotor System. Verlag Paul Parey. Springer Verlag. Berlin and Hamburg, Germany.
12. Petrov, I., Gerassimov, S., Nikolov, H. (1990) Metric characteristics and sexual dimorphism of cranial sighnsin Wild cat (*Felis silvesris* Schreber 1777) (Mammalia,Felidae) from Bulgaria. Acta Zool Bulg. 40: 44-54.
13. Sarma, K., Nasiruddulah, N., Islam, S. (2001) Anatomy of the skull of leopard cat (*Felis bengalencis*). Indian J Anim Sci. 71: 1011-1013.
14. Sarma, K. (2006) Morphological and craniometrical studies on the skull of Kagani Goat

(*Capra hircus*) of Jammu Region. Int J Morphol. 24: 449-455.

15. Tiwari, Y., Taluja, J.S., Vaish, R. (2011) Biometry of Mandible in Tiger (*Panthera tigris*). Ann Rev Res Biol. 1: 14-21.

16. Singh, I. (1997) Anatomical study on the skull of tiger. Indian J Anim Sci. 67: 777- 778.

17. Yamaguchi, N., Kitchener, A., Gilissen, E., MacDonald, D. (2009) Brian size of lion (*Panthera leo*) and tiger (*P.tigris*): implications for intragenic phylogeny, intraspecific differences and the effects of captivity. Biol J Linn Soc Lond. 98: 85-93.

4

Cutaneous neuro-myofibroblastic sarcoma induced by avian leukosis virus subgroup J in a rooster (*Gallus gallus domesticus*)

Norouzian, H.[1*], Dezfoulian, O.[2], Hosseini, H.[3]

[1]*Department of Clinical Sciences, School of Veterinary Medicine, Lorestan University, Khorramabad, Iran*
[2]*Department of Pathobiology, School of Veterinary Medicine, Lorestan University, Khorramabad, Iran*
[3]*Department of Clinical Sciences, School of Veterinary Medicine, Islamic Azad University, Karaj, Iran*

Key words:

avian leukosis, cutaneous sarcoma, *Gallus gallus*, myofibroblastic tumor, rooster

Correspondence

Norouzian, H.
Department of Clinical Sciences, School of Veterinary Medicine, Lorestan University, Khorramabad, Iran

Email: noroozianh@yahoo.com

Abstract:

An adult native cock (*Gallus gallus domesticus*) referred to the aviary clinic with multiple different sizes of round dermal nodules. The bird died few days later, and was then submitted for further evaluation. Macroscopic and microscopic examinations as well as a PCR test were done to identify type and cause of the tumor. In histopathological assessment of biopsy specimen, it consisted of interlacing bundles of fibroblasts that orientated in different directions with plump or elongated spindle shaped nuclei and fairly abundant cytoplasm. At necropsy several large white nodules were implanted in lung and liver. Microscopically the proliferated fibroblastic cells were invaded to both organs, and were similar to those described for skin lesion. The tumor cells had immunoreaction for alpha smooth muscle actin, vimentin and S100 protein, whereas they were negative for desmin and pancytokeratin, suggesting a diagnosis of metastatic neuro-myofibroblastic sarcoma. A PCR test specific for avian leukosis virus subgroup J (ALV-J) confirmed the presence of that virus in tumor specimens. Sequencing and phylogenetic analysis showed a relatively low similarity in the LTR segment (90%) of the studied virus with other ALV-J strains. It might be the first report of cutaneous neuro-myofibroblastic sarcoma, potentiated to metastasis to other organs induced by ALV-J.

Case History

The etiology of neoplastic diseases, specifically those appearing in exotic or wild birds is not well-defined, conversely the oncogenesis in poultry is more commonly identified, in which the most documented causes are infective. Avian leukosis/sarcoma viruses (ALSVs; subgroups A-E and J) related to the oncogenic retroviruses, are involved in the pathogenesis of numerous classified tumors originated from either mesenchymal or epithelial cells (Hafner et al. 1998; Ono et al. 2004; Ochi et al. 2012; Wang et al. 2013).

Among the ALV-encoded proteins, the envelope glycoprotein (env) on the surface of retroviral particles is the major determinant of the subgroup phenotype, host range and antigenicity. The env gene sequence of the prototype virus of subgroup J, HPRS-103, differs extremely from other ALV subgroups and has high identity (75%) to env-like sequences of some members of the EAV family of the endogenous avian retroviruses. Moreover, a novel EAV related sequence, designated EAV-HP, demonstrated in the chicken genome, has revealed about 97% homology to that of HPRS-103 env gene (Bai et al., 1995). Multiple copies of EAV-HP elements were present in the genome of all the lines of chickens and the ancestral jungle fowl (Smith et al., 1999). The above mentioned researches suggest that the emergence of ALV subgroup J might be the result of recombination with env-like sequences of avian leukosis E family. In the present study, the first report of neuromyofibroblastic sarcoma in chicken induced by ALV subgroup J in Iran has been described.

Clinical Presentation

A 2-year-old cock (*Gallus domesticus*) referred to birds' clinic in the School of Veterinary Medicine of Loretan university was examined with raised dermal multicentric nodules, locating on both left and right knee region, left lateral shank region, and right radial region of wing from single to multiple, clustered together, but the largest singular mass was 3.5 cm in diameter. The bird was being kept in a free-range grazing environment with several poultry, however, others had no similar signs. The firm nodules had no attaching to their underlying tissue, and it was possible they originated from the skin.

The biopsy sample obtained from knee was presented for pathologic examination. It was fixed in 10% neutral buffered formalin, routinely processed and stained with hematoxylin and eosin (HE).

Three weeks later the general condition of bird deteriorated progressively and it died before returning to clinic.

Diagnostic Testing

Macroscopic examination: In addition to nodules which were described previously, a few small skin nodules were also unveiled in post mortem evaluation, deeply embedded and firmly adherent to their adjacent subcutaneous fascia and muscles. The nodules were well-circumscribed, firm with gray/white color and smooth on cut surface. Of the internal organs, only liver and lung were affected with white spherical nodular growths, fairly invariable in size (Fig 1 and 2).

Microscopic examination (Biopsy specimen histopathology): The lesion was well-circumscribed but it had no true capsule. The cells were either arranged in broad interwoven bundles of highly cellular fibroblast-type cells, with moderately collagenous fibrous tissue, or to a lesser extent were present in loose-ground substance like- whorl pattern. Most of them had oval to elongated vesicular nuclei which contained one or two prominent nucleoli. Although many were markedly pleomorphic, nuclear hyperchromatism was occasionally present. The cells had considerable amounts of cytoplasm, but their boundaries were ill-defined. Moreover, moderate population of cells with typical eosinophilic granules were dispersed among the neoplastic cells.

Mild acanthosis, but extensive hyperkeratosis were striking features of epidermal layer. It was characterized by the formation of intraepidermal spongiosis of keratinocytes which differed from micro-size to moderate. Basophilic stained colonies of bacteria were striking in epidermal layer; however, inflammatory cell did not increase.

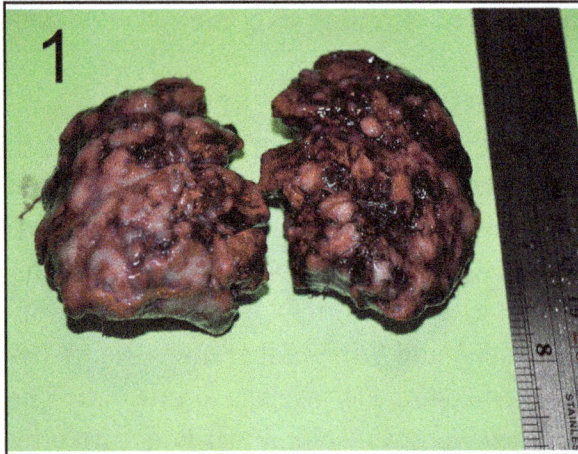

Figure 1. Multiple white nodules are implanted in the lung parenchyma.

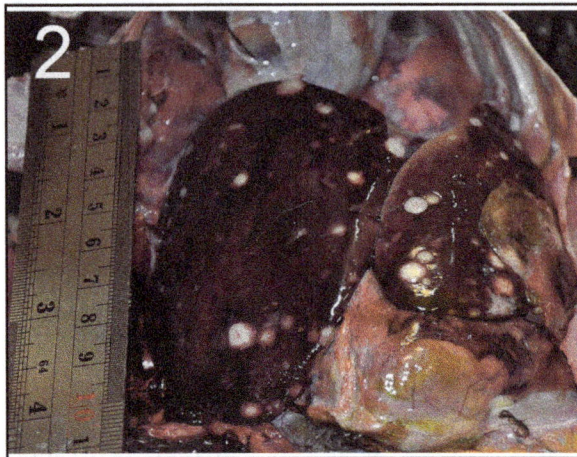

Figure 2. Multiple white nodules are implanted in the liver.

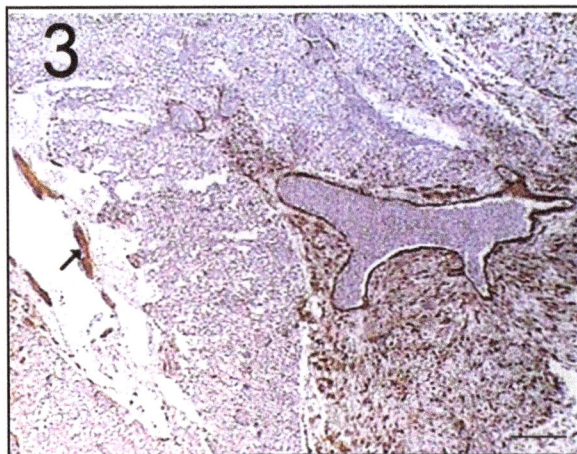

Figure 3. Pulmonary positive immunoreaction of neoplastic cells to alpha smooth muscle actin. The sm ooth muscle cells in the vascular wall as well as in the bronchus (arrow) are also immunolabled consistently as internal positive control. (200μm).

Post mortem histopathology: Microscopic examination in liver and lung was exactly the same as the description stated for subcutaneous mass, in which tumor cells invaded their parenchyma.

Immunohistochemistry: The following antibodies were applied in appropriate dilutions on tissue targets: vimentin (Dako, Glostrup, Denmark), S-100 protein (Dako), neuron-specific enolase {NSE (Dako)}, pan-cytokeratin (Dako), alpha-smooth muscle actin (Dako) and desmin (Dako) by use of Envision kit (Dako). Moreover, S-100 and alpha-SMA were also used on normal skin of chicken. Neoplastic cells were strongly immunoreacted for alpha-smooth muscle actin, vimentin, S100 and NSE (Fig.3-6), but they had no reaction to desmin and pancytokeratin. The smooth muscle cells of blood vessel walls were considered as internal positive controls for actin and vimentin, but control skin of chicken was not immunolabeled at all to alpha-SMA and S100. S100 and NSE antibodieshad cross reaction with intestine and brain of chicken respectively and for pituitary adenocarcinoma of budgie. Based on histopathology results, the type of tumor was neuro-myofibroblastic sarcoma.

Polymerase chain reaction. RNA was extracted from tumor tissues (liver, lung and skin) by using RNeasy Mini Kit, according to the manufacturer's instructions (Qiagen, Germany), and was stored at -80 C.

Specific reverse transcription Polymerase chain reaction (RT-PCR) for subgroup J of ALV was performed directly on tumor tissues. RT-PCR analysis with the primers, forward primer DU5F 5'-GGGCGGG-GCTTCGGTTGTA-3' and reverse primer DU5R 5'-TCGCTCATGCAGGTGCTC-GTAGTT-3' was performed (Zavala et al. 2002). These primer sets for ALV-J amplified the 517 base pair (bp) segment specific

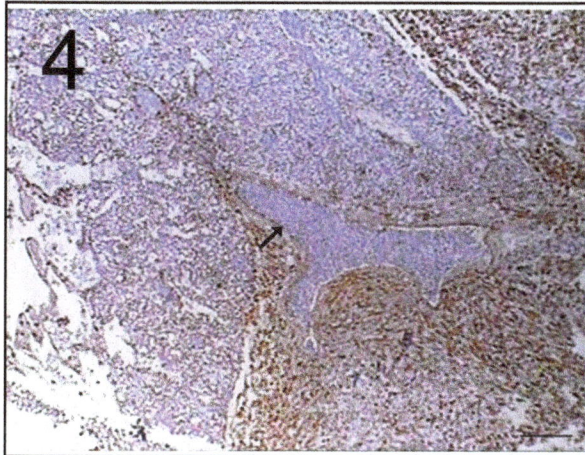

Figure 4. The tumor cells in lung are displaying positive staining for vimentin. The rim of large vein is unevenly stained (arrow). (200μm).

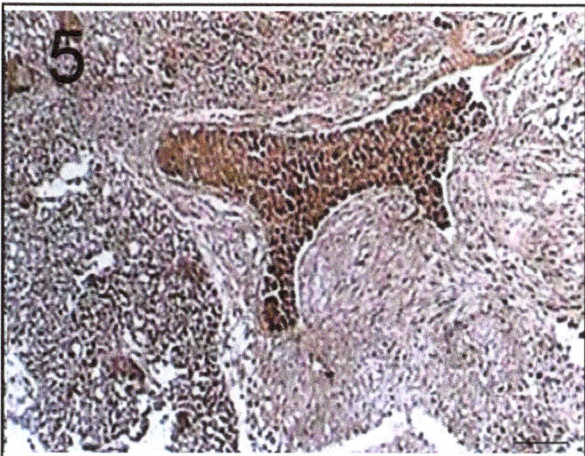

Figure 5. expression of S100 protein in Schwann tumor cells, those positive cells are more dispersed than alpha-sma and vimentin. The red blood cells are also false positive stained.

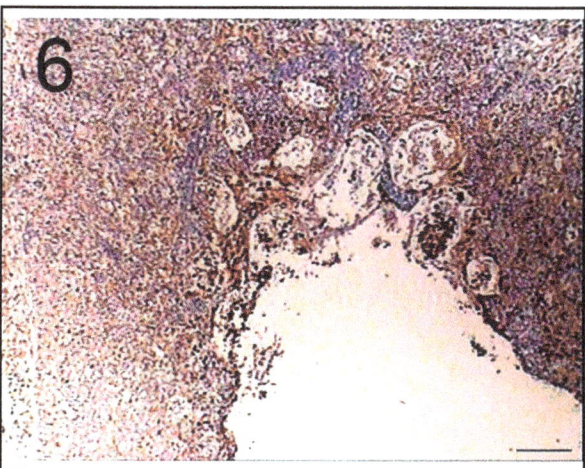

Figure 6. immunopositive neoplastic cells to NSE, are more condensed around parabronchus. (E-J; 200μm).

for the LTR region of ALV subgroup J. For

positive control, positive DNA was kindly provided by Dr. K. Venugopal and for negative control DEPC treated water was used. The PCR mixture was heated at 93C for 3 minutes, then subjected to 35 cycles of PCR amplification (93C for 10 seconds, 54C for 10 seconds, and 72C for 20 seconds) and finally at 72C for 5 minutes using a T100 TM Thermal Cycler (Bio-Rad, USA).

In another PCR for ALV, the primers' H5 (5-GGATGAGGTGACTAAGAAAG-3) and AJ1 (5-ATGAACGGCCCATTC(T/C) CCTATTCC- 3) amplified the hyper variable region in the env gene of ALV subgroups A to E (Venugopal et al. 2008).The PCR mixture was heated to 94 C for 1 minute and then subjected to 30 cycles of PCR amplification (94C for 60 seconds, 60C for 60 seconds, decreasing to 48c during 30 cycles, and 72C for 2 minutes, followed by an extra 10 minutes at the end of the last cycle), which produced 1758 bp DNA fragments from the tumors of the affected chicken. To determine any role of Marek's disease virus 1 (MDV1) in tumor lesions, PCR was performed on the same materials (Handberg et al. 2001). The positive control was positive DNA, obtained from Dr. K. Venugopal.

PCR products were detected after 1.5% agarose gel electrophoresis and were purified by the Gene JET Gel Extraction Kit (Fermentas, Canada), according to the manufacturer's instructions. The purified DNA fragments were cloned into the pTZ57R/T cloning vector (Fermentas, Canada). Three clones of each fragment were sequenced using M13 forward and M13 reverse primers (Promega, USA) at Sequetech Co. Ltd., USA. Nucleotide sequence alignment and phylogenetic analysis were carried out by the Clustal W method in MegAlign of DNASTAR program (Madison, WI). The

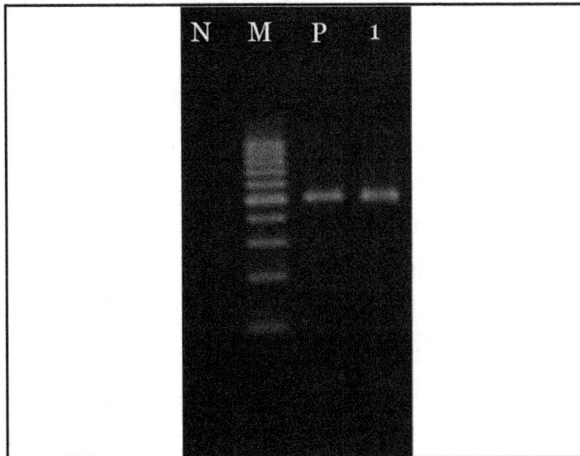

Figure 7. PCR result for detection of ALV subgroup J. Lane N: Negative control; M: 100 bp Marker (Fermentas, Canada); Lane P: Positive control; Lane 1: tumor sample.

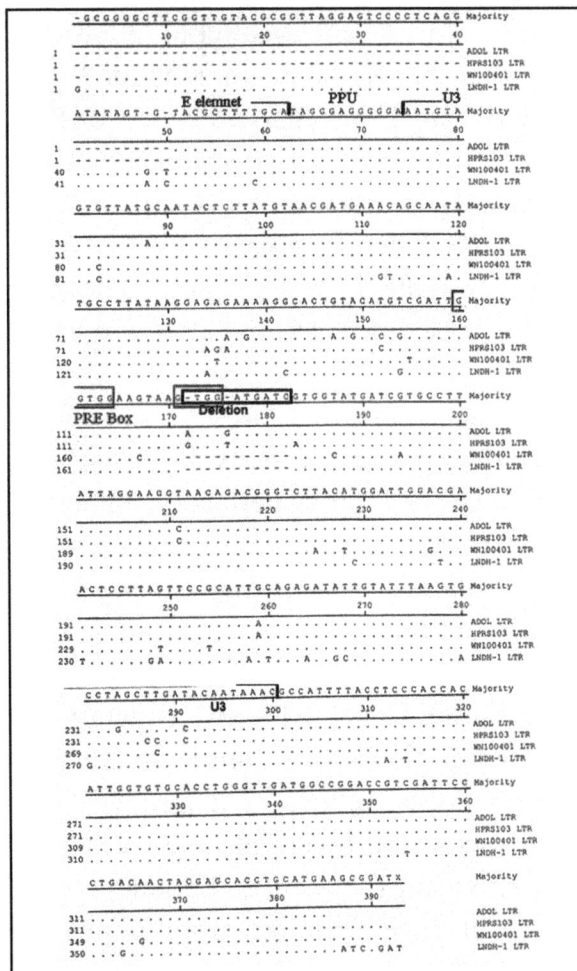

Figure 8. Sequence Comparison of the LTR of ALV subgroup J strains ADOL-7501, HPRS-103, WN100401 and the sequence obtained in this study (LNDH-1). Dashes are equal to homology among compared sequences; substitutions are shown by the nucleotide symbol in related positions. Deletions and PRE boxes are showed with black and red triangles, respectively.

sequences determined in this study are available in GenBank (accession numbers KT326192 and KT326193).

Using primers specific for ALV subgroup J (DU5F and DU5R), a positive result could be detected in all examined tumor tissues (Fig. 7), although the MDV-1 specific sequence was detected in positive control but not in the tissues. A segment of about 1.8 bp of env gene was detected in the other PCR test.

Molecular characterization of LTR. The nucleotide sequence of the LTR region of the studied ALV subgroup J was compared with strains ADOL-7501, HPRS-103 and WN100401 (Fig. 8). A total number of 26 base substitutions were found in the LTR region of the studied ALV subgroup J in comparison to the prototype strain HPRS-103.

The sequence analysis of LTR of the studied virus revealed that its U3 region has only 215 bp, because of an 11 bp deletion. The R and U5 regions of the studied ALV subgroup J wereconserved compared with other ALV subgroup J isolates.

Some sequences regulating transcription of the ALV have been identified in the U3 region of the LTR, including CArG, Y, and PRE, C/EBP, CAAT, and TATA boxes (Gao et al. 2012). In most ALV subgroup J isolates (including HPRS-103 and ADOL-7501), there are two PRE boxes (GGTGG motif), flanking the nucleotide sequence AAGTAA. One of the PRE boxes was omitted at position 171 to 174, for the deletion (Fig. 8).

Phylogenetic analysis and sequence similarity. Based on results of phylogenetic analysis, the LTR sequence of the studied virus belonged to a new branch (Fig. 9) and has the least (82.2%) and the most (88.1 %) sequence similarity with GD1109

Percent Identity	1	2	3	4	5	6	7	8	9	10	11	12	13		
1		91.0	95.8	94.5	91.0	92.6	86.7	89.1	95.3	93.2	92.3	90.0	89.6	1	ADOL LTR
2	9.0		92.1	93.2	95.0	96.6	85.1	92.1	92.2	91.4	98.5	89.2	90.9	2	GD1109 LTR
3	4.3	7.7		97.8	92.0	93.7	89.6	91.1	99.0	95.6	93.1	91.8	94.1	3	HPRS103 LTR
4	5.7	7.1	2.2		92.4	93.6	86.7	94.6	98.3	95.1	93.6	93.2	93.2	4	JS nt LTR
5	9.7	4.5	8.6	8.1		98.7	83.7	87.7	91.9	90.7	97.0	89.0	88.0	5	JS09GY2 LTR
6	7.9	3.5	6.6	6.7	1.3		88.3	92.4	93.2	91.7	98.2	90.1	93.2	6	JS09GY3 LTR
7	12.5	16.3	13.0	14.5	15.6	15.3		86.4	85.8	86.0	86.4	89.6	88.9	7	LNDH-1 LTR
8	8.6	7.7	6.5	5.6	9.6	8.0	14.4		90.2	92.4	92.1	90.2	95.1	8	NHH LTR
9	4.9	7.6	1.0	1.7	8.7	7.2	12.4	6.7		95.6	92.9	91.9	89.2	9	NX0101 LTR
10	7.2	9.3	4.6	5.1	10.9	9.6	15.1	8.1	4.6		91.7	91.4	91.2	10	SD07LK1 LTR
11	8.2	1.6	7.3	6.7	3.1	1.9	15.8	8.4	7.5	9.6		90.1	92.5	11	sdau1002 LTR
12	10.9	11.6	8.8	7.5	12.1	11.1	10.6	9.6	8.7	9.6	11.1		89.3	12	SVR807 LTR
13	8.9	9.1	6.1	7.2	9.2	7.2	13.6	5.1	7.8	9.4	8.3	11.3		13	WN100401 LTR
	1	2	3	4	5	6	7	8	9	10	11	12	13		

(Divergence, lower-left triangle)

Figure 9. Comparison of the nucleotide sequence identity of the LTR gene of LNDH-1 and other ALV-J strains.

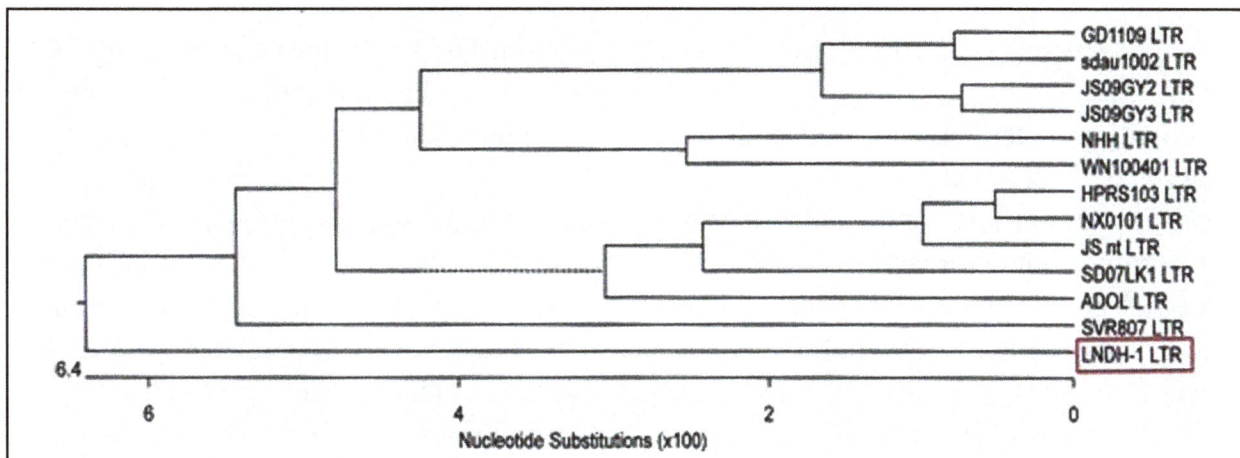

Figure 10. Phylogenic analysis of the LTR region of ALV subgroup J isolates (including the studied ALV-J).

and WN100401 strains, respectively (both isolates from China). In the phylogenetic tree (Fig. 10) of the LTR, the studied virus (LNDH-1) is placed in a separate branch.

A BLAST search revealed that the LTR and 1.8 bp env fragments of the studied ALV subgroup J were 90% and 99% homologous to the region of LTR of the ALV subgroup J isolate WN100401 and env of the endogenous virus strain ALVE-B11, respectively (GenBank accession numbers KC11043 and KC610517).

Assessments

Alpha-smooth muscle actin is one of actin isoform, found basically in smooth muscle cells, but it exists in largest amounts within vascular smooth muscle cells and has a function in development of fibrogenesis (Cherng and Young, 2008; Kawasaki et al. 2008). The expression of alpha-SMA occurs specifically in activated myofibroblasts, which differentiate from cutaneous fibroblasts and also contains some biological characteristics of smooth muscle cells (Cherng and Young, 2008; Elberg et al. 2008; Nakatani et al. 2008). These cells are present in tissue injury for wound repair by its contraction and their appearance and proliferation are provisional and dependent on exposure to chemical substances or cytokines (Park et al. 2007; Cherng and Young, 2008). However, after repair completion, these cells disappear through apoptosis (Darby and Hewitson, 2007; Cherng and Young, 2008). Alpha-SMA is present in mouse subcutaneous fibroblasts (Storch et al. 2007; Cherng and Young, 2008), but in present study it was absent in normal skin tissue of chicken. Therefore, it might be concluded that presence of neoplastic myofibroblasts is a process in response to permanent mutated fibroblasts which are motivated by ALV-subgroup j.

Myofibroblastic tumors which are also designated as myofibrosarcoma and myofibroblastic sarcoma are documented in a few reports in veterinary literature (Bell et al. 2011, Newman et al., 1999, Silva et al., 2012).

According to the case, in one study the authors concluded that positive labeling of alpha-smooth muscle actin and vimentin and negative immunoreactions for desmin and S100 protein were suggestive of myofibroblastic sarcoma in the limb of a horse (Silva et al . 2012). In another report in a horse, desmin was also positive, similar to alpha-SMA and vimentin but negative for S-100 which the authors believed that the originated tumor based on diagnostic criteria of human being was myofibroblastic sarcoma and such tumors are consistently negative to S-100 (Newman et al. 1999).

According to the investigation of 10 feline orbital tumors, Bell et al. (2011) realized that all myofibroblastic sarcomas immunostained with smooth muscle actin and vimentin, whereas interestingly, in contrast to previous reports all tumors reacted to S-100 which is probably related to origination of cells from neural crest in facial mesenchyme. As mentioned, other tumors of myofibroblastic sarcomas whether in animal or human being were negative for S-100, therefore, presumably its expression in rooster skin tumor pertains to two distinct lines of tumor cells.

Among tumor types the prevalence of fibrosarcoma in chickens is significantly lesser than other tumors which were exposed by infected ALV-J(Cheng et al. 2010). The low incidence of connective tissue neoplasms in chickens indicates that the origin and histogenesis of such lesions are not defined exactly and their appearance sporadic (Strafuss and Ladds, 1970; Reece, 1996).

Based on the PCR results, genome of the studied rooster has been affected by an ALV of subgroup J. In the tumor tissues, MDV proviral DNA was not detected using PCR, but a 1.8- kbp fragment of the env region was amplified and it was most similar to ALVE-B11. ev loci are inheritable proviral elements and ubiquitously identified in chicken cells. Normally, few or no endogenous ALVs (EAV) are expressed from ev loci in chickens. The reason behind this inefficient viral particle production is that the locus has a (+1) frame shift mutation in the pol RT-β region, which results in a truncated RT-β subunit and integrase (Johnson and Heneine, 2001). Hatai et al. (2008) isolated a strain of ALV (TymS_90) from layer chickens with fowl glioma that was a recombinant ALV derived from ev-1 and other strains of avian leukemia and sarcoma viruses. Although such hypothesis could be assumed for the ALV subgroup J sequenced in the present study, it could not be clarified whether the detected fragment was derived from an EAV or such a recombinant ALV. More detailed study, using primers specific to ALV subgroup J should be performed in the future.

The pathogenicity and oncogenesis potential of ALVs are not merely concerned with changes in the env gene, although they are the most important known factors. Two non-coding segments in the genome of ALV subgroup J, including U3 region of LTR and E element, also have a significant role in the pathogenicity of the virus (Hue et al. 2006; Gao et al. 2012). The LTR sequences of the ALV subgroup J strains have been previously compared (Gao et al. 2012). The phylogenetic analysis indicated that the LTR sequence of the studied isolate has approximately low homology with each of the other strains presented in the phylogenetic analysis. Twenty-six nucleotide substitutions in the U3 region were found in the studied isolate. Other scientists also mentioned that the U3 region of LTR evolves rapidly (Gao et al. 2012). A deletion of 11 bp was seen in our studied ALV subgroup J. Such a deletion is relatively rare among ALVs of subgroup J and is seen in only some Chinese strains, e.g. WN100401 (accession number HQ271447). The U3 region of the LTR contains transcriptional regulating elements and determines both the level of viral transcription and the oncogenic potential of ALVs (Gao et al. 2012).The nucleotide deletions in the U3 region of LTR in our studied virus caused omission of PRE box (Fig. 8).

This report is the first of ALV subgroup J, obtained for a chicken's tumor in Iran. The LTR region of the ALV subgroup J isolate, studied in this article, formed a separate branch from the prototype strain HPRS-103, a strain from the US (ADOL-7501) and other Chinese ALV subgroup J strains, including those isolated from broiler or layer chickens (Fig. 10). According to the sequence identity, the homology among LTR region of the studied ALV subgroup J and other ALV-J strains is relatively low (maximum 88.1%) (Fig. 9). Although it is not determined whether this information is related to changes in functional characteristics

of LTR gene, some interesting points on the molecular characteristics of the studied ALV subgroup J isolate were revealed. Such information together with more comprehensive future studies on the virus will contribute to a better understanding of the genetic differences of the studied ALV subgroup J with other countries' isolates.

Acknowledgements

We gratefully acknowledge the Deputy of Research Office of Lorestan University for their financial support.

References

1. Bai, J., Payne, L.N., Skinner, M.A. (1995) HPRS-103 (exogenous avian leukosis virus, subgroup J) has an env gene related to those of endogenous elements EAV-0 and E51 and an E element found previously only in sarcoma viruses. J Virol. 69: 779-784.

2. Bell, C.M., Schwarz, T., Dubielzig, R.R. (2011) Diagnostic features of feline restrictive orbital myofibroblastic sarcoma. Vet Pathol. 48: 742-750.

3. Cheng, Z., Liu, J., Cui, Z., Zhang, L. (2010) Tumors associated with avian leukosis virus subgroup J in layer hens during 2007 to 2009 in China. J Vet Med Sci. 72: 1027-1033.

4. Cherng, S., Young, J., Ma, H. (2008) Alpha smooth muscle actin (alpha-SMA). J Am Sci. 4: 7-9.

5. Darby, I.A., Hewitson, T.D. (2007) Fibroblast differentiation in wound healing and fibrosis. Int Rev Cytol. 257: 143-179.

6. Elberg, G., Chen, L., Elberg, D., Chan, M.D., Logan, C.J., Turman, M.A. (2008) MKL1 mediates TGF-{beta} 1- induced {alpha}-smooth muscle actin expression in human renal epithelial cells. American J Renal Physiol. 294: 1116-1128.

7. Hafner, S., Goodwin, M.A., Smith, E.J., Fadly, A., Kelley, L.C. (1998) Pulmonary Sarcomas in a Young Chicken. Avian Dis. 42: 824-826.

8. Handberg, K.J., Nielsen, O.L., Jørgensen, P.H. (2001) The use of serotype 1- and serotype 3-specific polymerase chain reaction for the detection of Marek's disease virus in chickens. Avian Pathol. 30: 243-249.

9. Hatai, H., Ochiai, K., Nagakura, K., Imanishi, S., Ochi., A., Kozakura, R., Ono, M., Goryo, M., Ohashi, K., Umemura, T. (2008) A recombinant avian leukosis virus associated with fowl glioma in layer chickens in Japan. Avian Pathol. 37: 127-137.

10. Johnson, J.A., Heneine, W. (2001) Characterization of endogenous avian leukosis viruses in chicken embryonic fibroblast substrates used in production of measles and mumps vaccines. J Virol. 75: 3605-3612.

11. Kawasaki, Y., Imaizumi, T., Matsuura, H., Ohara, S., Takano, K, Suyama, K., Hashimoto, K., Nozawa, R., Suzuki H., Hosoya, M. (2008) Renal expression of alpha-smooth muscle actin and c-Met in children with Henoch-Schönleinpurpura nephritis. Pediatr Nephrol. 23: 913-919.

12. Nakatani, T., Honda, E., Hayakawa, S., Sato, M., Satoh, K, Kudo, M., Munakata, H. (2008) Effects of decorin on the expression of alpha-smooth muscle actin in a human myofibroblast cell line. Mol Cell Biochem, 308: 201-207.

13. Newman, S.J., Cheramie, H., Duniho, S.M., Scarratt, W.K. (1999) Abdominal spindle cell sarcoma of probable myofibroblastic origin in a horse. J Vet Diagn Invest. 11: 278-282.

14. Ochi, A., Ochiai, K., Nakamura, S., Kobara, A., Sunden, Y., Umemura, T. (2012) Molecular characteristics and pathogenicity of an avian leukosis virus isolated from avian neurofibrosarcoma. Avian Dis. 56: 35-43.

15. Ono, M., Tsukamoto, K., Tanimura, N., Haritani, M., Kimura, K.M, Suzuki, G., Okuda, Y., Sato, S. (2004) An epizootic of subcutaneous tumors associated with subgroup a avian leukosis/sarcoma virus in young layer chickens. Avian Dis. 48: 940-946.

16. Park, S., Bivona, B.J., Harrison-Bernard, L.M (2007) Compromised renal microvascular reactivity of angiotensin type 1 double null mice. American J Physiol Renal Physiol. 293: 60-67.

17. Reece, R.L (1996) Some observations of naturally occurring neoplasms of domestic fowls I the state of Victoria, Australia (1997-87). Avian Pathol. 25: 407-447.

18. Silva, J.F., Palhares, M.S., Maranhão, R.P.A., Gheller, V.A., Boeloni, J.N., Serakides, R., Ocarino, N.M. (2012) Myofibroblastic Sarcoma in the Limb of a Horse. J Equine Vet Sci. 32: 197-200.

19. Smith, L.M., Toye, A.A., Howes, K, Bumstead, N., Payne, L.N., Venugopal, K. (1999) Novel endogenous retroviral sequences in the chicken genome closely related to HPRS-103 (subgroup J) avian leukosis virus. J Gen Virol. 80: 261-268.

20. Storch, K.N., Taatjes, D.J., Bouffard, N.A., Locknar, S., Bishop, N.M., Langevin, H.M. (2007) Alpha smooth muscle actin distribution in cytoplasm and nuclear invaginations of connective tissue fibroblasts. Histochem Cell Biol. 127: 523-530.

21. Strafuss, A.C., Ladds, P.W. (1970) Fibrosarcoma in a young chicken. Avian Dis. 14: 406-409.

22. Venugopal, K., Smith, L.M., Howes, K., Payne, L.N. (1998) Antigenic variants of J subgroup avian leukosis virus: sequence analysis reveals multiple changes in the env gene. J Gen Virol. 79: 757-764.

23. Wang, G., Jiang, Y., Yu, L., Wang, Y., Zhao,

X. (2013) Avian leukosis virus subgroup J associated with the outbreak of erythroblastosis in chickens in China. Virol J. 10: 92.

24. Zavala, G., Jackwood, M.W., Hilt, D.A. (2002) Polymerase chain reaction for detection of avian leukosis virus subgroup J in feather pulp. Avian Dis. 46: 971-978.

5

Thyroid hormones profile in Holstein calves following dexamethasone and isoflupredone administration

Chalmeh, A.*, Pourjafar, M., Nazifi, S., Zarei, M.R.

Department of Clinical Sciences, School of Veterinary Medicine, Shiraz University, Shiraz, Iran

Key words:

glucocorticoids, Holstein calves, metabolism, side effects, thyroid hormones

Correspondence

Chalmeh, A.
Department of Clinical Sciences, School of Veterinary Medicine, Shiraz University, Shiraz, Iran

Email: achalmeh81@gmail.com

Abstract:

BACKGROUND: Glucocorticoids are the steroidal drugs which are very widely used in large animal medicine. These agents have advantages in large animals but they have also been associated with many potential adverse effects, especially at high doses or prolonged use. **OBJECTIVES:** The present experimental study was designed to clarify the effects of dexamethasone (DEXA) and isoflupredone (ISO), as the most common glucocorticoids in large animal medicine, on bovine thyroid hormones. **METHODS:** Ten clinically healthy Holstein calves (6-8 months old) were assigned into 2 equal groups. Dexamethasone (1 mg/kg) and isoflupredone (1 mg/kg) were administered intramuscularly in DEXA and ISOgroups, respectively, for two consecutive days. Blood samples were taken at days 0 (before the 1stdose), 1 (before the 2 nd dose), 2, 3, 5 and 7, from all studied animals and serum concentrations of T3, T4, fT3 and fT4 were determined in all specimens. **RESULTS:** Levels of T3 and T4 were decreased significantly after administration of both drugs. The concentrations of T3 and T4 in Iso group were significantly lower than the DEXA one ($p < 0.05$). There were no significant changes in serum fT3 and fT4 levels following drug administration. **CONCLUSIONS:** Pharmacological doses of dexamethasone and isoflupredone have suppressive actions on the circulating levels of thyroid hormones in Holstein calves possibly via inhibition of TSH production at hypothalamic-pituitary-thyroid level.

Introduction

Several therapeutic agents can affect thyroid function at different levels (Betty, 2000; Bryan, 2009). These agents can alter circulating values of thyroid hormone by changing the levels of binding proteins or by competing for their hormone binding sites. Drugs may affect the synthesis or secretion of thyroid hormones. Pharmacological agents may also alter thyroid hormone metabolism and cellular uptake. Furthermore, drugs may interfere with hormone action at the target sites (Uma and Mihir, 2006). Hence, evaluating the circulating levels of thyroid hormones profile following the use of any medications can assist veterinarians to monitor the patients in order to prevent the side effects of drugs.

Glucocorticoids such as dexamethasone and isoflupredone are the steroidal drugs which are very widely used in large animal medicine. These agents have anti-inflammatory and immunosuppressant properties which are critical for the treatment of a variety of diseases (Radostits et al., 2007). However, besides their benefits, glucocorticoids, especially at high doses or for prolonged period, have been associated with many potential adverse effects (Plumb, 2008). Researchers mentioned that if large doses of these agents are given for a long period of time it may reduce thyroid stimulating hormone secretion from anterior pituitary thereby decreasing thyroid hormone secretion by different mechanisms (Wilke and Utiger, 1969). Thyroid cell function can be regulated by glucocorticoids via changes in the concentrations of the pivotal bioregulators such as thyroid stimulating hormone (Kaminsky et al., 1994).

Literatures mentioned the effects of glucocorticoids on thyroid functions in human beings (Burr et al., 1976; Hosur et al., 2012), laboratory (Nyborg et al., 1984; Stachoń et al., 2014) and farm animals (Messer et al., 1995) but in spite of the common use of glucocorticoids in bovine medicine, information regarding the effects of these agents on thyroid hormones profile is rare in these animals. Hence, the present experimental study was performed to clarify the effects of dexamethasone and isoflupredone on circulating levels of triiodothyronine (T3), thyroxine (T4), free triiodothyronine (fT3) and free thyroxine (fT4) in clinically healthy Holstein calves.

Materials and Methods

In October 2013, 10 clinically healthy Holstein calves (6-8 months old) were selected from two different dairy farms around Shiraz, Iran. The animals were examined prior to study and were proved to be clinically healthy. Calves were assigned into 2 equal groups (n=5). Dexamethasone (Vetacoid® 0.2%, Aburaihan Pharmaceutical Co, Tehran, Iran, 1 mg/kg, intramuscularly) and isoflupredone (Vetapredone® 0.2%, Aburaihan Pharmaceutical Co, Tehran, Iran, 1 mg/kg, intramuscularly) were administered in DEXA and ISO groups, respectively, for two consecutive days. Blood samples were taken at days 0 (before the 1stdose), 1 (before the 2nddose), 2, 3, 5 and 7 from all calves through the jugular vein in plain tubes. Immediately after blood collections, sera were separated by centrifugation (10 minutes at 3,000×g) and stored at −22°C until assayed.

Serum T3 concentrations were determined using a competitive enzyme immunoassay kit (Padtan Elm Co., Tehran, Iran). The intra- and inter-assay CVs were 12.6% and 13.2%, respectively. The sensitivity of the test was 0.2 ng/mL. Serum T4 concentrations were measured using a competitive enzyme immunoassay kit (Monobind Inc., CA, USA). The intra- and inter-assay CVs were 3.0% and 3.7%, respectively. The sensitivity of the test was 0.4 mg/dl. Serum fT3 and fT4 concentrations were determined by the fT3 and the fT4 ELISA kits (DiaPlus Inc., San Francisco, CA, USA). The intra- and inter-assay CVs of the fT3 assays were 4.1% and 5.2%, respectively. The sensitivity of the test was 0.05 pg/ml. The intra- and inter-assay CVs of the fT4 assays were 4.5% and 3.7%, respectively. The sensitivity of this test was 0.05 ng/dl, too.

Data were expressed as mean ± standard error (SE). Statistical analysis was performed using two independent samples t-test to compare mean concentrations of thyroid hormones within similar hours between experimental groups. Repeated mea-

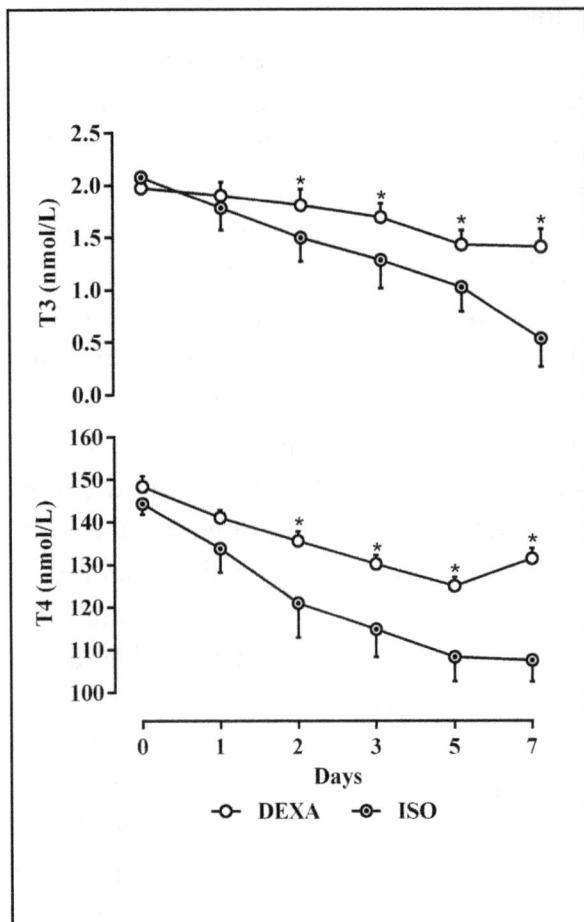

Figure 1. Effects of dexamethasone and isoflupredone (both at 1 mg/kg, injected intramuscularly for two consecutive days) on serum T3 and T4 levels in clinically healthy Holstein calves. Stars indicate significant differences between groups on similar days ($p < 0.05$).

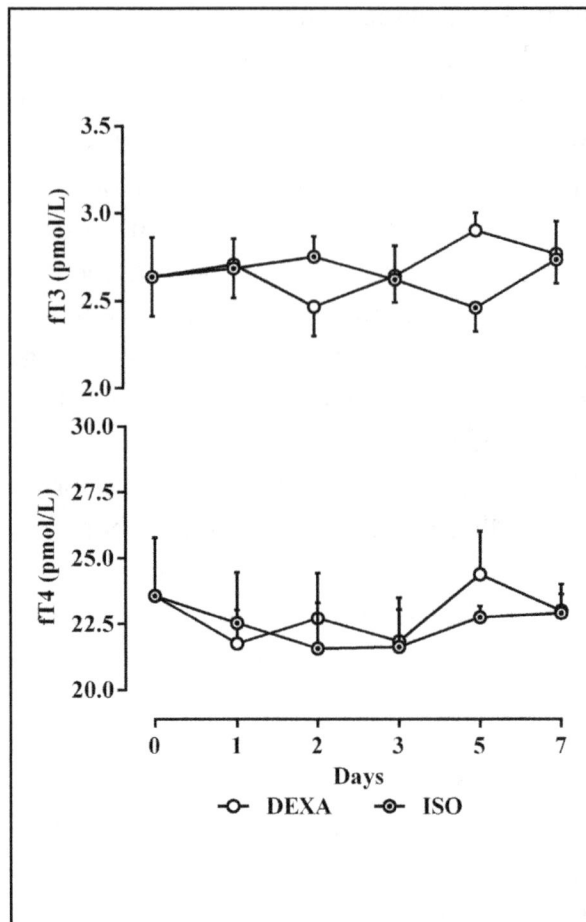

Figure 2. Effects of dexamethasone and isoflupredone (both at 1 mg/kg, injected intramuscularly for two consecutive days) on serum fT3 and fT4 levels in clinically healthy Holstein calves. Stars indicate significant differences between groups on similar days ($p < 0.05$).

sures ANOVA was also used in order to study the changes in pattern of serum thyroid hormones in each group, using SPSS software (SPSS for Windows, version 11.5, SPSS Inc, Chicago, Illinois). The level of significance was set at $p < 0.05$.

Results

Effects of dexamethasone and isoflupredone on serum thyroid hormones of clinically healthy Holstein calves are presented in Figs. 1 and 2. Levels of T3 and T4 were decreased significantly after both drugs were administrated ($p < 0.05$). The decreasing pattern of T3 and T4 were continued to last blood sampling at day 7 and their concentrations did not reach base line values at day zero. The concentrations of T3 and T4 in ISO group were significantly lower than those of DEXA group ($p < 0.05$; Figure 1). There were no significant changes in patterns in serum fT3 and fT4 levels following drug administration. Furthermore, no significant differences were seen between groups at all similar hours ($p > 0.05$; Figure 2).

Discussion

Thyroid gland produces the thyroid hormones containing T3 and its prohormone, T4, which are tyrosine-based hormones.

Thyrotropes of the anterior pituitary gland secrete thyroid stimulating hormone (TSH) and this hormone regulates the production of T3 and T4 by follicular cells of the thyroid gland. T4 is the major circulating thyroid hormone which has a longer half-life than T3. T4 is changed to T3 which is more potent than T4. fT3 and fT4 represent the amount of T3 and T4 that are not bound to proteins. Evaluating the fT3 and fT4 can be used to assess and manage disorders of the thyroid gland (Yen, 2001).

Thyroid hormones are primarily responsible for metabolism regulation. They increase the metabolic rate, change protein synthesis, regulate osteoblasts and nervous system maturation and increase the sensitivity to catecholamines. The proper circulating levels of thyroid hormones are necessary to develop and differentiate all of the cells. These hormones are also responsible for regulation of protein, fat, carbohydrate and vitamin metabolism. Numerous physiological, pathological and pharmacological stimuli influence thyroid hormone metabolism (Taylor et al., 1997; Tan et al., 1998).

We hypothesized that glucocorticoids, as a common pharmacological agent in large animals, can potentially affect the thyroid hormones profile. Hence the present experimental study was performed to compare the effects of dexamethasone and isoflupredone on the metabolism of thyroid hormones in clinically healthy Holstein calves. The results of the current research showed that circulating levels of T3 and T4 in both DEXA and ISO groups were decreased significantly after glucocorticoids administration.

All of the researchers mentioned that administration of glucocorticoids suppress the thyroid hormones. Glucocorticoids decreased blood serum TSH concentrations in euthyroid women (Bános et al., 1979). Dexamethasone administration to hypothyroid rats decreased serum TSH. Dexamethasone augmented a T3-induced decrease of TSH. However, changes in pituitary TSH α- and β-subunit mRNA concentrations were not found (Ahlquist et al., 1989).

Kakucska et al. (1995) obtained clearer results on the effects of glucocorticoids on the hypothalamo-pituitary-thyroid axis. In the paraventricular hypothalamic nuclei of adrenalectomized rats, an increase in corticotropin releasing hormone mRNA occurred in parallel to the increase in pro-thyrotropin releasing hormone mRNA. On the contrary, administration of corticosterone or dexamethasone caused a marked decrease in corticotropin releasing hormone mRNA and pro-thyrotropin releasing hormone mRNA (Kakucska et al., 1995).

Administration of a single dose of hydrocortisone (500 mg) increased both TSH production and stimulation by thyrotropin releasing hormone in normal subjects and patients with Cushing's syndrome (Rubello et al., 1992). Only long-term hypocorticism may be a cause for decreased TSH level. The earlier recovery of the diurnal rhythm of TSH than that of cortisol suggests that the TSH rhythm is not under the direct control of circulating cortisol (Azukizawa et al., 1979). Fang and Shian (1981) suggested that adrenal glands may not be directly involved in the hypothalamic control of the pituitary content of TSH. They also revealed that physiological levels of glucocorticoids clearly exert an inhibitory effect on TSH release by the pituitary gland in response to provocative stimulation.

Administration of a high dose of dexamethasone not only suppressed TSH but also decreased the TSH response to thyrotropin releasing hormone administration (Re et al., 1976).The inhibitory effect of dexamethasone is used for monitoring of subclinical hypothyroidism in obese patients. Administration of thyrotropin releasing hormone after dexamethasone increased the TSH level only in hypothyroid patients but not in euthyroid obese patients (Coiro et al., 2001). Results of the Ghadhban and Jawad's study (2013) revealed a significant decrease in the serum concentrations of T3 and T4 during administration of dexamethasone in rabbits at 0.5 mg/kg BW. This decrease in the thyroid hormones of rabbit circulation may be due to dexamethasone action as suppression of hypothalamic-pituitary-thyroid activity.

In conclusion, it can be stated that pharmacological doses of dexamethasone and isoflupredone have suppressive actions on the circulating levels of active thyroid hormone in Holstein calves. Based on the findings of other researchers it may be suggested that the common pathway of this action is at hypothalamic-pituitary-thyroid level to inhibit TSH production and hence reduce thyroidal T3 and T4 release. The results of the present experimental study showed that decreasing the serum T3 and T4 levels can be considered as a side effect of glucocorticoids in Holstein calves and veterinarians should note the disadvantages of these pharmacological agents.

Acknowledgments

The authors would like to thank Shiraz University for financial support of this project.

References

Ahlquist, J., Franklyn, J., Ramsden, D., Sheppard, M. (1989) The influence of dexamethasone on serum thyrotrophin and thyrotrophin synthesis in the rat. Mol Cell Endocrinol. 64: 55-61.

Azukizawa, M., Mori, S., Ohta, H., Matsumura, S., Yoshimoto, H., Uozumi, T., Miyai, K., Kumahara, Y. (1979) Effect of a single dose of glucocorticoid on the diurnal variations of TSH, thyroxine, 3,5,3'-triiodothyronine, 3,3',5'-triiodothyronine and cortisol in normal men. Endocrinol Jpn. 26: 719-723.

Bános, C., Takó, J., Salamon, F., Györgyi, S., Czikkely, R. (1979) Effect of ACTH-stimulated glucocorticoid hypersecretion on the serum concentrations of thyroxine-binding globulin, thyroxine, triiodothyronine, reverse triiodothyronine and on the TSH response to TRH. Acta Med Acad Sci Hung. 36: 381-394.

Betty, J.D. (2000) How medications affect thyroid function. West J Med. 172: 102-106.

Bryan, R.H. (2009) Drugs that suppress TSH or cause central hypothyroidism. Best Pract Res Clin Endocrinol Metab. 23: 793-800.

Burr, W.A., Ramsden, D.B., Griffiths, R.S., Hottenberg, R., Meinhold, H., Wenzel, K.W. (1976) Effects of a single dose of dexamethasone on serum concentration of thyroid hormone. Lancet. 308: 58-61.

Coiro, V., Volpi, R., Capretti, L., Speroni, G., Pilla, S., Cataldo, S., Bianconcini, M., Bazzani, E., Chiodera, P. (2001) Effect of dexamethasone on TSH-secretion induced by TRH in human obesity. Investig Med. 49: 330-334.

Fang, V., Shian, L. (1981) Adrenal influence on pituitary secretion of thyrotropin and prolactin in rats. Endocrinology. 108: 1545-1551.

Ghadhban, R.F., Jawad, A.D.H. (2013) Effects of dexamethasone, estrogen administration on leptin, thyroid, reproductive hormone concentration and lipid profile of female rabbit's serum. Bas J Vet Res. 12: 41-53.

Hosur, M.B., Puranik, R.S., Vanaki, S., Puranik, S.R. (2012) Study of thyroid hormones free triiodothyronine (FT3), free thyroxine (FT4) and thyroid stimulating hormone (TSH) in subjects with dental fluorosis. Eur J Dent. 6: 184-190.

Kakucska, I., Qi, Y., Lechan, R. (1995) Changes in adrenal status affect hypothalamic thyrotropin-releasing hormone gene expression in parallel with corticotropin-releasing hormone. Endocrinology. 136: 2795-2802.

Kaminsky, S., Levy, O., Salvador, C., Dai, G., Carrasco, N. (1994) Na(+)-I- symport activity is present in membrane vesicles from thyrotropin-deprived non-I(-)-transporting cultured thyroid cells. Proc Natl Acad Sci. 91: 3789-3793.

Messer, N.T., Ganjam, V.K., Nachreiner, R.F., Krause, G.F. (1995) Effect of dexamethasone administration on serum thyroid hormone concentrations in clinically normal horses. J Am Vet Med Assoc. 206: 63-66.

Nyborg, J.K., Nguyen, A.P., Spindler, S.R. (1984) Relationship between thyroid and glucocorticoid hormone receptor occupancy, growth hormone gene transcription, and mRNA accumulation. J Biol Chem. 259: 12377-12381.

Plumb, D.C. (2008) Plumb's Veterinary Drug Handbook. (6th ed.) Blackwell Publishing. Iowa, USA. p. 457-639.

Radostits, O.M., Gay, C., Hinchcliff, K.W., Constable, P.D. (2007) Veterinary Medicine: A Textbook of the Diseases of Cattle, Horses, Sheep, Pigs and Goats. (10th ed.) Saunders. London, UK. p. 53-60.

Re, R., Kourides, I., Ridgway, E., Weintraub, B., Maloof, F. (1976) The effect of glucocorticoid administration on human pituitary secretion of thyrotropin and prolactin. J Clin Endocrinol Metab. 43: 338-346.

Rubello, D., Sonino, N., Casara, D., Girelli, M., Busnardo, B., Boscaro, M. (1992) Acute and chronic effects of high glucocorticoid levels on hypothalamic-pituitary-thyroid axis in man. J Endocrinol Invest. 15: 437-441.

Stachoń, M., Gromadzka-Ostrowska, J., Lachowicz, K., Fürstenberg, E., Pałkowska, E., Gajewska, D., Myszkowska-Ryciak, J., Kozłowska, L., Rosołowska-Huszcz, D. (2014) Interdependence of the peripheral metabolism of glucocorticoids and thyroid hormones under calorie deficit in rats at different ages. J Anim Feed Sci. 23: 167-176.

Tan, K.C., Shiu, S.W., Kung, A.W. (1998) Effect of thyroid dysfunction on high-density lipoprotein subfraction metabolism: roles of hepatic lipase and cholesteryl ester transfer protein. J Clin Endocrinol Metab. 83: 2921-2924.

Taylor, A.H., Stephan, Z.F., Steele, R.E., Wong, N.C. (1997) Beneficial effects of a novel thyromimetic on lipoprotein metabolism. Mol Pharmacol. 52: 542-547.

Uma, K.S., Mihir, S. (2006) Drug induced thyroid disorders. J Indian Med Assoc: 104, 583, 585-587, 600.

Wilke, J.F., Utiger, R.D. (1969) The effect of glucocorticoids on thyrotropin secretion. J Clin Invest. 48: 2086-2090.

Yen, P.M. (2001) Physiological and molecular basis of thyroid hormone action. Physiol Rev. 81: 1097-1142.

6

Comparison of required induction dose, induction and recovery characteristics, and cardiorespiratory effects of co-administration of ketofol with diazepam and midazolam in healthy dogs

Imani, H.*, Baniadam, A., Mosallanejad, B., Shabani, Sh.

Department of Clinical Science, Faculty of Veterinary Medicine, Shahid Chamran University of Ahvaz, Ahvaz, Iran

Key words:

co-administration, diazepam, dog, ketofol, midazolam

Correspondence

Imani, H.
Department of Clinical Science, Faculty of Veterinary Medicine, Shahid Chamran University of Ahvaz, Ahvaz, Iran

Email: h.imani@scu.ac.ir

Abstract:

BACKGROUND: Co-administration of anesthetics has been employed to decrease potential unpleasant effects associated with single drug. OBJECTIVES: This study was designed to evaluate the effects of co-administration of ketofol with diazepam or midazolam in healthy dogs. METHODS: Six adult mixbreed male dogs were used. After sedation with acepromazine (0.1 mg/kg), anesthesia was induced with keteofol (KF; 1 ml contained 5 mg ketamine and 5 mg propofol), ketofol-diazepam (KFD), or ketofol-midazolam (KFM) (1 ml contained 5 mg KF and 2.5 mg diazepam or midazolam) randomly. All the dogs received the three treatments with at least one week interval. RESULTS: The total dose of ketofol used for induction of anesthesia in KF (4.2±0.44 mg/kg) was significantly higher than KFD (2.27±0.6 mg/kg) and KFM (1.68±0.25 mg/kg). The total dose of diazepam and midazolam used in KFD and KFM was 1.00±0.25 and 0.73±0.10 mg/kg, respectively (p>0.05). The time needed for sternal recumbency, standing position and normal walking was longer in KFD and KFM compared to KF (p<0.05). Heart rate (HR) showed significant increase in KF at several time points (p<0.05). Respiratory rate (fr) in KF showed a significant decrease during the anesthesia period compared to the base (p<0.05). HR and fr were more stable in KFD and KFM. Induction and recovery quality in the three treatments were acceptable. CONCLUSIONS: Co-administration of ketofol with diazepam and midazolam reduced the required induction dose and prolonged recovery in dogs. Diazepam and midazolam could attenuate the unfavorable effects of ketofol in some cardiorespiratory variables.

Introduction

General anesthesia is frequently used in dogs in various occasions from minimally invasive procedures to the most complicated surgeries. Induction as well as recovery of anesthesia are two critical conditions during general anesthesia due to the occurrence of certain life-threatening hazards in these stages. An optimum induction and recovery is calm and has fewer undesirable effects. Since no drug has been introduced without unfavorable effects, co-administration of various drugs is employed to reduce potential side effects and to produce anesthesia with more satisfactory outcomes (Martinez-Taboada and Leece, 2014).

Propofol, an alkyl phenol, is a popular induction agent which is used widely in the anesthesia of dogs (Covey-Crump and Murison, 2008). The smooth induction with rapid and complete recovery have been proved as the most valuable characteristics of propofol in dogs (Watkins et al., 1987). The main complications associated with propofol are dose dependent respiratory and cardiovascular depression as well as hypotension (Kennedy and Smith, 2014). Ketamine, an NMDA antagonist, is another anesthetic that can be used for induction in dogs. In contrast to propofol, ketamine has some cardiovascular stimulatory effects which result in an increase in heart rate (HR) and cardiac output (Abbasivash et al., 2014). Ketamine can also be associated with muscle rigidity, convulsions, and violent recovery; it is therefore recommended that ketamine be used in conjunction with other drugs such as benzodiazepines (Kennedy and Smith, 2014). It has been suggested that ketamine may compensate the cardiovascular depression induced by propofol (Abbasivash et al., 2014). Co-administration of ketamine and propofol, used in separate syringes, has resulted in higher HR and less occurrence of apnea compared to propofol alone in dogs (Lerche et al., 2000). Ketofol, a mixture of propofol and low dose ketamine into the same syringe, has also been evaluated in dogs (Henao-Guerrero and Riccó, 2014; Kennedy and Smith, 2014; Martinez-Taboada and Leece, 2014). Ketofol is of interest as it requires administration of only a single infusion. In addition, ketofol may lead to more hemodynamic stability than other combinations of ketamine and propofol (Martinez-Taboada and Leece, 2014).

Benzodiazepines are commonly used as co-induction agents with conventional anesthetics. The three main benefits of these drugs are rapid onset of action, minimal negative cardiovascular effects, and anticonvulsant prop-erties (Hopkins et al., 2014). It has also been shown that co-administration of diazepam and midazolam could reduce the induction dose of propofol in dogs (Braun et al., 2007; Fayyaz et al., 2009; Hopkins et al., 2014; Ko et al., 2006). Diazepam and midazolam have been used with ketamine as the co-induction agent mostly to reduce the central excitatory effects of ketamine (Ilkiw et al., 1996; White et al., 2001). To the best of the authors' knowledge, no study has yet evaluated the effects of co-administration of ketofol with diazepam or midazolam combined into the same syringe in dogs.

The present investigation was designed to evaluate required induction dose, induction and recovery characteristics, and cardiorespiratory variables in dogs sedated with acepromazine and induced with a single infusion of ketofol with diazepam and midazolam.

Materials and Methods

Six adult mix-breed male dogs, weighing 20 ± 1 kg and aged 22 ± 3 months were used. The animals were transferred to Veterinary Hospital of Shahid Chamran University of Ahvaz at least two weeks prior to the beginning of study. Health status was established based on a complete blood count (CBC), total protein (TP), and thorough physical examination. The animals were housed in individual cages with free access to water and feeding twice a day. The dogs were fasted 12 hours prior to any experiment. They had no access to water for two hours before any experiment. All procedures in this study were approved by the Animal Care and Research Committee of Shahid Chamran University of Ahvaz.

In the present study, the dogs received one of the three treatments of keteofol (KF), keto-fol-diazepam (KFD), and ketofol-midazolam (KFM), randomly in each session. All the animals received all three treatments with at least one week interval (6 dogs per group). Preparation of ketofol in this study was based on the study of Andofatto and Willman (2010). In brief, ketamine 5% (Ketamine hydrochloride, Rotexmedica, Trittau, Germany; 50 mg/mL) was attenuated to ketamine 1% (1 mg/mL) by normal saline. Then, an equivalent volume of ketamine and propofol (Anesia, Alleman, Germany; 10 mg/mL) was combined into the same syringe (each mL ketofol contained 5 mg ketamine and 5 mg propofol). The syringe of ketofol admixture was kept for maximum 6 hours after preparation. For preparing KFD and KFM, diazepam (Zepadic, Caspian Tamin, Iran; 5 mg/mL) or midazolam (Midamax, Tehran Chemie, Iran; 5 mg/mL) were added to previously prepared ketofol admixture in the ratio of 1:1 (each mL KFD and KFM contained 5 mg ketofol and 2.5 mg diazepam or midazolam). The time of KFD and KFM preparation was immediately prior to injection.

To conduct the experiment, the animals were transferred to the place of the study. Thirty min was given to allow animals to acclimatize to the environment. After recording the temperament of the animals and recording heart rate (HR), respiratory rate (fr), and rectal temperature (RT), acepromazine (Neurotranq, Alfasan, Netherland; 10 mg/mL) at 0.1 mg/kg was administered intramuscularly (IM). Thirty min later and after scoring the quality of sedation (Appendix), and recording HR, fr and RT, the animals were transferred onto a surgery table and positioned in sternal recumbency. A 20 gauge catheter was placed into the left cephalic vein and normal saline was administered at the rate of 10 mL/kg/hr for five minutes. To induce anesthesia, treatments were injected via a syringe connected to the cephalic catheter at a rate of about 0.2 mL/kg/min. All injections were performed via hand and the person who applied injections was unaware of the treatments. Nonetheless, the color of KF and KFM was milky and the color of KFD was yellowish. Another researcher was responsible for placement of the tracheal tube, concomitantly. The

dogs were intubated when chewing and licking were stopped. After ensuring the correct placement of the tracheal tube, the administration of the drugs was discontinued immediately. The animals were allowed to breathe the room air, spontaneously. At this time, induction quality was scored (Appendix).

After induction of anesthesia, the animals were positioned in the right lateral recumbency and immediately connected to a multiparameter monitoring system (Burtons, Guardian Industrial Estate, UK) for measurement of hemoglobin oxygen saturation (SPO2), noninvasive systolic, diastolic and mean arterial blood pressure (SAP, DAP, and MAP, respectively), end-tidal carbon dioxide tension (ETCO2), HR, fr, and RT. All data were recorded one minute after intubation, then at every three minutes, and at just before extubation. Extubation was done when the animal was chewing continuously and could not tolerate tracheal tube any more. The animal received normal saline intravenously (IV) at the rate of 10 mL/kg/hr, until the extubation was done. After extubation, HR, fr, and RT were recorded every five min till 30 min post induction and then every 10 min till the full recovery of the animal. During the recovery period, the times of head upraising, sternal recumbency, standing position and normal walking were recorded. Full recovery was defined as when the dogs started walking normally. Recovery was scored at this time (Appendix). All the scores for sedation, intubation and recovery were given by the same researcher who was not aware of the treatments.

Statistical analysis: Statistical analysis was performed using SPSS software version 22 for windows (IBM SPSS statistic, IBM Corporation, NY, USA). Values of HR, fr, and RT were expressed at seven sections including base (prior to premedication), sedation (30 minutes after premedication), after induction, anesthesia period (the mean values during the anesthesia till extubation), before extubation, recovery period (the mean values during the recovery till normal walking), and recovery point (when the dog was able to walk normally). Data related to SPO2, SAP, DAP, MAP, and ETCO2 were reported at three sections including after induction, anesthesia period (the mean values during the anesthesia till extubation), and before extubation. The normality of data was analyzed using Kolmogrov-Smirnov test. All normally distributed data were expressed as mean ± standard deviation (SD) and nonparametric data were reported as median (range). A repeated measure ANOVA followed by Bonferoni test was used for the comparison of sequences during recovery, and variables of HR, fr, RT, SPO2, SAP, DAP, MAP, and ETCO2. Friedman tests were employed for the comparison of sedation score, induction score, and recovery score. $p < 0.05$ was considered statistically significant.

Results

There were no differences in the temperaments of the dogs and all the dogs were seemingly normal prior to beginning the study. The sedation score following administration of acepromazine did not show any significant differences among the three groups ($p > 0.05$; Table 1).

The induction time in KFM (1.63±0.10 min) was significantly faster in comparison to KF (2.14±0.11 min) and KFD (2.25±0.23 min) ($p < 0.05$). The total dose of ketofol used for induction of anesthesia in KF (4.2±0.44 mg/kg) was significantly greater than KFD (2.27±0.6 mg/kg) and KFM (1.68±0.25 mg/kg) ($p < 0.05$). The total dose of ketofol was significantly higher in KFD versus KFM ($p < 0.05$). The total dose of diazepam and midazolam used in KFD and KFM was 1.00±0.25 and 0.73±0.10 mg/kg, respectively, with no significant differences between them ($p > 0.05$). The time needed for chronological sequences of events in the recovery period is presented in Table 2. Sig-

Table 1. Median (upper-lower range) of scores that were given for quality of sedation, induction, and recovery in dogs (n = 6) that received KF (ketofol), KFD (ketofol-diazepam), and KFM (ketofol-midazolam).

	Sedation score	Induction Score	Recovery score
KF	1 (1-2)	1 (1-1)	1 (1-1)
KFD	1 (0-2)	1 (1-1)	1 (1-2)
KFM	1 (1-2)	1 (1-2)	2 (1-2)

nificant swallow reflex was seen later in KFD compared to KF and KFM ($p < 0.05$). The time to the sternal recumbency, standing position and normal walking was longer in KFD and KFM compared to KF ($p < 0.05$).

HR, fr, and RT values were presented in Table 3. Comparison of HR among the groups showed significant lower values in KFD compared to KF at anesthesia period, before extubation, and recovery period ($p < 0.05$). HR in KFM before extubation was significantly higher than KFD ($p < 0.01$). HR in KFM in the recovery period was significantly lower in comparison to KF ($p < 0.05$). HR within KF showed a significant increase during the entire evaluation period compared to the base ($p < 0.05$). HR in KFD was significantly higher at normal walking than the base ($p < 0.01$). HR in KFM was significantly higher at recovery period compared to the base ($p < 0.05$). fr was significantly higher in KFM compared to KF at anesthesia period ($p < 0.05$). fr Showed a significant difference at normal walking in KF compared to KFD ($p < 0.05$) and KFM ($p < 0.01$). The comparison of fr in KF showed a significant decrease after induction and anesthesia period compared to the base ($p < 0.05$).

Values related to SPO2, SAP, DAP, MAP, and ETCO2 were presented in Table 4. SPO2 in KFM was significantly higher in anesthesia period and before extubation in comparison to after induction ($p < 0.05$). SPO2 before extubation was significantly higher than in anesthesia period in this group ($p < 0.05$). SAP in KFM showed a significant decrease before extubation compared to after induction ($p < 0.05$).

Table 2. Time (min) needed for various chronological sequences of recovery events in dogs (n = 6) that received KF (ketofol), KFD (ketofol-diazepam), and KFM (ketofol-midazolam). * Significantly different from KF values (p<0.05).

	Swallow reflex (Extubation)	Head upraising	Sternal recumbency	Standing position	Normal walking
KF	8.67 ± 2.50	13.00 ± 3.74	13.83 ± 3.65	18.00 ± 7.51	27.00 ± 7.01
KFD	15.17 ± 4.83 *	19.50 ± 7.17	22.00 ± 7.26 *	27.50 ± 8.16 *	42.00 ± 11.11 *
KFM	12.33 ± 5.42	16.17 ± 7.33	19.83 ± 4.44 *	31.17 ± 8.56 *	46.83 ± 8.83 *

Table 3. Mean ± SD of HR (beats/min), *fr* (breaths/min), and RT (°C) in dogs (n = 6) that received KF (ketofol), KFD (ketofol-diazepam), and KFM (ketofol-midazolam). HR: heart rate, fr: respiratory rate, RT: rectal temperature. * Significantly different from KF values (p<0.05). † Significantly different from KFD values (p<0.05). a Significantly different from base values (p<0.05).

	Base	Sedation	After induction	Anesthesia period	Before extubation	Recovery period	Normal walking
KF							
HR	94 ± 7	93 ± 16	128 ± 29 a	122 ± 22 a	120 ± 18 a	133 ± 18 a	135 ± 13 a
fr	24 ± 7	19 ± 6	11 ± 5 a	11 ± 3 a	24 ± 11	24 ± 7	23 ± 7
RT	38.8 ± 0.3	38.4 ± 0.4	36.8 ± 0.9 a	37.3 ± 0.9	37.5 ± 0.8	38 ± 0.5	37.9 ± 0.7
KFD							
HR	99 ± 13	78 ± 15	108 ± 9	91 ± 7 *	92 ± 8 *	112 ± 11 *	132 ± 9 a
fr	24 ± 7	18 ± 5	15 ± 8	17 ± 6	23 ± 11	25 ± 7	27 ± 7 *
RT	38.7 ± 0.5	38.3 ± 0.5	37.4 ± 0.2	37.5 ± 0.8	37.3 ± 0.8	37.4 ± 0.5	37.4 ± 0.6
KFM							
HR	88 ± 16	86 ± 14	117 ± 18	101 ± 21	105 ± 9 †	114 ± 13 * , a	125 ± 26 a
fr	23 ± 9	22 ± 7	18 ± 7	22 ± 5 *	27 ± 10	31 ± 8	28 ± 8 *
RT	38.7 ± 0.4	38.3 ± 0.4	37.5 ± 0.6	37.6 ± 0.5	37.5 ± 0.6	37.5 ± 0.8	37.4 ± 0.9

Table 4. Mean ± SD of SPO2 (%), SAP (mmHg), DAP (mmHg), MAP (mmHg), and ETCO2 (mmHg), in dogs (n = 6) that received KF (ketofol), KFD (ketofol-diazepam), and KFM (ketofol-midazolam) treatments. SPO2: hemoglobin oxygen saturation, SAP: systolic arterial pressure, DAP: diastolic arterial pressure, MAP: mean arterial pressure. ETCO2: end-tidal carbon dioxide tension. a significantly different from after induction (p < 0.05).

	After induction	Anesthesia period	Before extubation
KF			
SPO2	90 ± 6	92 ± 3	95 ± 2
SAP	125 ± 14	126 ± 15	123 ± 18
DAP	76 ± 8	77 ± 12	81 ± 12
MAP	91 ± 12	93 ± 13	91 ± 16
ETCO2	26 ± 10	29 ± 6	30 ± 7
KFD			
SPO2	89 ± 5	92 ± 4	94 ± 4
SAP	137 ± 10	135 ± 17	136 ± 34
DAP	90 ± 18	81 ± 13	79 ± 9
MAP	107 ± 16	95 ± 16	94 ± 14
ETCO2	30 ± 9	31 ± 5	28 ± 6
KFM			
SPO2	88 ± 3	93 ± 1 a	96 ± 2 a
SAP	125 ± 10	127 ± 15	122 ± 13
DAP	80 ± 5	73 ± 8	72 ± 4 a
MAP	98 ± 11	91 ± 10	85 ± 5
ETCO2	30 ± 8	31 ± 5	27 ± 5

Table 5. Appendix. Description of scoring system used to categorize sedation and quality of induction and recovery in dogs (n = 6) that received KF (ketofol), KFD (ketofol-diazepam), and KFM (ketofol-midazolam). * Source: Adapted from Mair A.R., Pawson P., Courcier E., Flaherty D.: A comparison of the effects of two different doses of ketamine used for co-induction of anaesthesia with a target-controlled infusion of propofol in dogs. Vet Anesth Analg 2009, 36, 532-538. †Source: Adapted from Muir W., Gadawski J.: Respiratory depression and apnea induced by propofol in dogs. Am J of Vet Res 1998, 59, 157-161.

Sedation *	0	No sedation
	1	Mild sedation (i.e. quieter, but still bright and active)
	2	Moderate sedation (i.e. quiet, reluctant to move, possibly ataxic but still able to walk)
	3	Profound sedation (i.e. unable to walk)
Induction †	1	No outward sign of excitement, rapidly assumes lateral recumbency, good muscular relaxation, easily intubated within 60 seconds of finishing dosing
	2	Mild signs of excitement, some struggling, may or may not be intubated within 60 seconds of finishing dosing
	3	Hyperkinesis, obvious signs of excitement, vocalization, defecation or urination, cannot be intubated
Recovery †	1	Assumes sternal recumbency with little or no struggling, and attempts to stand and walk with little or no difficulty
	2	Some struggling, requires assistance with sternal recumbency or standing, responsive to external stimuli, becomes quiet in sternal recumbency
	3	Prolonged struggling, unable to assume sternal recumbency or difficulty in maintaining sternal or standing position, becomes hyperkinetic when assisted, prolonged paddling and swimming motion

Median (upper-lower range) of scores for induction and recovery was shown in Table 1. There were no significant differences in induction scores as well as recovery scores among the three treatments (p>0.05). Overall, induction and recovery were smooth in all of the dogs, except for the two dogs in KFD that showed some twitching in the recovery period. Although it was not measured, imbalance in walking was more apparent in KF than KFD and KFM.

Discussion

In this study the total dose of ketofol required for tracheal intubation was smaller in KFD and KFM compared to KF. Ketofol was introduced to anesthesiologists in an attempt to reduce the doses of ketamine and propofol to avoid or lessen the unfavorable effects associated with the use of each of these two drugs. Previous studies in dogs have shown a significant reduction in the amount of ketamine and propofol when used together, and necessary for induction and/or maintenance of anesthesia compared to propofol alone (Henao-Guerrero and Riccó, 2014; Kennedy and Smith, 2014; Lerche et al., 2000; Mannarino et al., 2012; Seliskar et al., 2007). Similar findings have been observed when ketofol was employed for induction of anesthesia in humans (Andolfatto and Willman, 2010; Erdogan et al., 2013). The total dose of ketofol used for induction of anesthesia in the current study was 4.2±0.44 mg/kg in KF, which is comparable to 4.0±1.0 mg/kg and 3.6±1.8 mg/kg in dogs reported by Kennedy and Smith (2014) and Martinez-Taboada and Leece (2014), respectively. Addition of diazepam and midazolam to ketofol in the current study showed an approximately 46% and 60% reduction in the dose of ketofol, respectively (2.27±0.6 mg/kg and 1.68±0.25 mg/kg, respectively). Co-administration of various anesthetics with benzodiazepines with the aim of reducing the dose of anesthetics and employing cardiovascular benefits of benzodiazepines has already been reported in dogs (Covey-Crump and Murison, 2008; Henao-Guerrero and Riccó, 2014; Hopkins et al., 2014; Riccó and Henao-Guerrero, 2014). The clinical efficacy of co-induction of propofol-ketamine-midazolam in humans has also been shown by Abbasivash et al. (2014). To the best of the authors' knowledge, the current study is the first experimental investigation aimed at evaluation of combination of diazepam and midazolam with ketofol into the same syringe, as the co-administration agents.

Diazepam is a poorly water soluble drug and therefore requires being prepared in a solution of an organic solvent such as propylene glycol and ethanol (Rankin, 2015). In the current study, diazepam was added to previously prepared ketofol. Because of the possible unwanted interaction of drugs, we prepared the admixture immediately prior to injection. Addition of diazepam to ketofol into the same syringe resulted in changing the color of the admixture from white to yellowish; nevertheless, no precipitation or biphasic state was observed prior to or during the injection period.

The results of the present study showed the prolongation of recovery period in KFD and KFM compared to KF. Although benzodiazepines have been used in dogs to ameliorate the central excitatory effects, reduce the dose, and to minimize hemodynamic changes associated with anesthetics (Rankin, 2015), these drugs have also been used to prolong anesthesia in horses (Brock and Hildebrand, 1990; Butera et al., 1978).

HR showed a trend to increase one minute post administration of all three treatments; however, it was not statistically significant in KFD and KFM. Ketofol has been associated with higher HR values compared to baseline in dogs (Henao-Guerrero and Riccó, 2014; Kennedy and Smith, 2014; Martinez-Taboada and Leece, 2014). Similar results have been observed when ketamine and propofol, in separate syringes, were employed for induction of anesthesia in dogs (Lerche et al., 2000; Seliskar et al., 2007). Ketamine could indirectly stimulate the cardiovascular system and subsequently increase HR and MAP (Tweed et al., 1972; Wong and Jenkins, 1974). Furthermore, it is speculated that addition of ketamine to propofol could attenuate dose-dependent depression of sympathetic tone produced

by propofol (Martinez-Taboada and Leece, 2014). Higher values of HR during anesthesia in KF could be explained by the stimulating effects of ketamine on the cardiovascular system (Henao-Guerrero and Riccó, 2014; Riccó and Henao-Guerrero, 2014). HR showed greater decrease in KFD and KFM compared to KF at several time points. Use of diazepam has been associated with decreasing myocardial contractility, systemic blood pressure, and HR in anesthetized cats (Chai and Wang, 1966). It has also been reported that administration of diazepam prior to ketamine minimizing the cardiovascular stimulation produced by ketamine (Haskins et al., 1986). It is likely that decreases in HR in KFD and KFM could be produced by diazepam and midazolam via the same mechanism.

Combination of ketamine and propofol has attenuated the decrease of MAP associated with administration of propofol alone in dogs (Henao-Guerrero and Riccó, 2014; Kennedy and Smith, 2014; Lerche et al., 2000; Martinez-Taboada and Leece, 2014). In the present study MAP did not show any significant differences among groups and all values were in the second half of the normal range reported in dogs (Haskins et al., 2005). MAP was also not statistically different in the evaluation period in all three treatments; nevertheless, MAP tended to decrease over time in KFD and KFM. As mentioned above, this trend could be explained by the effects of benzodiazepines on stimulatory effects of ketamine.

Propofol is known as a dose-dependent respiratory depressant in humans and dogs (Muir and Gadawski, 1998; Smith et al., 1994; Smith et al., 1993). It has been reported that ketamine in clinically applicable or sub-anesthetic doses can cause respiratory depression in dogs (Haskins et al., 1985). Respiratory depression is also a relatively common finding in studies that evaluated the respiratory effects of ketofol or ketamine and propofol combination in dogs (Kennedy and Smith, 2014; Lerche et al.,

2000; Mair et al., 2009; Martinez-Taboada and Leece, 2014; Seliskar et al., 2007). It seems that ketamine could exacerbate respiratory depression produced by propofol (Lerche et al., 2000; Seliskar et al., 2007). In the present study *fr* in KF showed a significant decrease after induction and anesthesia period in comparison with base. *fr* decreased after induction in KFD and KFM, however, in contrast to KF this decrease was not significant. SPO2 in all the treatments showed a trend to increase over time; nonetheless, the differences were not significant. The decrease of fr and lower values of SPO2 after induction could be interpreted as the occurrence of respiratory depression after the treatments. In the study reported here, in all the three treatments, ETCO2 was lower than the normal range for dogs (Haskins, 2015). Oxygen supplementation and/or assisted ventilation to resolve respiratory depression have been recommended in dogs anesthetized with ketofol (Kennedy and Smith, 2014).

Selisker et al. (2015) reported stiffness as well as some excitement and disorientation in dogs that received propofol/ketamine. In contrast, recovery has obtained a better score in ketofol treatments in comparison with propofol alone in the study of Kennedy and Smith 2014; still, the difference was not significant. In the current study, all recoveries were quiet and satisfactory, except for the two dogs in KFD that showed some twitching. Both dogs eventually recovered without any sequelae. However, it was not recorded, imbalance in walking was more common in KF than KFD and KFM.

Conclusion: Co-administration of ketofol with diazepam and midazolam reduced the required induction dose and prolonged recovery in dogs. Induction and recovery quality in the three treatments were acceptable; however, more attention is needed for recovery in using the combination of ketofol and midazolam. In the present study, diazepam and midazolam attenuated unfavorable effects of ketofol in HR

and *fr*. Oxygen supplementation in dogs receiving ketofol with or without diazepam and midazolam is recommended.

Acknowledgments

The authors are grateful to the Research Council of the Shahid Chamran University of Ahvaz for financial support of this study. Authors would also like to thank Mr. Norouzi and Mr. Tab, the technicians of the Department of Clinical Science, for their valuable support.

References

1. Abbasivash, R., Aghdashi, M.M., Sinaei, B., Kheradmand, F. (2014) The effects of propofol-midazolam-ketamine co-induction on hemodynamic changes and catecholamine response. J Clin Anesth. 26: 628-633.
2. Andolfatto, G., Willman, E. (2010) A prospective case series of pediatric procedural sedation and analgesia in the emergency department using single-syringe ketamine-propofol combination (Ketofol). Acad Emerg Med. 17: 194-201.
3. Braun, C., Hofmeister, E.H., Lockwood, A.A., Parfitt, S.L. (2007) Effects of diazepam or lidocaine premedication on propofol induction and cardiovascular parameters in dogs. J Am Anim Hosp Assoc. 43: 8-12.
4. Brock, N., Hildebrand, S. (1990) A comparison of xylazine-diazepam-ketamine and xylazine-guaifenesin-ketamine in equine anesthesia. Vet Surg. 19: 468-474.
5. Butera, T., Moore, J., Garner, H., Amend, J., Clarke, L., Hatfield, D. (1978) Diazepam/xylazine/ketamine combination for short-term anesthesia in the horse. Vet Med Small Anim Clin. 73: 490,495-496,499.
6. Chai, C., Wang, S. (1966) Cardiovascular actions of diazepam in the cat. J Pharmacol Exp Ther. 154: 271-280.
7. Covey-Crump, G.L., Murison, P.J. (2008) Fentanyl or midazolam for co-induction of anaesthesia with propofol in dogs. Vet Anesth An-

alg. 35: 463-472.

8. Erdogan, M.A., Begec, Z., Aydogan, M.S., Ozgul, U., Yucel, A., Colak, C., Durmus, M. (2013) Comparison of effects of propofol and ketamine-propofol mixture (ketofol) on laryngeal mask airway insertion conditions and hemodynamics in elderly patients: a randomized, prospective, double-blind trial. J Anesth. 27: 12-17.

9. Fayyaz, S., Kerr, C.L., Dyson, D.H., Mirakhur, K.K. (2009) The cardiopulmonary effects of anesthetic induction with isoflurane, ketamine-diazepam or propofol-diazepam in the hypovolemic dog. Vet Anesth Analg. 36: 110-123.

10. Haskins, S., Farver, T., Patz, J. (1986) Cardiovascular changes in dogs given diazepam and diazepam-ketamine. Am J Vet Res. 47: 795-798.

11. Haskins, S., Pascoe, P.J., Ilkiw, J.E., Fudge, J., Hopper, K., Aldrich, J. (2005) Reference cardiopulmonary values in normal dogs. Comp Med. 55: 156-161.

12. Haskins, S.C. (2015) Monitoring Anesthetized Patients, In: Veterinary Anesthesia and Analgesia. The Fifth Edition of Lumb and Jones. Grimm, K.A., Lamont, L.A., Tranquilli, W.J., Greene, S.A., Robertson, S.A. (eds.). John Wiley & Sons, Pondicherry, India, p. 86-113.

13. Haskins, S.C., Farver, T.B., Patz, J.D. (1985) Ketamine in dogs. Am J Vet Res. 46: 1855-1860.

14. Henao-Guerrero, N., Riccó, C.H. (2014) Comparison of the cardiorespiratory effects of a combination of ketamine and propofol, propofol alone, or a combination of ketamine and diazepam before and after induction of anesthesia in dogs sedated with acepromazine and oxymorphone. Am J Vet Res. 75: 231-239.

15. Hopkins, A., Giuffrida, M., Larenza, M.P. (2014) Midazolam, as a co-induction agent, has propofol sparing effects but also decreases systolic blood pressure in healthy dogs. Vet Anesth Analg. 41: 64-72.

16. Ilkiw, J., Suter, C., McNeal, D., Farver, T., Steffey, E. (1996) The effect of intravenous administration of variable-dose midazolam after fixed-dose ketamine in healthy awake cats. J Vet Pharmacol Ther. 19: 217-224.

17. Kennedy, M.J., Smith, L.J. (2014) A comparison of cardiopulmonary function, recovery quality, and total dosages required for induction and total intravenous anesthesia with propofol versus a propofol-ketamine combination in healthy Beagle dogs. Vet Anesth Analg. 42: 350-359.

18. Ko, J.C., Payton, M.E., White, A.G., Galloway, D.S., Inoue, T. (2006) Effects of intravenous diazepam or microdose medetomidine on propofol-induced sedation in dogs. J Am Anim Hosp Assoc. 42: 18-27.

19. Lerche, P., Nolan, A., Reid, J. (2000) Comparative study of propofol or propofol. Vet Rec. 146: 571-574.

20. Mair, A.R., Pawson, P., Courcier, E., Flaherty, D. (2009). A comparison of the effects of two different doses of ketamine used for co-induction of anaesthesia with a target-controlled infusion of propofol in dogs. Vet Anesth Analg. 36: 532-538.

21. Mannarino, R., Luna, S.P., Monteiro, E.R., Beier, S.L., Castro, V.B. (2012) Minimum infusion rate and hemodynamic effects of propofol, propofol-lidocaine and propofol-lidocaine-ketamine in dogs. Vet Anesth Analg. 39: 160-173.

22. Martinez-Taboada, F., Leece, E.A. (2014) Comparison of propofol with ketofol, a propofol-ketamine admixture, for induction of anaesthesia in healthy dogs. Vet Anesth Analg. 41: 575-582.

23. Muir, W., Gadawski, J. (1998) Respiratory depression and apnea induced by propofol in dogs. Am J Vet Res. 59: 157-161.

24. Rankin, D.C. (2015) Sedatives and Tranquilizers, In: Veterinary Anesthesia and Analgesia. The Fifth Edition of Lumb and Jones. Grimm, K.A., Lamont, L.A., Tranquilli, W.J., Greene, S.A., Robertson, S.A. (eds.). John Wiley & Sons, Pondicherry, India, p. 196-207.

25. Riccó, C.H., Henao-Guerrero, N. (2014) Cardiovascular effects of orotracheal intubation following anesthetic induction with propofol, ketamine-propofol, or ketamine-diazepam in premedicated dogs. J Am Vet Med Assoc. 244: 934-939.

26. Seliskar, A., Nemec, A., Roskar, T., Butinar, J. (2007) Total intravenous anaesthesia with propofol or propofol/ketamine in spontaneously breathing dogs premedicated with medetomidine. Vet Rec. 160: 85-91.

27. Smith, I., White, P.F., Nathanson, M., Gouldson, R. (1994) Propofol. An update on its clinical use. Anesthesiology. 81: 1005.

28. Smith, J., Gaynor, J., Bednarski, R., Muir, W. (1993) Adverse effects of administration of propofol with various preanesthetic regimens in dogs. J Am Vet Med Assoc. 202: 1111-1115.

29. Tweed, W., Minuck, M., Mymin, D. (1972) Circulatory responses to ketamine anesthesia. Anesthesiology, 37: 613-619.

30. Watkins, S., Hall, L., Clarke, K. (1987) Propofol as an intravenous anaesthetic agent in dogs. Vet Rec. 120: 326-329.

31. White, K.L., Shelton, K., Taylor, P.M. (2001) Comparison of diazepam-ketamine and thiopentone for induction of anaesthesia in healthy dogs. Vet Anesth Analg. 28: 42-48.

32. Wong, D.H., Jenkins, L.C. (1974) An experimental study of the mechanism of action of ketamine on the central nervous system. Can Anesth Soc J. 21: 57-67.

7

Evaluation of antioxidant potential of *Aloe vera* and pituitary sexual hormones after experimental diabetes in male rat

Behmanesh, M.A.[1*], Erfani Majd, N.[1], Shahriari, A.[2], Najafzadeh, H.[3]

[1]*Department of Histology, Faculty of Veterinary Medicine, Shahid Chamran University, Ahvaz, Iran*

[2]*Department of Biochemistry, Faculty of Veterinary Medicine, Shahid Chamran University, Ahvaz, Iran*

[3]*Department of Pharmacology and Toxicology, Faculty of Veterinary Medicine, Shahid Chamran University, Ahvaz, Iran*

Key words:

Aloe vera, anti oxidant, diabetes, pituitary – sexual hormones, rat

Correspondence

Behmanesh, M.A.
Department of Histology,
Faculty of Veterinary Medicine,
Shahid Chamran University,
Ahvaz, Iran

Email: behmanesh.ma@yahoo.com

Abstract:

BACKGROUND: Diabetes is a metabolic disease that is associated with hyperglycemia and infertility. Previous studies indicate that *Aloe vera* may positively affect the blood glucose and fertility. **OBJECTIVES:** The present study was carried out to evaluate the effect of *Aloe vera* on serum oxidant/antioxidant activity and reproductive hormones following experimental diabetes. **METHODS:** Sixty adult male Wistar rats were divided to 5 groups. Control group(A) was kept without treatment. Group(E) only received *Aloe vera* gel(400 mg/kg-orally). Experimental diabetes mellitus was induced in 3 groups of rats by streptozotocin(65 mg/kg-Ip). One diabetic group was kept without treatment (B). Another diabetic group received *Aloe vera* gel (400 mg/kg-orally) (C) and another received insulin (10 units)(D). *Aloe vera* gel and insulin was administrated for 30 days, then the rats were anesthetized and the blood collected. The amount of malondialdehid (MDA), antioxidant activity(AOA), glutathion peroxidase activity(GPX), thiol protein(TSH), testosterone, LH and FSH was determined in serum. **RESULTS:** Level of testosterone was significantly decreased while amount of MDA, TSH, GPX and AOA was significantly increased in non-treated diabetic rats. *Aloe vera* increased antioxidant defense. **CONCLUSIONS:** *Aloe vera* improves antioxidant activity and reduces diabetic complications.

Introduction

Diabetes mellitus is a disease which affects the endocrine system and is considered to be one of the most serious health problems to modern global health (Basmatzou, 2016). Concurrent with the development of diabetes, hyperglycemia can cause structural and functional changes in various organs and tissues(Cai,2000). The existing evidence suggests that diabetes causes disturbances in the reproductive system and reduces fertility in humans and in animal models (Carlos,2001).

Spermatogenesis is highly affected by the activity of Leydig cells. Diabetes causes changes in Leydig cells activity and thus reduces the level of testosterone in the blood. The reduction of testosterone is one of the main factors affecting the performance of blood testis barrier (Gautam,2006).

Many mechanisms have been proposed to explain the changes of testicular structure in diabetic conditions. In recent years more attention has been paid to the mechanisms that affect the performance of gonadotropin cells and their secretion. Some reports indicate that the lack of proper activities of hypothalamic–pituitary axis decreases the hormonal levels of gonadotropin cells in blood and this reduction is involved in the structural changes of testis tissue (Ricci, 2009). Testicular function is controlled by pituitary hormones. Follicle-Stimulating Hormone (FSH) regulates the spermatogenesis while Luteinizing Hormone (LH) controls the activity of Leydig cells. In these researches a decreased serum level of FSH and LH following diabetes has also been reported (Hutson,1983).

On the other hand enough evidence exists about the increased oxidative stress in diabetic patients, due to the excessive production of reactive oxygen (ROS) and a reduction in the performance of the antioxidant defense (Jakus, 2004. Maiti, 2004 and Oksanen, 1975). The high concentration of free radicals in diabetes may be due to the increased glucose autoxidation (Ricci,2009). The ROS varieties are caused by cell damage through some mechanisms involving lipid peroxidation, oxidative damage of proteins and DNA through the induction of oxidative stress (Aitken,1989). In normal conditions the removal mechanisms of free radicals inhibit the ROS production and consequently reduce the damages caused by them (Jakus,2004). *Aloe vera* (Aloe barbadensis) has long been used for treating a range of certain diseases.

Aloe vera extract has been proved to have anti-diabetic and anti-cancer function. *Aloe vera* is also used as a substitute to antibiotics (Kianfard, 2011). It is often recommended for diabetic patients due to its hypoglycemic effects (Oksanen, 1975). Anthraquinine are the constituents of *Aloe vera* which have laxative effects and the hypoglycemic properties of *Aloe vera* may be related to these compounds (Okyar, 2001). *Aloe vera* is enriched with the antioxidants that can reduce lipid peroxidation and the eliminated free radicals (Noor, 2008).

Materials and Methods

In order to accomplish the goals of this study, 60 healthy Wistar male rats weighing 200 ± 50 g were purchased from the Experimental Animal Center, in the Medical University of Ahvaz and were transferred to the Histology department of the Faculty of Veterinary Medicine in Shahid Chamran University. The purchased rats were kept in the same environmental conditions (12 h light/ 12 h of darkness), constant temperature and same amount of nutrition intake for two weeks in order for them to adapt to the environment. Following the adjustment phase, the rats were randomly divided into the following groups:

1- Control group (A): received the normal nutrition and were kept in normal conditions (15 male rats).

2- *Aloe vera* Group (B): received 400 mg/kg *Aloe vera* gel orally for 30 days (10 male rats).

3- Non treated Diabetic group: in this group in order to induce diabetes, streptozotocin (STZ) was intraperitoneally injected at dose 65 mg/kg. One week after STZ injection, in order to detect the presence of diabetes, the rats were evaluated in terms of blood glucose levels, through the tail vein blood and glucometer test. The rats with glucose levels more than 250 Mm/lit were-known as diabetic rat group (15 male rats).

4- *Aloe vera*-treated Diabetic group: In this group the diabetic rat received 400 mg/kg *Aloe vera* gel for 30 days by gavage (10 male rats).

5- Insulin-treated group: in this group diabetic rats received 10 IU insulin per day for 30 days (10 male rats).

During the course of the experiment, blood glucose was measured once every two weeks. At the end of the experiment after anesthesia with chloroform, vein section was performed in order to isolate the serum and measure the stress biomarkers and hormones. Malondialdehyde (MDA) was measured as a trailing indicator of lipid peroxidation through TBARS method. Based on this method the concentration of malondialdehyde was obtained based on MDA-TBA complex optical density at 532 nanometer wavelength in comparison with MDA standard curves (Pitton,1987). The measurement of thiolprotein was done based on the resuscitation of Elman reagent (DTNB) through the reduced glutathione and the formation of the yellow complex. The color intensity was measured proportionally to the amount of G-SH at 405 nm (Ellman,1959). Protein carbonyl was measured through the dinitrophenyl hydrazine reaction with this protein, and also by measuring the absorbance of the hydrazone protein complex at 370 nm wavelength (Kosif, 2008). The total antioxidant defense was measured by FRAP assay (Iris, 1996). FSH, LH and the testosterone amount were measured using Elisa method. Data analysis was performed using SPSS version 22 and the one-way analysis of variance (ANOVA) and post-hoc LSD with significance level of (p≤ 0.05).

Results

The highest blood sugar levels were observed within three days in diabetic rats and this can be considered as a significant increase compared with other groups. In days 15 and 30, level of blood sugar in diabetic rats showed a significant increase compared with control and *Aloe vera* groups, the diabetic group, the diabetic group which received insulin and the diabetic group that received *Aloe vera*. Comparing the blood sugar level of the diabetic rats which received insulin and the diabetic group who received *Aloe vera*, a significant increase is observed in the control group and the control group which received *Aloe vera* (Table 1).

The most antioxidant activity was observed in the diabetic rats in all three days which signified a significant increase in the control group and the control group who received *Aloe vera* for fifteen days. Furthermore, there is a meaningful decrease in the control group that received *Aloe vera* compared to the diabetic group that received insulin (Table 2). A significant decrease was observed in the protein carbonyl levels at day 15 in the diabetic rats compared to the diabetic group that received *Aloe vera* and the group which received *Aloe vera*. At day 30, a significant increase was observed in the protein carbonyl levels in the control group who received *Aloe vera* compared to the diabetic group and the group which received insulin (Table 2). Malondialdehyde increased in the first day of diabetes induction and compared to the control group this increase can be considered significant. On day 15 and 30, after the induction of diabetes, the amount of this factor in the diabetic

Table 1. The mean and standard deviation of blood sugar of rats in different groups. Letters a, b, c, d, e in each column indicate significant differences at p≤0.05.

Blood sugar / Groups	The first day of diabetes	15 days after diabetes	30 days after diabetes
Control (A)	118±7.3 [b]	110±8.2 [bcd]	112±5.7 [bcd]
Diabetics (B)	445±6.3 [a]	407±8.2 [acde]	439±3.7 [acde]
Diabetes + *Aloe vera* (C)	-	264±5 [abe]	190±2.6 [abe]
Diabetic + insulin (D)	-	255±4.7 [abe]	184±4.2 [abe]
Aloe vera (E)	-	107±6.7 [bcd]	108±8.1 [bcd]

Table 2. Serum levels (mean ± SD) total antioxidant activity, malondialdehyde, protein carbonyl in diabetic rats treated with *Aloe vera* (n = 10). Letters a, b, c, d, e in each column indicate significant differences at p≤0.05.

Indicators / Groups	Total antioxidant activity			Malondialdehyde			Protein carbonyl		
	The first day of diabetes	15 days after diabetes	30 days after diabetes	The first day of diabetes	15 days after diabetes	30 days after diabetes	The first day of diabetes	15 days after diabetes	30 days after diabetes
Control (a)	488±5	507±8.5 [b]	356.1±8.2	319±9 [b]	426±8 [b]	419±6.8	14.5±1.2	13.56±1.05	13.6±0.4
Diabetics (b)	558±7.5	679±6.6 [ac]	429.9±7.4	858±8 [a]	772±7 [ad]	765.9±4 [ad]	13.4±0.24	11.98±1.07 [ce]	12.73±0.69 [e]
Diabetes + *Aloe vera* (c)	-	627.6±8.1 [e]	395.1±9	-	656.6±8.1	520.2±5.2	-	14.03±0.24 [b]	14.48±0.56
Diabetic + insulin (d)	-	599.2±7.1 [e]	468.6±7	-	499.2±8.6 [b]	439.1±7 [b]	-	13.58±0.88	12.81±0.16 [E]
Aloe vera (e)	-	434.2±6.5 [bcd]	432.2±7.3	-	663.6±5.6	533.9±4.3	-	13.97±1.6 [b]	15.22±0.16 [Bd]

Table 3. Serum levels (mean ± SD) of markers of oxidative stress in diabetic rats treated with *Aloe vera* (n = 10). Letters a, b, c, d, e in each column indicate significant differences at p≤0.05.

Indicators / Groups	Protein thiols			Glutathione peroxidase		
	The first day of diabetes	15 days after diabetes	30 days after diabetes	The first day of diabetes	15 days after diabetes	30 days after diabetes
Control (a)	30.11±7.8	37.09±8 [C]	24.03±2.8 [b]	60.56±7.9	52.8±4.9 [C]	41.35±8.8 [bc]
Diabetics (b)	19.07±4.1	47.12±6.1 [C]	46.26±7.1 [ace]	162.16±7.5	161.23±8.3 [C]	541.78±8.8 [acde]
Diabetes + *Aloe vera* (c)	-	21.92±6.3 [Abe]	29.01±9.4 [b]	-	651.93±8.5 [Abde]	341.03±5.1 [abde]
Diabetic + insulin (d)	-	35.12±7.8	32.09±3.1	-	170.57±9.1 [C]	122.9±5.2 [bc]
Aloe vera (e)	-	43.09±2.8 [C]	29.88±7.7 [b]	-	81.31±6.1 [c]	63.09±5.5 [bc]

rats shows a significant increase compared with the control group who received insulin and the control rats (Table 2). The thiol proteins levels have a significant decrease in the diabetic and *Aloe vera* recipients compared with the control group, the control group who received *Aloe vera* and the diabetic rats, also on day 30. A significant increase was observed in thiol proteins levels in diabetic rats compared to the control group, the control group who received *Aloe vera* and the diabetic recipients of *Aloe vera* (Table 2). A significant increase of Glutathione peroxidase was also observed in diabetic rats that received *Aloe vera*. On day 15 and 30, after the diabetes induction a significant increase of this factor was observed in diabetic and diabetic recipients of *Aloe vera* compared to the other groups (Table 2).

The calculated amounts of the FSH, LH

Table 4. Average of FSH, LH and testosterone hormones in rats. Letters a, b, c, d, e in each column indicate significant differences at p≤0.05.

Hormones \ Groups	FSH (mIU/ml)			LH (mIU/ml)			Testosterone (ng / dL)		
	The first day of diabetes	15 days after diabetes	30 days after diabetes	The first day of diabetes	15 days after diabetes	30 days after diabetes	The first day of diabetes	15 days after diabetes	30 days after diabetes
Control (a)	406.35±6.3 B	439.91±8.38 b	499.21±6.81 b	8.18±0.62 b	8.56±0.81 B	7.38±0.63 b	9.38±0.47 b	10.2±0.96 b	9.01±0.07 b
Diabetics (b)	251.55±4.63 A	250.34±6.45 ae	268.48±9.98 a	3.3±0.19 a	3.41±0.59 acde	3.34±0.18 acde	4.75±0.84 a	4.85±0.39 a	4.58±0.78 ae
Diabetes + Aloe vera (c)	-	307.41±9.2	400.79±6.5	-	7.15±16 B	8.34±0.38 b	-	7.66±0.92	7.64±0.23
Diabetic + insulin (d)	-	367.19±9.63	394.81±7.94	-	7.33±0.26 B	7.93±0.58 b	-	7.46±0.85	8.3±0.46
Aloe vera (e)	-	419.75±7.7 b	365.47±9.5	-	8.47±0.53 B	7.37±0.18 b	-	8.75±0.77	9.51±0.43 b

and testosterone in serum blood were significantly different in the first 15 and 30 days after the development of diabetes. FSH levels on the first day of diabetes in diabetic rats had a significant reduction compared to the control group. On day 15 after diabetes induction, FSH decreased in diabetic rats and this reduction can be considered meaningful in control group and recipients of *Aloe vera* (ml/ miu). Moreover, on day 30 after diabetes induction FSH levels reduction was statistically significant in diabetic group compared with the control group (Table 3).

In the first day of diabetes induction a significant decrease was observed in LH levels in blood serum of diabetic rats. LH reduction on day 15 and 30 after diabetes induction was statistically significant in diabetic rats compared to the other groups (Table 3).

In the first day of diabetes induction a significant decrease was observed in testosterone levels, of the diabetic rats compared to the control group. Testosterone reduction on day 15 of diabetes induction was also statistically significant in diabetic rats. On day 30 of the diabetes induction, a significant decrease in testosterone level was observed in the diabetic group (Table 3).

Discussion

The increased blood glucose levels in diabetes leads to structural and functional changes in tissues and organs, including reproductive organs (Cai, 2000). In this study, the mean glucose levels in streptozotocin induced diabetic rats significantly increased in diabetic rats compared to the control group and that is because of the reduction of β-cells in the pancreatic islets after the onset of diabetes. A significant decrease was observed in the amount of blood sugar of the diabetic rats that received insulin and the diabetic rats which received *Aloe vera* with doses of 400 mg/kg for about 15 and 30 days after diabetes induction. Josias and colleagues(Josias,2008) and Rajasekaran et al (Rajasekaran, 2006) administered *Aloe vera* gel with dosage of 300 mg/kg orally per day for rats for 21 days and reported a significant reduction in the glucose levels of their blood which is consistent with the findings of the present study. Helal et al (Helal,2003) and Noor et al in 2008 achieved similar results about blood sugar reduction after *Aloe vera* administration (Helal, 2003; Noor, 2008). Noor et al in 2008 stated that blood sugar reduction after using *Aloe vera* may be due to the prevention of the pancreatic β-cell death by the *Aloe vera*, or by a similar function of insulin, through the glucose uptake by peripheral tissues, and inhibiting glucose production via gluconeogenesis in the liver and muscles (Noor, 2008).

In this study, serum levels of FSH, LH and testosterone in the blood of rats in different groups were compared. In this case a significant decrease was observed in serum levels of FSH, LH and testosterone, in diabetic rats which can be due to the increased oxidative stress after diabetes induction. Furthermore, it was observed that the amount of LH in the serum of diabetic rats that received *Aloe vera* increased compared to other diabetic rats. This can indicate *Aloe vera* potentials to reduce the damaging effects of diabetes and its antioxidant effects. Ricci and colleagues reported the reduction of plasma levels of testosterone following diabetes and stated that it is affected by the reduction in the number of Leydig cells and an increase in oxidative stress after diabetes induction (Ricci, 2009). They also stated that the reduction of testosterone is responsible for the changes in epithelium of tubules in diabetic animals. Stephan and colleagues stated that the Leydig cell reduction and morphological changes that occur in the testis of the diabetic rats was a result of the increased oxidative stress induced by hyperglycemia and the reduction of the antioxidant defense (Stephan, 2007).

Howland and Zebrowski reported that serum testosterone level in diabetic rats was significantly reduced compared to the control group. They also reported that the concentrations of FSH and LH increased in the pituitary gland of diabetic rats (Howland and Zebrowski,1976). Ballester et al reported that the reduction of serum levels of FSH, LH, testosterone and insulin subsequent to diabetes (Ballester, 2004). These results are compatible with the findings obtained in this study. In this study biochemical factors such as malondialdehyde, thiolprotein, glutathione peroxidase and total antioxidant activity were examined in order to investigate the role of *Aloe vera* in dealing with the oxidative stress which is caused by diabetes. In this study it was observed that the level of malondialdehyde in the first, 15 and 30 days of induction in diabetic group significantly increased compared to the control group by stimulating the immune system to cope with the oxidative stress (Ballester, 2004). These results were compatible with the results obtained from Stephen et al's study which measured the malondialdehyde levels 60 days after diabetes induction. They also stated that the oxidative stress-induced hyperglycemia after diabetes induction decreases antioxidant defense and increases the malondialdehyde (Stephan, 2007). Mohasseb and colleagues noted the increase in amount of malondialdehyde 8 weeks after diabetes induction (Mohaseb, 2010).

It was also observed that the thiol protein, the glutathione peroxidase and the total antioxidant activity increased significantly in the diabetic rats compared with control group. This fact confirms the stimulation of the immune system to cope with oxidative stress induced by hyperglycemia after diabetes induction. The higher levels of antioxidant activity and other biochemical factors that are involved in the elimination of the reactive oxygen types (ROS) in the diabetic rats which received Aloe era shows *Aloe vera* potentials and its antioxidant compounds, and further, the stimulation of the immune system that could lead to a reduction in the damaging effects of diabetes, following *Aloe vera* administration.

Acknowledgements

The authors wish to express their gratitude to the research council of Shahid Chamran University for their financial support.

References

Aitken, R.J., Clarkson, J.S., Fishel, S. (1989) Generation of reactive oxygen species, lipid peroxidation, and human sperm function. J Biol Reprod. 41: 183–197.

Amaral, S., Oliveira, P.J., Ramalho-Santos, J. (2008) Diabetes and the impairment of reproductive function: possible role of mitochondria and reactive oxygen species. Curr Diabetes Rev. 4: 46-54.

Ballester, J., Munoz, M.C., Dominguez, J., Rigau, T., Guinovart, J.J., Rodriguez-Gil, JE. (2004) Insulin-dependent diabetes affects testicular function by FSH- and LHlinked mechanisms. J Androl. 25: 706-719.

Basmatzou, T., Hatziveis, K. (2016) Diabetes mellitus and influence on human fertility. International Journal of Caring Sciences. 9: 371-380.

Cai, L., Chen, S., Evans, T. (2000) Apoptotic germ cell death and testicular damage in experimental diabetes: prevention by endothelium antagonism. Urol Res. 28: 342-347.

Carlos, M., Palmeira, Dario, L., Santos, Raquel Seiça, António, J., Moreno and Maria S. santos. (2001) Enhanced mitochondrial testicular antioxidant capacity in Goto-Kakizaki diabetic rats: role of coenzyme Q, Am J Physiol. 281: 1023-1028.

Chen, C.S., Chao, H.T., Pan, R.L., Wei, Yh.

(1997) Hydroxyl radicalinduced decline in motility and increase in lipid peroxidation and DNA modification in human sperm. Biol Mol J. 43: 291–303.

Ellman, G.l. (1959) Tissue sulfhydryl groups. Arch Biochem Biophys. 82: 70-7.

Ghafari, S., Kabiri Balazadeh, B., Golalipour, M.J. (2011) Effect of *Urtica dioica* L. (Uriticaceae) on testicular tissue in STZ-induced diabetic rats. Pak J Biol Sci. 14: 798-804.

Gamal, M.A., Hassan' and Tarek Abdel Moneium. (2001) Structural Changes in the Testes of Streptozotocin-Induced Diabetic Rats. Suez Canal University Med J. 4: 17-25.

Gautam, D.K., Misro, M.M., Chaki, S.P., Sehgal, N. (2006) H2O2 at physiological concentrations modulates Leydig cell function inducing oxidative stress and apoptosis. Apoptosis. 11: 39–46.

Gavin, J.R., Alberti, K.G.M.., Davidson, MB., Defronzo, RA., Drash, A., Gabbe, SG., et al. (1997) Report of the expert committee on the diagnosis and classification of diabetes mellitus. Care Diabetes J. 20: 1183-97.

Helal, E.G.E., Hasan, M.H.A., Mustafa, A.M., Al-Kamel, A. (2003) Effect of *Aloe vera* extract on some physiological parameters in diabetic albino rats. Egy J Hospital Med. 12: 53-61.

Hutson, J.C., Stocco, D.M., Campbell, G.T., Wagoner, J. (1983) Sertoli cell function in diabetic, insulin-treated diabetic, and semi-starved rats. J Diabetes. 32: 112 -116.

Iris, F.F., Benzi Strain, J.J. (1996) The ferric reducing ability of plasma (FRAP) as a Measure of "Antioxidant Power": The FRAP Assay. Anal Biochem J. 239: 70-76.

Jakus, V., Rietbrock, N. (2004) advanced glycation end products and the progress of diabetic vascular complacations. Physiol Res. 53: 131-142.

Josias, H. (2008) Composition and application

of *Aloe vera* leaf gel. Molecules. 13: 1599-1616.

Kaemmerer, H., Mitzkat, H.J. (1985) Ion-exchange chromatography of amino acids in ejaculates of diabetics. Andrologia. 17: 485–487.

Karimi Jashni, H., Najmadini, N., Hooshmand, F. (2012) Effect of alcoholic extract of *Aloe vera* plant on serum testosterone and gonadotropin levels in rats. Journal of Jahrom University o Medical Medical Science. 10: 1-7.

Kianfard, D., Sadrkhanlou, R., Hasanzadeh, SH. (2011) The histological, histomorphometrical and histochemical changes of testicular tissue in the metformin treated and untreated streptozotocin induced adult diabetic rat. Vet Res. 2: 13-24.

Kosif, R., Akta, G., Öztekin, A. (2008) Microscopic examination of placenta of rats prenatally exposed to *Aloe barbadensis*: A Preliminary Study International J Morphol. 26: 275-281.

Levine, R.L., Williams, J., Stadtman, E.R., Shacter, E. (1994) Carbonyl assays for determination of oxidatively modified proteins. Methods Enzymol. 233: 346-57.

Mohasseb, M., Ebied, S., Yehia, M.A.H., Hussein, N. (2010) Testicular oxidative damage and role of combined antioxidant supplementation in experimental diabetic rats. J Physiol. 67: 185–194.

Maiti, R.D., Jana, U.K., Ghosh, D. (2004) Antidiabetic effect of aqueous extacts of seed of Tamarindus indica- tamarind seed in streptozotocin induce diabetic rats. Ethnopharmacol J. 92: 85-91.

Maritim, A,C., Sandres, R.A., Watkins, J.B. (2003) Diabetes, oxidative stress and antioxidants: A review. J. J Biochem Mol Toxicol, 17: 24-38.

Noor, A., Gunasekaran, S., Soosai Manickam, A., Vijayalakshmi, M.A. (2008) Antidiabetic activity of *Aloe vera* and histology of organs in streptozotocin induced diabetic rats. Curr Sci. 94: 8-25.

Nwanjo, H.U. (2006) Antioxidant activity of the exudate from Aloe barbadensis leaves in diabetic rats. J Biochem. 18: 77-81.

Okamura, M., Watanabe, T., Kashida, Y., Machida, N., Mitsumori, K. (2004) Possible mechanisms underlying the testicular toxicity of oxfendazole in rats. Toxicol Pathol J. 32: 1- 8.

Oksanen, A. (1975) Testicular lesion of streptozotocin diabetic rats. Hormon Res. 6: 138-144.

Okyar, A., Can, A., Akev, N., Baktir, G., Sutlupinar, N. (2001) Effect of *Aloe vera* leaves on blood glucose level in type I and type II diabetic rat models. Phytother Res. 15: 157-161.

Oyewopo, A.O., Oremosu, A.A., Akang, E.N., Noronha, C.C., Okanlawon, A.O. (2011) Effects of *Aloe vera* (*Aloe barbadensis*) aqueous leaf extract on testicular weight, sperm count and motility of adult male sprague-dawley rats. J Am Sci. 7: 31-34.

Pitton, I., Bestetti, G.E., Rossi, G.L. (1987) The changes in the hypothalamo- pituitary- gonadal axis of streptozotocin treated male rats depend from age at diabetes onset. 19: 464-473.

Plaser, Z.A., Cushman, L.L., Johnson, B.C. (1966) Estimation of product of lipid peroxidation (malondialehyde) in biochemical systems. Anal Biochem. 16: 359-64.

Reavan, E., wright, D. (1983) Effect of age and diet on insulin secretion and insulin action in the rat. Diabetes. 32: 175- 180.

Rajasekaran, S., Sivagnanam, K., Subramanian, S. (2005) Antioxidant effect of *Aloe vera* gel extract in streptozotocin-induced diabetes in rats. Pharmacol Rep. 57: 90-96.

Ricci, G., Catizone, A., Esposito, R., Pisanti, F. A., Vietri, M.T., Galdieri, M. (2009) Diabetic rat testes: morphological and functional alterations. Int J Andrologica. 41: 361-368.

Rossi, G.L., Bestetti, G. (1981) Morphological changes in the hypothalamic-hypophyseal-gonadal axis of male rats after twelve months of streptozotocin-induced diabetes. diabetologia. 21: 476-481.

Serpa, R.F.B., Jesus, E.F.O., Anjos, M.Y. (2000) Cognitive impairment related changes in the elemental concentration in the brain of old rat. Spectrochem Acta. 61: 1219-1223.

Stephen, O., Adewole, A., Abdulkadir, A., Salako oladepo, W., Thajasrarie, N. (2007) Effect of oxidative stress induced by streptozotocin on the morphology and trace mineral of the testes of diabetic wistar rats. Pharmacology online. 2: 478- 497.

Vornberger, W., Prins, G., Musto, N.A., Suarez-quian, C.A. (1994) androgen receptor distribution in rat testis: new implications for androgen regulation of spermatogenesis. Endocrinology. 134: 2307-2316.

Ward, D.N., Bousfiald, G.R., Moore, K.H. (1991) Gonadotropins reproduction domestic animals. Academic press, San Diego California, USA.

8

Preparation and in vitro evaluation of a novel chitosan-based hydrogel for injectable delivery of enrofloxacin

Khanamani Falahatipour, S.[1], Rassouli, A.[1*], Hosseinzadeh Ardakani Y.[2], Akbari Javar, H.[2], Kiani, K.[1], Zaharei Salehi, T.[3]

[1]Department of Pharmacology, Faculty of Veterinary Medicine, University of Tehran, Tehran, Iran

[2]Department of Pharmaceutics, Faculty of Pharmacy, Tehran University of Medical Sciences, Tehran, Iran

[3]Department of Microbiology, Faculty of Veterinary Medicine, University of Tehran, Tehran, Iran

Key words:

beta-glycerophosphate, chitosan, enrofloxacin, hydrogel, sustained release

Correspondence

Rassouli, A.
Department of Pharmacology, Faculty of Veterinary Medicine, University of Tehran, Tehran, Iran

Email: arasooli@ut.ac.ir

Abstract:

BACKGROUND: The development of injectable sustained-release products are of great interest to veterinary pharmaceuticals and animal health business. Recently, great attention has been paid to in situ gel-forming chitosan/beta-glycerophosphate (chitosan/β-GP) solutions due to their good biodegradability and thermosensitivity. **OBJECTIVES:** The general aim of this study was to prepare a novel in situ gel-forming drug delivery system with a sustained release profile for enrofloxacin. **METHODS:** Chitosan, β-GP and enrofloxacin were used in different concentrations and six formulations of chitosan/β-GP were prepared. The properties of the hydrogels including the pattern of drug release, gelation time, syringeability, morphology, FTIR spectra, and in vitro antimicrobial activity were evaluated. **RESULTS:** The release rate of enrofloxacin from the hydrogels and syringeability of the final solutions were decreased by increasing in β-GP and chitosan concentrations. All formulations could release the drug up to 120 hours but formulation 1 (chitosan-2%, β-GP-5% and enrofloxacin-1%) gave the best results based on its optimal drug release profile and viscosity. The FTIR studies showed that there were no interactions between enrofloxacin and hydrogel excipients. Scanning electron microscopy showed that the formed gel had a continuous texture, while the swelled gel in phosphate buffer had a porous structure. Microbiological tests revealed high bactericidal activities for this enrofloxacin- loaded hydrogel which were comparable to those of positive control (enrofloxacin suspension) in terms of inhibition zone, MIC and MBC values. **CONCLUSIONS:** Because of simple preparation and sustained release profile of the drug, this hydrogel could be a promising delivery system for enrofloxacin in animals.

Introduction

Hydrogels are cross-linked, three-dimensional hydrophilic networks that swell but do not dissolve when brought into contact with water (Khodaverdi, et al. 2012). Hydrogels can be formulated in a variety of physical forms, including slabs, microparticles, nanoparticles, coatings and films (Kuhwasha, et al., 2013). Their highly porous structure can easily be tuned by controlling the density of cross-links in the gel matrix and the affinity of the hydrogels for the aqueous environment in which they are swollen (Khan, 2014). If a drug is incorporated into the polymer solution, it becomes entrapped within polymer matrix as it solidifies. Drug release occurs over time as polymer biodegrades (Pandya, et al., 2014). The development of injectable sustained-release formulations for intramuscular/subcutaneous (IM/ SC) use has become an increasingly important issue in the animal health business during the last two decades. Such products are of interest in both the farm and companion animal business areas (Matschke, et al. 2002). Injectable hydrogels have attracted much attention during the past decade, due to their rapid gelation from flowable aqueous solution when injected into the desired tissue or organ (Qiu, et al. 2011).

Chitosan, a natural copolymer produced by the deacetylation of chitin, is especially interesting for pharmaceutical application because of its high solubilized capacity, biodegradability, and desired safety profile (Li, et al. 2014). Chitosan is widely used in food and pharmaceutical industries as well as in biotechnology (Parida, et al. 2011). The in situ gelation mechanism involves neutralization of the ammonium groups in chitosan, allowing strengthened hydrophobic and hydrogen bonding between the chitosan chains at elevated temperatures (Chen, et al. 2011). Chitosan solutions that are physically mixed with glycerol-2-phosphate (β-GP) can be injected into the body in liquid form, forming a gel in situ at the body temperature. The rate of gelation depends on the degree of chitosan deacetylation, the concentration of β-GP, and the temperature and pH of the final solution (Chenite, et al. 2000). Chitosan hydrogels can be produced by cross-linking of chitosan macromolecules. These hydrogels can easily swell in water or biological fluids, therefore, they have become a potential candidate for carriers of bioactive macromolecules, wound dressing, and controlled release of drugs in their swollen state (Mirzaei, et al. 2013).

Enrofloxacin is a fluoroquinolone antimicrobial agent developed exclusively for use in animals (Kumar, et al. 2015). It inhibits prokaryotic topoisomerase II (DNA gyrase), which is an important enzyme for bacterial replication (Vancutsem, et al. 1990). It has broad spectrum antibacterial activity, especially against gram negative bacteria, such as Pseudomonas spp (Udomkusonsri, et al. 2010). Enrofloxacin has the maximal lipid solubility among fluoroquinolones. This lipophilicity promotes its diffusion into biological tissues, including bacterial cells (Martinez, et al. 2006).

The pharmacokinetics of enrofloxacin are characterized in general terms by high bioavailability in most species and rapid absorption after IM, SC or oral administration. However, several studies reported that enrofloxacin showed low bioavailability after oral administration in ruminants. This drug has a wide volume of distribution in the organism, excellent tissue penetration and a serum half-life in the range of 3 to 6 hours (López-Cadenas, et al. 2013, Anadon, et al. 1999) Other important characteristics of enrofloxacin include few adverse effects, good therapeutic index and good tolerance in animals (Anadon, et al. 1999).

Major motive forces for the development of innovative veterinary sustained release products include the reductions in the frequency of drug administration, duration of medical treatment and the imposed stress to the animals. As a consequence, an increased ease of drug use by the veterinarians and the pet's owner as well as a decrease in treatment costs seems to be typical for these products. These factors have stimulated the expansion of modified releasing drug delivery systems for use in both companion and farm animals. While oral drug delivery continues to be the main route of administration, the parenteral route suggests an absorbing alternative when oral administration is difficult or cumbersome. The development of new injectable drug delivery systems has received considerable attention over the past few decades. The minimization of dosing frequency enhances patient compliance and comfort. Therefore, injectable drug delivery systems capable of releasing an active ingredient in a controlled manner for a desired period have a high priority. Additionally, biodegradable systems allowing the administration without the need for a subsequent medical procedure to remove the device, contribute to higher patient compliance. However, these innovative therapies are developed at the expense of increased complexity, often leading to issues such as high development and production costs (Sautter 2006).

The focus of the present investigation is to prepare and evaluate beta glycerophosphate-chitosan system as in situ gelling vehicle for controlled delivery of enrofloxacin in a slow release manner. Then, in vitro release profiles of enrofloxacin from the prepared formulations as well as antibacterial activities were investigated.

Materials and Methods

Medium molecular weight chitosan with degree of deacetylation (DDA) of 75-85% and β-glycerophosphate disodium salt pentahydrate were purchased from Sigma-Aldrich (St. Louis, MO). Enrofloxacin standard (99.57%) was purchased from TEMAD Pharmaceutical Co. (Iran). Acetic acid was purchased from Merck (Darmstadt, Germany). Other chemicals were reagent grade.

Preparation of in situ gel: Six formulations were prepared by dissolving different amounts of chitosan powder in 0.1 mol/l diluted acetic acid to achieve concentrations of 2.0 and 3.0% (w/v) along with 5.0, 7.5 and 10.0% (w/v) β-GP and using 5 or 10 g/l enrofloxacin to form hydrogels (Table 1).

Briefly, chitosan powders (200mg/300mg) were dissolved in 8mL of 0.1M acetic acid and gently stirred for 3h to make a homogeneous solution. 50 mg/100 mg enrofloxacin was added to the chitosan solution and stirred for another 1h. Different concentrations of β-GP were dissolved in deionized water. The chitosan and β-GP solutions were placed in an ice-water bath at 4°C. The β-GP solution was added to chitosan and drug solution for 10 min drop-wise. The final 10.0 ml solution was maintained at 4°C for further studies.

Determination of gelation time and syringeability: In this study, gelation was assessed using the inverted tube test, as described by Zhou and coworkers (Zhou, et al. 2011). When a test tube containing a solution is titled, it is defined as a sol phase if the solution deforms by flow, or a gel phase if there is no flow (Fig 1). Firstly, 2 ml of chitosan/ β-GP solutions were maintained for 12 h at 4°C in 5 ml vials with inner diameter of 10 mm to remove air bubbles. The vials were then incubated in a temperature-controlled bath. The sol-gel transition time was determined by inverting the vials horizontally every minute. The time at which the gel did not flow was recorded as the gelation time. The syringeability of the chitosan/ β-GP solutions is how easy it is to expel sample from a syringe and an important parameter for practical administration of gels was also tested.

In vitro drug release studies: In vitro release was performed under sink conditions using the molded 1.0 g gel immersed at 37°C in 500 ml of phosphate buffer pH =7.4 containing 0.5% Tween 80. The dissolution system was shaken at 100 rpm. Samples were removed periodically and the medium was replenished. Because of drug instability, all of the release medium was substituted every 24 hours. The absorbance of the samples was measured at 273 nm by using UV-Vis spectrophotometer. All measurements were performed in triplicate. Data are reported as means ± SD.

Drug release kinetics: To analyze the in vitro release data, various kinetic models were used to describe the release kinetics. The zero order rate in Eq. (1) describes the system where the drug release rate is independent of its concentration (Pandian, et al. 2012). The first order Eq. (2) describes the release from system where release rate is concentration dependent (Shoaib, et al. 2006). Higuchi (1963) described the release of drugs from insoluble matrix as a square root of time dependent process based on Fickian diffusion Eq. (3). The Hixson-Crowell cube root law Eq. (4) describes the release from systems where there is a change in surface area and diameter of particles or tablets (Hixson and Crowell 1931).

$$C = K^0 t \quad (1)$$

Where, K0 is zero-order rate constant expressed in units of concentration/time and t is the time.

$$\text{Log } C = \text{Log } C^0 - Kt / 2.303 \quad (2)$$

Where, C^0 is the initial concentration of drug and K is first order constant and t is the time [9]

$$Q = Kt^{1/2} \quad (3)$$

Where, K is the constant reflecting the design variables of the system. Hence drug release rate is proportional to the reciprocal of the square root of time.

$$Q^0 1/3 - Qt^{1/3} = KHC \, t \quad (4)$$

Where, Qt is the amount of drug released in time t, Q0 is the initial amount of the drug in tablet and KHC is the rate constant for Hixson-Crowell rate equation as the cube root of the percentage of drug remaining in the matrix vs time.

The kinetic analysis of the release profile was calculated according to the Peppas equation:

$$Mt / M\infty = kt^n \quad (5)$$

where 'Mt' is the cumulative amount of drug released at time 't'; 'M∞' is the total amount of drug incorporated; 'k' is the proportionality constant, the value of which depends on the structural and geometrical properties of the matrix; and 'n' is the release exponent, its value depends on the mechanism of drug release. 'R' regression coefficient was also calculated in a set of data; the model showing highest R value was taken as the best model. If 'n' value is < 0.5, the polymer relaxation does not affect the molecular transport, hence diffusion is Fickian. If n > 0.5, the solid transport will be non-Fickian and will be relaxation controlled. If n=1, release follows case II transport (zero order release) and if n > 1, indicates super case II transport (Venkatesh, 2012).

The method that best fits the release data was evaluated by the regression coefficient (r^2). Criteria for selecting the most appropriate model was based on the ideal fit indicated by the values of r^2 near to 1 (Ranjha and Qureshi, 2014).

Morphological studies: For SEM studies, gels containing 5 different chitosan/β-GP ratios were fabricated. For sample preparation, all formulations were initially placed in a freezer at -20°C as a short-term storage and then freeze-dried overnight. Dried gels were cut with a sharp blade to expose internal microstructure and sputter coated with platinum-gold for SEM imaging at 30 kV using scanning electron microscope (FESEM, Hitachi. S4160, Japan).

FTIR spectra: FTIR spectra of enrofloxacin, chitosan, β-GP, dried chitosan/β-GP gel and formulation F1 were recorded in KBr pellets (the samples were triturated with KBr in the ratio of 1:100 and pressed to form pellets) in the range of 400-4000cm-1 using a FTIR spectrophotometer (Nicolet, Model Impact 410; Madison, WI) at room temperature.

Microbiological studies: To determine the antibacterial activity of enrofloxacin hydrogel, the "well diffusion test" was carried out by using *Escherichia coli*, *E.coli* ATCC35218, Pseudomonas aeruginosa, *P. aeruginosa* ATCC10145 and Klebsiella pneumonia, *K. pneumoniae* ATCC13883 as gram-negative pathogenic strains and Staphylococcus aureus ATCC29213 as gram-positive pathogenic strain. The bacterial suspensions with a cell density comparable to 0.5 McFarland (1.5 ×10^8 CFU/ml) were transferred onto the surface of Muller-Hinton agar plates by using sterile cotton swab. Wells with 8mm diameter were prepared by punching a sterile cork borer onto the solid agar medium. Aliquots of 20 μl of each solution were delivered into the wells (containing 20 μg/ml of enrofloxacin)

for enrofloxacin hydrogel, enrofloxacin suspension as positive control, and the blank preparation (formulated exactly the same as hydrogel but without adding enrofloxacin) were used as control to investigate the antimicrobial properties of vehicle. The plates were kept in non-upside down position for 30-60 min to facilitate the diffusion of formulations into the media. After incubation time of about 24h at 37°C, the zones of inhibition around the wells were measured in mm using a caliper (Jahangirian, et al. 2013). The development of a clear zone around the cylinders after 24 h of incubation indicated antibacterial activity against the test organisms. Zone of inhibition data was analyzed using independent t-tests. All experiments were carried out in triplicate.

Determination of MIC and MBC: The broth macrodilution tube method was used to determine MIC and MBC of the formulations against *E. coli* and *S. aureus* bacteria (Yilmaz 2012). A stock solution of enrofloxacin was prepared in sterile water (32μg/ml) that was further diluted in Muller-Hinton broth to reach a concentration range of 0.5 to 32 μg in 4 ml of Muller-Hinton broth. Enrofloxacin hydrogel and enrofloxacin were dispersed in Muller-Hinton broth to reach an equal concentration of enrofloxacin from 0.5 to 32 μg/ml (depending on the percentage of drug loading ratio). Final concentration of bacteria in individual tubes was adjusted to about 5×10^6 CFU/ml by adding 50 μl of *S. aureus* and *E. coli* inoculums. The blank preparations (formulated exactly the same as each formulation without adding enrofloxacin) were used as control and also prepared as above. Control tubes containing just Muller-Hinton broth without any antimicrobial agent and Muller-Hinton broth with enrofloxacin hydrogel formulations and enrofloxacin, both without bacteria, were used as negative control tubes for checking any probable contamination.

To determine MIC values, after 24h incubation at 37°C, the test tubes were examined for possible bacterial turbidity, MIC of each test compound was determined as the lowest drug concentration that could inhibit visible bacterial growth for 24 h The MBC was measured by sub-culturing the broths used for MIC determination onto fresh agar plates. The MBC is the lowest concentration of the drug that kills 99.9% of cells of a given bacterial strain. All experiments were conducted in triplicate (Lalitha 2004, Yilmaz 2012).

Results

Gelation time and syringeability: Chitosan/glycerophosphate gel exhibited thermosensitive property, which was liquid (solution) at refrigerated temperature and solidified into a white semi-transparent hydrogel at body temperature (Fig 1). The influence of Gp salt concentration on the gelation time of chitosan solution was also shown in Table 2. Apparently, by increasing the concentration of Gp salt, the required time for gelation decreases. F3 solution with 10% Gp salt took 17 min to form gel whereas for F1 with 5.0% Gp salt, the gelation time was 25 min. The same situation was observed for other pairs.

The syringeability of formulations has been presented in Table 2. The syringeability of the final solutions greatly decreased with the increase of chitosan concentration. The best syringeability was observed with chitosan concentration of 2% (w/v).

In vitro drug release studies: The cumulative amounts of enrofloxacin released

Table 1. The compositions of thermosensitive chitosan/ β-GP enrofloxacin formulations.

Ingredients	Formulation (10 ml)					
	F1	F2	F3	F4	F5	F6
Chitosan (mg)	200	200	200	300	300	200
β-GP (mg)	500	750	1000	500	1000	500
Enrofloxacin (mg)	100	100	100	100	100	50

from the hydrogel as a function of time are shown in Fig 2. It was found that cumulative percentage drug release for formulations prepared F1, F2, F3, F4, F5, F6 were 82.8%, 84.2%, 74.0%, 81.7%, 76.8%, 76.2%, respectively. All formulations sustained the drug release for 120h. Formulation F5 did not release enrofloxacin until about 48h, F2 and F3 did not release enrofloxacin until about 4h, whereas F1, F4 and F6 started the release of enrofloxacin within the first hour of the experiment.

Effect of chitosan concentration on enrofloxacin release behavior: The viscosity of the gel was low when the chitosan concentration was 2.0% (w/v) and grew higher at 3.0% (w/v). As can be seen in Fig 2, the release rates of enrofloxacin were 44.0% and 53.8% for CS/ β-GP thermo-sensitive hydrogels containing 2.0% (w/v) and 3.0% (w/v) CS, respectively along with 5.0% (w/v) β-GP during the first 24 h. It was found that, 41.7% % and 0 % of the trapped drugs were released during the first 24 h for hydrogels containing 2.0% (w/v) and 3.0% (w/v) CS, respectively along with 10.0% (w/v) β- GP. The final cumulative release rates were 82.8%, 74.0%, 81.7 and 76.8% for formulation F1, F3, F4, F5, respectively. CS/β-GP thermo-sensitive hydrogels containing 3.0% (w/v) (F4 and F5) CS showed the abrupt release. On the contrary, hydrogels containing 2.0% (w/v) CS presented the gradual release, which was desirable for controlled release.

Table 2. In vitro drug release kinetics parameters of different enrofloxacin hydrogels.

Hydrogel code	Zero Order	First Order	Higuchi	Hixson-Crowell	Korsmeyer-Peppas	
	r^2	r^2	r^2	r^2	n	r^2
F1	0.8788	0.9600	0.9754	0.9372	1.8923	0.5910
F2	0.8212	0.8923	0.9344	0.8693	1.8961	0.9190
F3	0.8203	0.8556	0.9316	0.8451	1.8327	0.9209
F4	0.8553	0.9264	0.9624	0.9048	0.3688	0.9836
F5	0.9276	0.9157	0.8210	0.9230	0.7834	0.7885
F6	0.9600	0.9935	0.9927	0.9886	0.6850	0.9545

Table 3. Gelation time and syringeability of formulated enrofloxacin hydrogels.

Formulation	F1	F2	F3	F4	F5
Gelation Time (min)	25	20	17	8	5
Syringeability	Easily	Drop-wise	Drop-wise	Drop-wise	Hardly

Table 4. Zone of inhibition of microbial growth around the cylinder containing enrofloxacin hydrogels and enrofloxacin suspension (positive control).

Bacteria	Zone of inhibition (mm ±SD)	
	Enrofloxacin hydrogel	Positive control
S. aureus	32.0±1.01	34.2±1.08
E. coli	35.5±1.26	38.1±1.31
P. aeruginosa	28.3±1.21	33.6±1.04
K. pneumonia	36.6±1.51	37.2±1.12

Table 5. The MIC and MBC of enrofloxacin hydrogels and enrofloxacin suspension (positive control) against S. aureus and E. coli bacteria. Data expressed as mean ±SD (n=3).

Bacteria		Enrofloxacin hydrogel	Positive control
S. aureus	MIC (µg/ml)	1.0±0.0	1.0±0.0
	MBC (µg/ml)	1.0±0.0	1.0±0.0
E. coli	MIC (µg/ml)	0.5±0.0	0.5±0.0
	MBC (µg/ml)	1.0±0.0	1.0±0.0

Effect of β-GP concentration on enrofloxacin release behavior: In vitro release behaviors of enrofloxacin from chitosan/β-GP hydrogels containing different amounts of β-GP (5.0% (w/v) and 10.0% (w/v)) were shown in Fig 1. The initial release rates of enrofloxacin were 3.14% and 17.5% for hydrogels F1 and F4 (containing 5.0% (w/v) β-GP), respectively. While for both hydrogels containing 10.0% (w/v) β-GP (F3 and F5) the initial release was 0.0%. The pH value of hydrogels increased and got close to the physiological pH by increasing the β-GP concentration. Among all the formulations, hydrogels F4 and F5 with 10.0% (w/v) β-GP showed the most prominent viscosity change during the phase transition.

Effect of drug concentration on enrofloxacin release behavior: The release behavior of chitosan /β-GP hydrogels containing different amounts (5 and 10 g/l) of enrofloxacin (F6 and F1) are shown in Fig 1. Results showed that in the first 24 h, the hydrogel containing 10 g/l enrofloxacin exhibited higher release rate than hydrogel containing 5 g/l enrofloxacin.

Kinetic modelling of drug release profiles: The model fitting for the release profile of formulations by using various models was shown in Table 3. By analyzing regression coefficient values of all formulations, it was found that formulation F6 hydrogel matrix exhibits almost first order kinetics. Formulation F5 followed zero order kinetics; F4 followed Korsmeyer-Peppas kinetics whereas the remaining formulations showed the release kinetic model of Higuchi. So, the predominant drug release mechanism was controlled release. Based on the results of syringeability, in vitro release tests and release profile of formulations, the

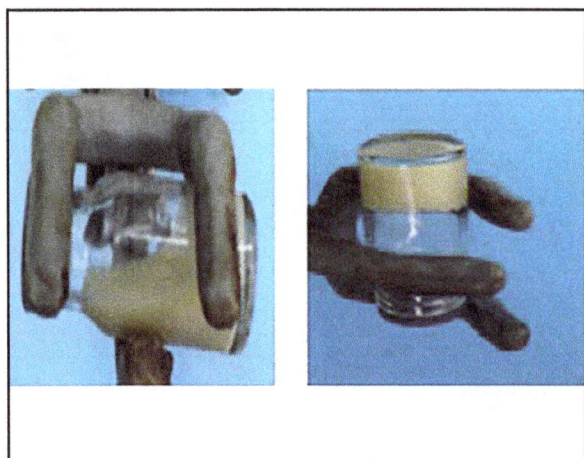

Figure 1. The chitosan/GP formulation at room temperature (left) and at 37°C (right).

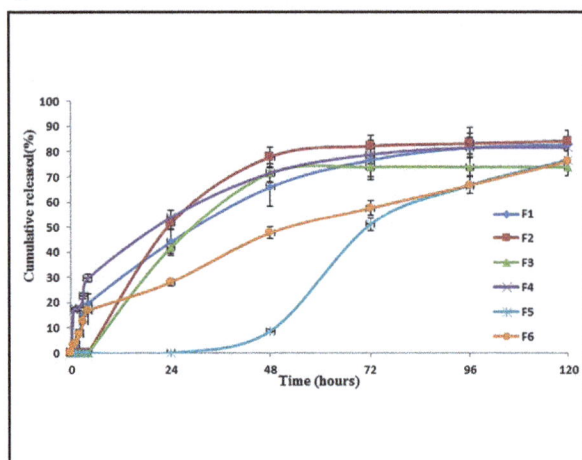

Figure 2. In vitro cumulative release of enrofloxacin (%) from different formulations of in situ gels in PBS + 0.5% Tween 80 at 37°C. Compositions of formulations (F1-F6) have been presented in Table 1. Each point represents the mean value ± SD (n = 3).

formulation F1 was chosen as the appropriate formulation for other tests.

For the drug release, the best fit model was "Korsmeyer-Peppas" model. The values of "n" were calculated from the drug release data (<70%). The obtained values of formulation F4 were between 0 and 0.5, indicating that the release of enrofloxacin was by Fickian diffusion. These values for Formulation F5 and F6 were > 0.5, indicating that the release of enrofloxacin was by non-Fickian diffusion and for other formulations was > 1, indicating that the release of enrofloxacin was by super case II transport.

Fourier Transform Infrared spectroscopy (FTIR) studies: The FTIR spectra of enrofloxacin, chitosan, β-GP, chitosan/β-GP and formulation F1 are shown in Fig 3. The FTIR studies showed that there were no interactions between enrofloxacin and excipients.

Enrofloxacin has two characteristic absorption peaks, 1736 cm^{-1} and 1628 cm^{-1}; the first is the C=O vibration absorption peak from carboxylic acid oxygen, and the second is assigned to keto C=O peak from the ring of enrofloxacin. For the enrofloxacin hydrogel system, the bands at 1736 and 1628 cm^{-1} were shifted to 1742 and 1629 cm^{-1}, respectively.

In the wavenumber range 800 - 1200 cm^{-1}, the FTIR spectrum of chitosan shows three bands at 1155, 1030 and 894 cm^{-1}. The wide band at 1030-1155cm^{-1} represents the bridge -O- stretch of the glucosamine residues. The spectrum of chitosan shows a band at 1595 cm^{-1} that is assigned to the NH_2 group of chitosan. These bands indicate that chitosan is a partially deacetylated product of chitin. The chitosan molecule shows four peaks at 1423, 1380, 1315 and 1255 cm^{-1}. The bands at 1423 and 1315 cm^{-1} are associated with oscillations characteristic for OH and C-H bending of CH2 groups. The band at 1380 cm^{-1} represents the C-O stretching of the primary alcoholic group -CH2-OH. Chitosan exhibited a broad peak at 3434 cm^{-1}, which was assigned to the stretching vibration of N-H and O-H bond. Peaks at 2924 cm^{-1} were due to the C-H stretch vibrations. A peak at 1653 cm^{-1} was due to the C=O stretch of amide bond.

Bands for wave numbers 1076 cm^{-1} and 782 cm^{-1} are characteristic for β-GP and correspond to stretching vibrations P-O-C. A band for wave number 971 cm^{-1} is char-

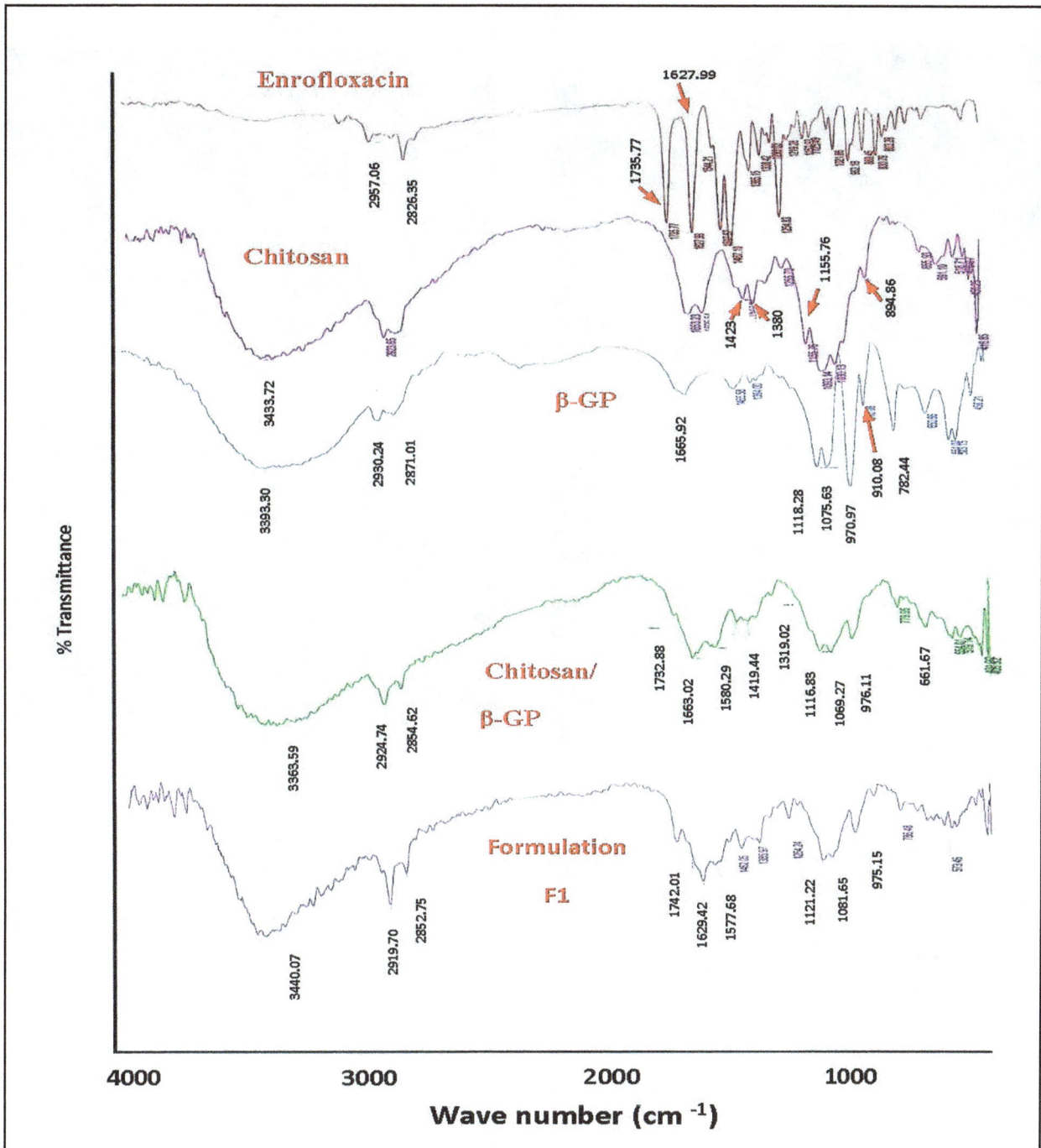

Figure 3. The FTIR spectra of enrofloxacin, chitosan, β-GP, chitosan/β-GP, formulation F1.

acteristic for (-PO4^{3-}). A band for wave number 910 cm^{-1} indicating the presence of groups (-HPO4^{2-}).

The FTIR spectrum of the chitosan/β-GP system after gelation indicates characteristic bands for chitosan and glycerol phosphate disodium salt. There are no additional bands observed. For the chitosan/β-GP system, the bands of chitosan at 1380 and 1315 cm^{-1} are shifted to 1385 and 1319 cm^{-1}, respectively and the bands of GP at 1076 and 971cm^{-1} are shifted to 1069 and 976 cm^{-1}. We can see from the FTIR spectra between mixture of enrofloxacin, chitosan and β-GP that no significant differences were shown.

Morphological studies: Scanning elec-

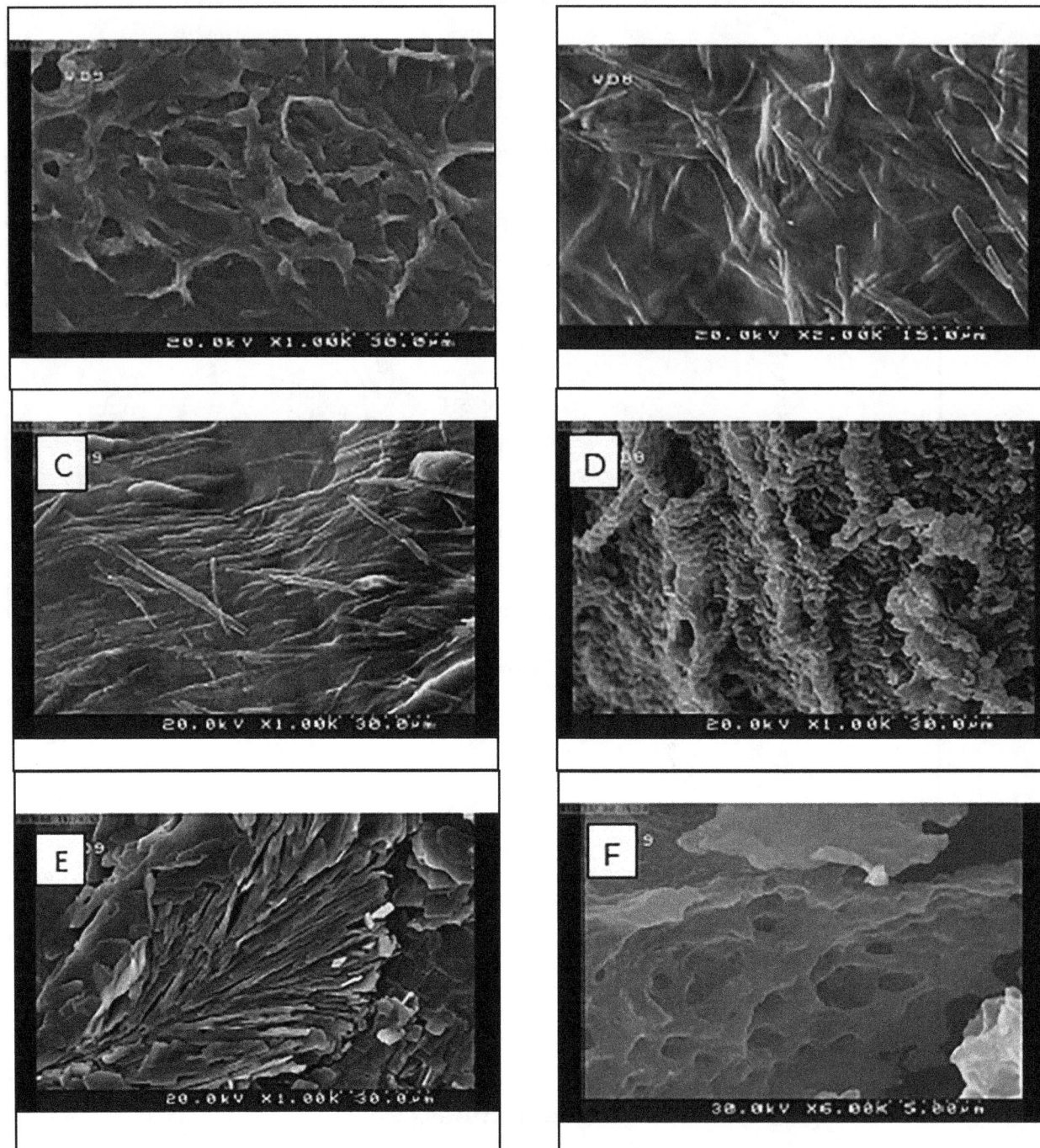

Figure 4. Scanning electron microscopy of freeze-dried chitosan based hydrogels. A:F1, B:F2, C:F3, D:F4, E:F5, F: Swelled hydrogel (F1) in phosphate buffer for 3 days.

tron microscopy was used to investigate morphology and porosity of produced chitosan hydrogels samples. The SEM photograph of the F1-F5 samples is shown in Fig 4 (A-E). It shows that the surface of Chitosan/ β-GP hydrogel is rough, obviously dense, non-porous and integrated. The formed gel had a continuous texture for the Chitosan/ β-GP hydrogel section (A-E), while the swelled gel in phosphate buffer (pH=7.4) had a porous structure as shown in Fig 4 (F). The SEM graphs of dried hydrogels roughly reflect the pores and water permeation in the hydrogels, because of the small difference of free water between the sol and gel state of poorly-swollen or non-swollen

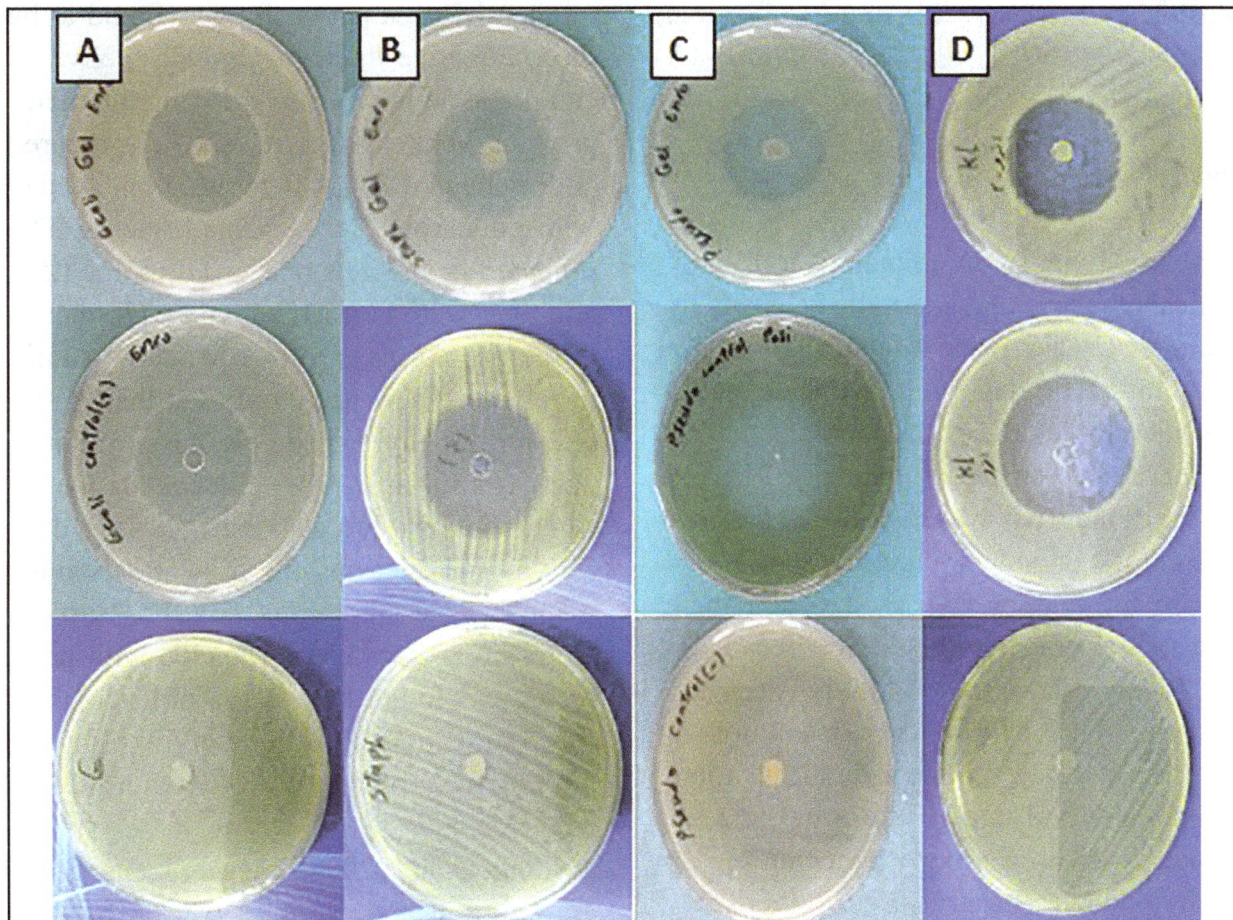

Figure 5. Antibacterial activity of enrofloxacin hydrogel (first row), free enrofloxacin as positive control (second row) and the blank hydrogel (third row) against different bacteria. Column A: *E. Coli*, Column B: *S. Aureus*, Column C: *P. aeruginosa*, Column D: *K. pneumonia*e.

chitosan hydrogels. The observed pores indicate that water once existed over there. The porous structure created a substantial water environment and resulted in burst release of drugs. The structure of the matrix clearly changed with composition. The higher the amount of β-GP salt added to the chitosan solution, the greater the increase in the amount of crystal precipitation, density and integrity of the formulation. The higher the concentration of chitosan added in the solution, the higher the density of polymer chains yielded.

Microbiological activities: The mean diameter of the inhibitory zones (mm) provided by enrofloxacin suspension (positive control) and enrofloxacin hydrogels are presented in Table 4. Both tested materials showed high antimicrobial activity against all microbial strains tested. The result of well diffusion assay showed that the inhibition zone of positive control was slightly greater than that of enrofloxacin hydrogel. However, no statistical differences in inhibitory zones were observed between the positive control and enrofloxacin hydrogels against *E. coli*, *K. pneumonia*, *P. aeruginosa* and *S. aureus* (p>0.05). No inhibition zone was observed for the drug-free hydrogel (the blank preparation), which demonstrates that our polymer-drug systems manifest an antibacterial activity and the blank preparation does not present any antimicrobial activity against tested bacteria.

MIC and MBC data of enrofloxacin suspension (positive control), and enrofloxacin hydrogels against *E. coli* and *S. aureus* are presented in Table 5.

Discussion

Infection control in animals is a primary clinical objective and is usually achieved by treatment once or twice a day for at least 3-5 days. In the present work, we evaluated a new thermosensitive formulation as the basis for antibacterial chemotherapy. The objective of the study was to prepare and evaluate enrofloxacin in situ gels as a sustained release formulation. We used enrofloxacin as a model drug for this study, because it is a widely used antimicrobial in veterinary medicine. The chitosan-based solution in the present study remained liquid at room temperature and turned into a gel as temperature increased to body temperature.

The polymeric matrix used in this study consisted of chitosan polymer and β-Glycerophosphate (β-GP). Addition of glycerol-2-phosphate (β-GP) to chitosan solution produces a hydrogel which undergoes sol-gel transition at a temperature close to 37°C, making the formulation a suitable vehicle for drug administration. Our results showed that formulation F4 had the highest burst release (17.5%) but in remaining formulations it was <10%. Drug release in all gel formulations was followed by a sustained release pattern over 120 h. The chitosan/β-GP system could sustain the delivery of hydrophobic drugs such as enrofloxacin for at least 4 days, which is a reasonable time span for antimicrobial therapy. Berrada et al. (2005) used the same chitosan/GP formulation to deliver intratumorally a hydrophobic anticancer agent campothecin by using a mouse tumor model. The implanted hydrogel con-

taining 4.5% campothecin was found to be more effective than systemically delivered campothecin in terms of delaying the tumor growth. Venkatesh et al. (2012) prepared and evaluated a C/GP formulation loaded with pilocarpine for sustained release. The prepared in situ gels released drug for 12 h, and they were non-irritant and well tolerated during the in vivo eye irritancy studies in rabbits. Their study revealed that in situ gels formulation was simple, easy to administer, comfortable, with reduced frequency of instillations and also enhanced the drug activity by releasing the drug in sustained manner. Ruel-Gariepy et al. (2004) used a chitosan/GP formulation loaded with paclitaxel and found it to be as efficacious as four intravenous injections of Taxol by inhibiting the growth of EMT-6 tumors in balb/c Mice.

Gong et al. (2009) prepared enrofloxacin chitosan nanoparticles (EFX-CS-NPs). They reported that the total drug release in 24 h was 79.9% with a sustained release pattern. In addition, Kumar et al. (2015) loaded enrofloxacin in solid lipid nanoparticles (SLNs) with sustained release profile which was characterized by an initial burst release of 18% within 2 h followed by a sustained release pattern up to 96 h.

Our results showed that concentration of chitosan affected the cumulative drug release. Formulations with higher percentage of chitosan retarded the onset of drug release. Similar trend was observed with glycerophosphate. It should be noted that chitosan/β-GP hydrogels containing 3.0% chitosan, retain more enrofloxacin during the sol-to-gel transformation process owing to low viscosity at the sol state but high viscosity at the gel state. The initial burst release decreased with increased polymer concentration. The initial burst effects also demonstrated that the higher the concentration of β-GP in the hydrogels, the lower the initial burst effect. Venkatesh et al. (2012) reported that concentration of chitosan affected the cumulative drug release. Formulations with higher percentage of chitosan retarded the drug release. Similar trend was observed with glycerophosphate, but not to the extent of chitosan.

The mechanisms of sol-gel transition in the chitosan/GP system include hydrophobic interactions, hydrogen bonding, electrostatic interactions, and molecular chain movement. At low temperature, the solubility of solute is probably due to hydration of the chitosan promoted by glycerophosphate. Upon heating, the chitosan chains lose their water of hydration, which promotes the bonding between chains and proceeds gelation. Three types of interactions may be involved in the process of gelation: (1) electrostatic attraction between the ammonium groups of chitosan and the phosphate group of glycerophosphate; (2) hydrogen bonding between polymer chains due to reduced electrostatic repulsion after neutralization of the chitosan solution with glycerophosphate; and (3) enhancement of chitosan-chitosan hydrophobic interactions by structuring action of glycerol. (John, et al. 1994; Song, et al. 2010).

Degree of deacetylation (DDA) of chitosan, pH of the chitosan/β-GP solution, pressure, ions and temperature are expected to control gel-forming process. DDA is the dominant parameter in controlling gelation time, because the deacetylation of chitosan can increase the hydrophilicity of the system. (Chenite, et al., 2000; Jia, et al. 2006, Purohit Kamlesh, et al. 2013). The primary action of β-GP is to rapidly take the proton

from the protonated amino groups of CS; thus, higher GP concentration induces higher pH (Ganji, et al. 2007). The addition of a glycerol-phosphate salt to aqueous chitosan solutions directly modulates the electrostatic and hydrophobic interactions, and hydrogen bonding between chitosan chains, which are the main molecular forces involved in gel formation (Chenite, et al. 2000). With the increase of β-GP salt concentration, more chitosan amino groups are neutralized. Therefore, electrostatic repulsive forces between chitosan chains are damaged and polymer chains are aggregated more easily. This leads to obvious reduction in gelation time (Khodaverdi, et al. 2012). In this study, we found that chitosan solution could be neutralized up to physiological pH by using β-GP due to the neutralizing effect of the phosphate groups (base). Our results apparently showed that by increasing the concentration of β-GP salt, the required time for gelation decreased. The short gelation time observed for formulation F4 and F5 may be attributed to DDA and concentration of chitosan and glycerophosphate. Our results are in agreement with the findings of Khodaverdi et al. 2012 who also reported that, by increasing the concentration of β-GP salt, the required time for gelation decreased. They reported that the Ch4 formulation solution with 0.55 M β-GP salt took 37 min to form gel whereas for Ch3 formulation with 0.45 M β-GP salt, the gelation time was 50 min. (Khodaverdi, et al. 2012). This result is in agreement with the findings of Kempe's group as well (Kempe, et al. 2008). They showed that higher β-Gp concentrations lead to faster gelation at constant temperature. Comparing the gelation behavior of chitosan/Gp solutions of various polymer concentrations, a reverse relationship between time of gelation and chitosan concentration could be found (F5 vs F3 or F4 vs F1). In other words, solutions with higher polymer concentrations which correspond to more -OH and -NH groups for intermolecular hydrogen binding; thereby, form gel faster than those with lower concentrations.

It was also demonstrated that the initial drug loading affected the release rate. The initial burst value was higher (3.79 vs 3.14%) for the 5 mg/ml-loaded gel vs 10 mg/ml-loaded gel. However, the following release rate was lower for the 5 mg/ml-loaded gel. Li et al. (2014) also reported that the initial burst effects for 1 mg/ml loaded gel and 4 mg/ml loaded gel were 22.06% and 17.56%, demonstrating that the higher the concentration of docetaxel in the hydrogels, the lower the initial burst effect (Li, et al. 2014).

The syringeability increased as the concentrations of β-GP and chitosan of solutions increased. Our results were in agreement with findings of Senyigit et al., 2014. They showed that significant decreases in syringeability observed as the molecular weight and viscosity of chitosan increased (p<0.05) (Şenyiğit, et al. 2014).

The higher value for regression coefficient (r^2) in Higuchi model indicates that the drug release mechanism is diffusion controlled (Ranjha and Qureshi 2014). High values of r^2 were obtained for formulations F1-F3 in Higuchi model, which illustrates that the rates of drug release were directly proportional to the square root of time (Murtaza, et al. 2012).

SEM pictures show a change in the gel structure after conditioning in water. Pores in the structure are seen in the micrometer range after conditioning in water. Modrazejewska et al. (2014) also showed that after

SEM evaluation of thermosensitive chitosan chloride gels following conditioning in water, the crystals resulting from chloride salt were washed and the pore sizes were about 10 μm (Modrzejewska, et al. 2014).

Regarding microbiological studies, our results indicated that the inhibition zones were rather small for the polymer drug system as compared to the free drug (positive control) but not significantly different (P >0.05). It seems that it is mainly due to the fact that the drug was not completely released after 24 hours. The hydrogels loaded with enrofloxacin presented high bactericidal activities. The enrofloxacin retained its antimicrobial activity after formulation into gelling solution. In a similar study, Bhushan et al. (2011) studied antimicrobial efficiency of a controlled release ciprofloxacin gel, CPXF6 hydrogel. The inhibitory effects of ciprofloxacin formulation on some microorganisms were evaluated using agar diffusion test. They showed that the values of zone of inhibition (ZOI) for *S. aureus* for conventional ciprofloxacin eye drop and CPXF6 hydrogel were 31.5 ± 1.1 and 34.4 ± 0.1, respectively. They reported that the higher ZOI values obtained for the formulations in comparison to the conventional eye drop could be attributed to the slow and prolonged diffusion of the ciprofloxacin from the polymeric solution due to its higher viscosity (Bhushan, et al. 2011). On the other hand, the ZOI values for in situ gel formulation were lower than those of a marketed eye drop (Wagh, et al. 2012).

Chitosan/β-GP gels of enrofloxacin showed appreciable in situ gelling properties in the present study. The in situ gels were found to be uniform, isotonic, thermosensitive and released the drug for 5 days. This study revealed that the novel in situ gel formulation was simple to prepare, easy to administer, comfortable due to reduced frequency of injections, and with enhanced drug activity due to sustained release profile. It was found that the release of enrofloxacin from chitosan/β-GP thermosensitive gel decreases by increasing in β-GP salt. The mechanism of gelation, which does not involve covalent cross-linkers, organic solvent or detergents, combined with a controllable residence time, renders this injectable biomaterial uniquely compatible with sensitive antimicrobial agents.

Conclusion: Chitosan/β-GP in situ gels revealed effective, homogeneous, injectable drug delivery for enrofloxacin and formulation F1 (chitosan-2%, β-GP 5% and enrofloxacin-1%) gave the best results based on its optimal drug release profile and syringeability. Microbiological findings suggest a good efficiency of the hydrogel in terms of antimicrobial activity. Because of simple preparation, easy administration and prolonged drug release, this approach represents an attractive platform for the delivery of enrofloxacin in animals.

Acknowledgments

Authors wish to thank Mr. Iraj Ashrafi for his contribution in the microbiological studies of this project.

References

Anadon, A., Martinez-Larra aga, M.R., Diaz, M.J., Fernandez-Cruz, M.L., Martinez, M.A., Frejo, M.T., Martínez, M., Iturbe, J., Tafur, M. (1999) Pharmacokinetic variables and tissue residues of enrofloxacin and ciprofloxacin in healthy pigs. Am J Vet Res. 60: 1377-1382.

Berrada, M., Serreqi, A., Dabbarh, F., Owusu, A., Gupta, A., Lehnert, S. (2005) A novel non-toxic camptothecin formulation for cancer chemotherapy. Biomaterials. 26: 2115-2120.

Bhushan, S., Agnihotri, V., Bodhankar, M. (2011) A Novel Thermoreversible Phase Transition System with Flux enhancers for ophthalmic application. Int J Pharm Pharm Sci. 3: 367-370.

Chen, M.C., Mi, F.L., Liao, Z.X., Sung, H.W. (2011) Chitosan: its applications in drug-eluting devices. Chitosan for Biomaterials I, Springer: 185-230.

Chenite, A., Chaput, C., Wang, D., Combes, C., Buschmann, M., Hoemann, C., Leroux, J., Atkinson, B., Binette, F., Selmani, A. (2000) Novel injectable neutral solutions of chitosan form biodegradable gels in situ. Biomaterials 21: 2155-2161.

Ganji, F., Abdekhodaie, M. (2007) Gelation time and degradation rate of chitosan-based injectable hydrogel. J Sol-Gel Sci Technol. 42: 47-53.

Gong, L.Y., Hu, K., Yang X.L. (2009) Preparation and release characteristics of enrofloxacin chitosan nanoparticles in vitro. Journal of Shanghai Ocean University. 3: 321-326.

Higuchi, T. (1963) Mechanism of sustained-action medication. Theoretical analysis of rate of release of solid drugs dispersed in solid matrices. J Pharm Sci. 52: 1145-1149.

Hixson, A., Crowell, J. (1931) Dependence of reaction velocity upon surface and agitation. Ind Eng Chem. 23: 1160-1168.

Jahangirian, H., Haron, M.J., Shah, M.H., Abdollahi, Y., Rezayi, M., Vafaei, N. (2013) Well diffusion method for evaluation of antibacterial activity of coper phenyl fatty hydroxamate synthesized from canola and palm kernel oils. Dig J Nanomater Biostruct (DJNB). 8: 1263-1270.

Jia, Z., Dequan, Z., Fengping, T., Jiang, G., Ying, L., Fuxin, D. (2006) Preparation of thermosensitive chitosan formulations containing 5-fluorouracil/poly-3-hydroxybutyrate microparticles used as injectable drug delivery system. Chin J Chem Eng. 14: 235-241.

John, H.D., Geoffrey, W., Herbert, C. (1994) Methods for the study of irritation and toxicity of substance applied topically to the skin and mucous membrane. J Pharmacol Exp Ther. 82: 377-390.

Kempe, S., Metz, H., Bastrop, M., Hvilsom, A., Contri, R.V., Mäder, K. (2008) Characterization of thermosensitive chitosan-based hydrogels by rheology and electron paramagnetic resonance spectroscopy. Eur J Pharm Biopharm. 68: 26-33.

Khan, S. (2014) In situ gelling drug delivery system: An overview. JIPBS. 1: 88-91.

Khodaverdi, E., Tafaghodi, M., Ganji, F., Abnoos, K., Naghizadeh, H. (2012). In vitro insulin release from thermosensitive chitosan hydrogel." AAPS Pharm Sci Tech. 13: 460-466.

Kumar, S., Arivuchelvan, A. Jagadeeswaran, A., Subramanian, N., Kumar, S., Mekala, P. (2015) Formulation, optimization and evaluation of enrofloxacin solid lipid nanoparticles for sustained oral delivery. Asian J Pharm Clin Res. 8: 231-236.

Kushwaha, S.K., Rai, A.K., Singh, S. (2013) Thermosensitive hydrogel for controlled drug delivery of anticancer agents. Int J Pharm Pharm Sci. 5: 547-552.

Lalitha, M. (2004) Manual on antimicrobial susceptibility testing. Performance standards for antimicrobial testing: 12th Informational Supplement. 56238: 454-456.

Li, C., Ren, S., Dai, Y., Tian, F., Wang, X., Zhou, S, Deng, S., Liu, Q., Zhao, J., Chen, X. (2014) Efficacy, pharmacokinetics, and biodistribution of thermosensitive chitosan/β-glycerophosphate hydrogel loaded with docetaxel. AAPS Pharm Sci Tech. 15: 417-424.

López-Cadenas, C., Sierra-Vega, M., García-Vieitez, J.J., Diez-Liébana, M.J., Sahagún-Prieto, A., Fernández-Martínez, N. (2013) Enrofloxacin: Pharmacokinetics and metabolism in domestic animal species. Curr Drug Metab. 14: 1042-1058.

Martinez, M., McDermott, P., Walker, R. (2006) Pharmacology of the fluoroquinolones: a perspective for the use in domestic animals. Vet J. 172: 10-28.

Matschke, C., Isele, U., van Hoogevest, P., Fahr, A. (2002) Sustained-release injectables formed in situ and their potential use for veterinary products. J Control Release. 85: 1-15.

Mirzaei, B.E.A., Ramazani, S.A., Shafiee, M., Danaei, M. (2013) Studies on glutaraldehyde crosslinked chitosan hydrogel properties for drug delivery systems. Int J Polym Mater Polym Biomater. 62: 605-611.

Modrzejewska, Z., Skwarczyńska, A., Maniukiewicz, W., Douglas, T.E. (2014) Mechanism of formation of thermosensitive chitosan chloride gels. Progress in the Chemistry and Application of Chitin and its Derivatives (19): 125-134.

Pandian, P., Kannan, K., Manikandan, M., Manavalan, R. (2012) Formulation and evaluation of oseltamivir phosphate capsules. Int J Pharm Pharm Sci. 4: 342-347.

Pandya, Y., Sisodiya, D., Dashora, K. (2014) Atrigel®, implants and controlled released drug delivery system. Int J Biopharm. 5: 208-213.

Parida, U.K., Nayak, A.K., Binhani, B.K., Nayak, P. (2011) Synthesis and characterization of chitosan-polyvinyl alcohol blended with cloisite 30B for controlled release of the anticancer drug curcumin. J Biomater Nanobiotechnol. 2: 414.

Qiu, X., Yang, Y., Wang, L., Lu, S., Shao, Z., Chen, X. (2011) Synergistic interactions during thermosensitive chitosan-β-glycerophosphate hydrogel formation. RSC Advances. 1: 282-289.

Ranjha, N.M. Qureshi, U.F. (2014) Preparation and characterization of crosslinked acrylic acid/hydroxy propyl methyl cellulose hydrogels for drug delivery. Int J Pharm Pharm Sci. 6: 400-410.

Ruel-Gariépy, E., Shive, M., Bichara, A., Berrada, M., Le Garrec, D., Chenite, A., Leroux, J.C. (2004) A thermosensitive chitosan-based hydrogel for the local delivery of paclitaxel. Eur J Pharm Biopharm. 57: 53-63.

Shoaib, M.H., Tazeen, J., Merchant, H.A., Yousuf, R.I. (2006) Evaluation of drug release kinetics from ibuprofen matrix tablets using HPLC. Pak J Pharm Sci. 19: 119-124.

Song, K., Qiao, M., Liu, T., Jiang, B., Macedo, H.M., Ma, X., Cui, Z. (2010) Preparation, fabrication and biocompatibility of novel injectable temperature-sensitive chitosan/glycerophosphate/collagen hydrogels. J Mater Sci: Mater Med. 21: 2835-2842.

Udomkusonsri, P., Kaewmokul, S., Arthitvong, S., Songserm, T. (2010) Use of enrofloxacin in calcium beads for local infection therapy in animals. Kasetsart J (Natural Science). 44: 1115-1120.

Vancutsem, P., Babish, J., Schwark, W. (1990) The fluoroquinolone antimicrobials: structure, antimicrobial activity, pharmacokinetics, clinical use in domestic animals and toxicity. The Cornell Veterinarian. 80: 173-186.

Venkatesh, M.P., Purohit Kamlesh, L., pramod Kumar, T.M. (2013) Development and evaluation of chitosan based thermosensitive in situ gels of pilocarpine. Int J Pharm Pharm Sci. 5: 164-169.

Wagh, V.D., Deshmukh, K.H., Wagh, K.V. (2012) Formulation and evaluation of in situ gel drug delivery system of Sesbania grandiflora flower extract for the treatment of bacterial conjunctivitis. J Pharm Res. 4: 1880-1884.

Yilmaz, M.T. (2012) Minimum inhibitory and minimum bactericidal concentrations of boron compounds against several bacterial strains. Turkish J Med Sci. 42: 1423-1429.

Zhou, H.Y., Zhang, Y.P., Zhang, W.F., Chen, X.G. (2011) Biocompatibility and characteristics of injectable chitosan-based thermosensitive hydrogel for drug delivery. Carbohydr Polym. 83: 1643-1651.

9

Preparation and evaluation of a thermosensitive liposomal hydrogel for sustained delivery of danofloxacin using mesoporous silica nanoparticles

Kiani, K.[1], Rassouli, A.[1*], Hosseinzadeh Ardakani, Y.[2], Akbari Javar, H.[2], Khanamani Falahatipour, S.[1], Khosraviyan, P.[2], Zahraee Salehi, T.[3]

[1]*Department of Pharmacology, Faculty of Veterinary Medicine, University of Tehran, Tehran, Iran*

[2]*Department of Pharmaceutics, Faculty of Pharmacy, Tehran University of Medical Sciences, Tehran, Iran*

[3]*Department of Microbiology, Faculty of Veterinary Medicine, University of Tehran, Tehran, Iran*

Key words:

danofloxacin, drug delivery, liposome, mesoporous silica nanoparticles, thermosensitive

Correspondence

Rassouli, A.
Department of Pharmacology,
Faculty of Veterinary Medicine,
University of Tehran, Tehran,
Iran

Email: arasooli@ut.ac.ir

Abstract:

BACKGROUND: Sustained release delivery system can reduce the dosage frequency and maintain the therapeutic level of drugs for a longer time. Biodegradable, biocompatible and thermosensitive chitosan-beta-glycerophosphate (C-GP) solutions can solidify at body temperature and maintain their physical integrity for a longer duration. **OBJECTIVES:** To develop a novel delivery system based on the integration of liposomes in hydrogel using mesoporous silica nanoparticles (MSNs) for sustained release of danofloxacin in farm animals. **METHODS:** The MSNs were prepared using N-cetyltrimethylammonium bromide and tetraethylortho silica. The liposomes were prepared by thin film hydration method. C-GP solution containing danofloxacin-loaded MSN liposomes underwent different in-vitro tests, including evaluation of the entrapment efficiency, gelation time, morphology, drug release pattern as well as antimicrobial activities against *S. aureus* and *E. coli*. **RESULTS:** The mean pore size of MSNs was 2.8 nm and the mean MSN entrapment efficiency was 45%. Kinetics of danofloxacin release from liposomal hydrogel followed the Higuchi's model. This formulation was capable of sustaining the danofloxacin release for more than 96 h. The FTIR studies showed that there were no interactions between danofloxacin and hydrogel excipients. Scanning electron microscopy (SEM) showed that the formed gel had a continuous texture, while the swelled gel in the phosphate buffer had a porous structure. Microbiological tests revealed a high antibacterial activity for lipomosal hydrogel of danofloxacin-loaded MSN comparable with danofloxacin solution. **CONCLUSIONS:** The liposomal hydrogel solidified at body temperature, effectively sustained the release of danofloxacin and showed in vitro antibacterial effects.

Introduction

Controlled release parenteral dosage forms of antibiotics have many applications in veterinary medicine since therapeutic levels of antibiotics could be maintained without the need for repeated injections (Medlicot et al., 2004). Recently, a considerable interest has focused on injectable, in situ forming gel for drug delivery. Hydrogels are three dimensional hydrophilic polymer networks capable of absorbing large amounts of water or biological fluids (Patois et al., 2009). Chitosan is obtained from chitin by alkaline acetylation, and it has many desirable properties including biocompatibility, biodegradability and high safety profile (Chang et al., 2009). The hydrogen bonding in chitosan chains due to the presence of amine and hydroxyl groups causes the chitosan solutions to be highly viscous (Bhupendra et al., 2011). A thermosensitive neutral solution based on chitosan/β-glycerophosphate was first reported by Chenite et al. (2001) and has recently become a major area of research. The neutral solution of chitosan and β-glycerophosphate remains liquid at room temperature but changes into a gel at body temperature (Khodaverdi et al., 2012). The in situ gelation mechanism involves neutralization of ammonium groups in chitosan, and strengthening of hydrophobic and hydrogen bonding between the chitosan chains at elevated temperatures (Chenite et al., 2001).

Since drug-loaded particles are suitable for controlled release and drug targeting, they have also been the focus of research in drug delivery systems. Among them, MSNs offer several attractive features, such as having a large surface area, being easily modified, pore size and volume, as well as being chemically inert and allowing easier functionalization of their surface. All of these features provide better control of drug loading and release profile. MSNs could be administered through parenteral and oral routes (Mohseni et al 2015).

Even though toxicity of silica nanoparticles is a concern, many studies have shown that this concern is not serious. For example, one study has shown that single and repeated intravenous doses in mouse caused no death (Liu et al., 2011).

Liposomes are colloidal vesicular structures of one or more lipid bilayers surrounding an aqueous compartment. A conventional drug injected into the blood stream typically achieves therapeutic level rapidly but keeps this level just for a short duration due to metabolism and excretion. Drug encapsulated by liposomes maintains its therapeutic level for a longer duration as the drug must first be released from the liposomes before being exposed to the metabolism and excretion processes (Shashi et al., 2013).

Danofloxacin, as a third fluoroquinolone antibacterial drug, acts by inhibition of bacterial DNA-gyrase. It has a rapid bactericidal activity against numerous Gram-negative and some Gram-positive bacteria, mycoplasmas and intracellular pathogens like *Brucella* and *Chlamydia* species (Yang et al., 2014). It has also shown excellent activity against respiratory pathogens of cattle, swine and poultry. Among the various drug delivery systems considered for pulmonary infections, nanoparticles have demonstrated several advantages, such as prolonged drug release, cell-specific targeted drug delivery or modified distribution of drugs, both at cellular and organ level (Beck-Broichsitter et al., 2009). For this purpose, MSNs with pore sizes in the range from 1 to 3 nm were synthesized. Due to high water solubility of danofloxacine, drug-loaded MSNs were encapsulated in liposomes and then added to chitosan/β-GP hydrogel. The release behavior of liposomal hydrogel containing danofloxacin-loaded MSNs as well as its morphology, gelation time and antibacterial activities were studied.

Materials and Methods

Medium molecular weight chitosan, with a degree of deacetylation (DDA) of 75-85% and β-Glycerophosphate disodium salt pentahydrate, were purchased from Sigma-Aldrich Chemical Co. (St. Louis, USA). Cetyltrimethylammonium bromide (CTAB, 98%) was purchased from Merck (Darmstadt, Germany). Tetraethyl orthosilicate (TEOS, 99%), egg phosphatidil choline and cholesterol were purchased from Sigma Aldrich (Seelze, Germany). Danofloxacin mesylate was provided by Kimiafaam Pharmaceutical Co. (Tehran, Iran). Acetic acid was purchased from Merck. All other chemicals were reagent grade.

Synthesis and characterization of MSNs: At first, N-cetyltrimethylammonium bromide (CTAB, 1.00 g, 2.75 mmol) was dissolved in 480 ml of deionized water, and then, 3.5 ml of NaOH (2.0 M) was introduced to the CTAB solution at 80 °C. After increasing the temperature to 80 °C, TEOS (5 mL, 21.9 mmol) was added drop-wise at a rate of 1mL/ min to the previous solution. The reaction mixture was stirred vigorously at 80 °C for 2 h. The white precipitate was isolated by filtration. Nanoparticles were washed with water and methanol and then dried under vacuum at 80 °C for 24 h. The surfactant was removed via calcination of the obtained powder. The powder was heated to 540 °C with a heating rate of 1 °C/min and then at 540 °C for 4 h. The surface area and pore size of MSNs were determined using a N2 adsorption-desorption instrument (Quanta chrome NOVA Automated Gas Sorption System, 2000e, USA).

Development of liposomes containing danofloxacin-loaded MSNs: Prior to liposome fusion, MSN (100 mg) was incubated with danofloxacin in 5.0 mL of water (10 mg/mL) for 24 h at room temperature. After stirring for 24 h under light-sealed conditions, the danofloxacin-loaded MSNs were centrifuged and washed with 20 mL of acetonitrile. To evaluate the danofloxacin loading efficiency, the supernatant was collected, and the residual danofloxacin content was determined by a UV spectrophotometer at 276.8 nm. The loading capacity of danofloxacin (Dano) was calculated by the following equation:

Loading capacity (%) = [(initial Dano (mg)- Dano in supernatant (mg)) / weight of formualation (mg)] * 100

The liposomes were prepared by a lipid-film based method (Sharma, 1997). Briefly, 50 mg of L-α-PC (phosphatidyl choline) and 10 mg of cholesterol were dissolved in 5 ml of chloroform and evaporated to form a thin lipid film with a rotary evaporator. Then, the formed lipid film was re-hydrated in 10 ml of distilled water prior to loading the danofloxacin in MSNs and was sonicated for 15 min. Finally, the mixture was centrifuged at 10,000 rpm for 30 min.

Preparation of hydrogel: Chitosan powders (250 mg) were dissolved in 6 ml of 0.1 M acetic acid and were gently stirred for 3 h to make a homogeneous solution. Then liposomes were fused with the chitosan solution and stirred for another 1 h. To make the β-GP solution, 1000 mg of β-GP was dissolved in deionized water. The chitosan and β-GP solutions were placed separately in an ice-water bath at 4 °C for 15 minutes. Then the β-GP solution was added drop-wise to the chitosan/liposome solution and stirred for 30 min.

Determination of gelation time: In the present study, gelation time was assessed using the inverted tube test, as described by Gupta and coworkers (Zhou et al., 2011). When a test tube containing a solution is titled, it is defined as a sol phase if the solution is deformed by the flow, or a gel phase if there is no flow. Firstly, 2 ml of the chitosan/ β-GP solutions was maintained for 12 h at 4°C in 5 ml vials with inner diameters of 10 mm to remove air bubbles. The vials were then incubated in a temperature-controlled bath. The sol-gel transition time was determined by inverting the vials horizontally every minute. The time at which the gel did not flow was recorded as the gelation time.

Standard calibration curve of danofloxacin: To construct the calibration curve, the danfloxacin solutions were prepared in a phosphate buffer, with a pH of 7.4, at a concentration range of 2.5 - 15.0 µg/ml. The absorbance of the solutions was measured at 276.8 nm using a UV-Vis spectrophotometer (Fig. 1).

In-vitro drug release study: The release profile of danofloxacin loaded in MSNs was investigated in phosphate buffer solution (PBS) as the test medium. Accurately weighed amounts of the prepared sample (1.0 g) were used under sink conditions at 37 °C. At predetermined time points up to 168 h, 1 ml of the release medium was collected and replenished with fresh buffer phosphate. The collected samples were analyzed with a UV spectrophotometer. The amount of the released drug (mg) was calculated by comparing its absorbance, at 276.8 nm, to the absorbance of a 10 mg/ml solution of danofloxacin in PBS. All measurements were performed in triplicate. Data are reported as means ± SD.

Morphological study: To maintain the porous structure of the hydrogels, they were freeze-dried first and then SEM was performed. The samples were plunged in liquid nitrogen, and the samples were cut with a cold knife. They were mounted on the plate base and coated with platinum-gold for SEM imaging, at 30 kV, using a scanning electron microscope (FESEM, Hitachi. S4160, Japan).

FTIR spectra analysis: The chitosan, β-GP, and dried chitosan/β-GP gel were placed in KBr pellets (the samples were mixed with KBr, with a ratio of 1:100, and pressed to form pellets) and were studied using an FTIR spectrophotometer (Nicolet, Model Impact 410; Madison, WI), in the range of 400-4000 cm-1 and at room temperature.

Microbiological tests: To determine the antibacterial activity of danofloxacin liposome hydrogel, the well diffusion test was carried out using *Escherichia coli* (*E.coli*) ATCC10145 as a Gram-negative pathogenic strain and *Staphylococcus aureus* (*S. aureus*) ATCC29213 as a Gram-positive pathogenic strain. The bacterial suspensions with a cell density of 0.5 McFarland (1.5×10^8 CFU/ml) were transferred onto the surface of Muller-Hinton agar plates using sterile cotton swabs. Wells with diameters of 8 mm were prepared by punching a sterile cork borer onto the solid agar medium. Aliquots (20 µl) of the danofloxacin gel (containing 20µg/ml of the drug) for danofloxacin hydrogel, danofloxacin suspension as positive control, the blank preparation (formulated exactly in the same way as the drug formulation but without adding danofloxacin) as a control to investigate the antimicrobial properties of chitosan and other ingredients were poured into the wells. The plates were kept for 30-60 min in an upward position to facilitate the distribution of the formulations in the media. After incubation for about 24 h, at 37 °C, the zones of inhibition around the wells were measured in mm using a caliper. All experiments were carried out in triplicate (Jahangirian et al., 2013).

Results

In-vitro drug release: As shown in Fig 2, a prolonged release pattern was observed for danofloxacin. About 27% of the drug was released within 24 h from the formulation and nearly 70% of the loaded drug was released within 96 hours. No burst effect was seen.

The release kinetic pattern of the drug from the prepared hydrogel was analyzed and the best method for this formulation was determined using a regression coefficient (r^2) close to 1. The values for r^2 were: Zero Order model, 0.90701; First Order model, 0.6645; Higuchii model, 0.9827; Hixon-Crowell model, 0.8339 and Korsmeyer-Peppas, 0.7574. According to the regression coefficient values, the drug release data best fit with Higuchi's kinetic model.

The most familiar form of Higuchi's model is the simplified Higuchi model, which relates drug concentration to the square root of time:

$$Mt^{gel}=kHt^{1/2}$$

where Mt^{gel} is the concentration of the drug in the drug matrix at time t and KH is the Higuchi dissolution constant (Singhvi et al., 2011)

Gelation time: The gelation process of liposomal hydrogel formulation was temperature- and time-dependent. By raising the temperature, the gelling process accel-

Table 1. In-vitro antibacterial activity of danofloxacin gel and danofloxacin solution as positive control (20μg/ml) against *S. aureus* and *E. coli* bacteria. * Data are expressed as mean ± standard deviation, n=3.

Bacteria	Zone of inhibition (mm)	
	Danofloxacin gel	Control positive
S. aureus	29.0±0.5	32.0±4.5
E. coli	36.0±1.0	40.0±2.9

erated; by increasing the temperature from 32 to 37°C the solidification time of the hydrogel was reduced from 30 to 15 min, and above 37°C, increasing the temperature did not change the time of gelling. The sol to gel transition at room temperature is illustrated in Fig 3.

Fourier transform infrared spectroscopy (FTIR) studies: The FTIR spectra of the lyophilized chitosan, β-GP, chitosan/β-GP, danofloxacin and liposomal hydrogel immediately after the gelation showed that there were no interactions between danofloxacin and excipients.

In the range of 2850- 2950 cm^{-1}, the spectrum of chitosan has one asymmetric band, at 2923 cm^{-1}. This band probably consists of two overlapping bands which represent the stretching vibrations in the aliphatic groups (-CH2 and -CH3) which are characteristic of the pyranose ring of chitosan.

The spectrum of chitosan shows a band at 16503 cm^{-1} which is assigned to the C=O stretch of the amide bond and at 1595 cm^{-1} which is assigned to the NH2 group of chitosan. These bands indicate that chitosan is a partially deacetylated product of chitin. In this range of frequency, no significant changes were observed.

In the range of 1200- 1500 cm^{-1}, the chitosan molecule showed four peaks, with the bands being 1255, 1315, 1380 and 1423cm^{-1}. The bands at 1423 and 1315 cm^{-1} are associated with the oscillations characteristic of C-H bending of CH2 groups. The band at

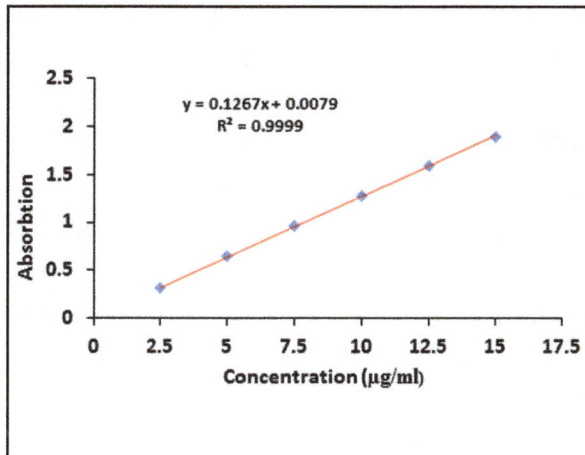

Figure 1. Calibration curve of danofloxacin in the phosphate buffer.

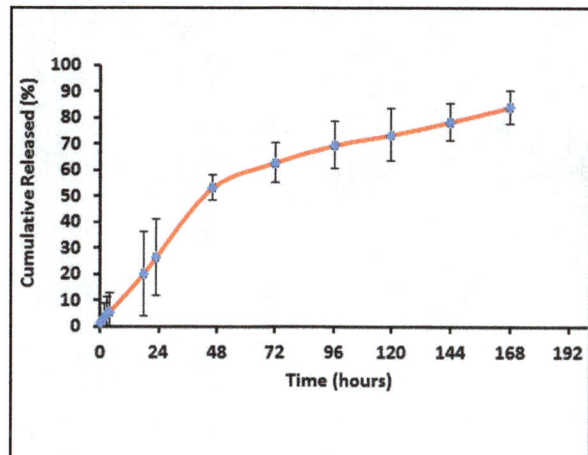

Figure 2. In vitro drug release profile of danofloxacin from the hydrogel.

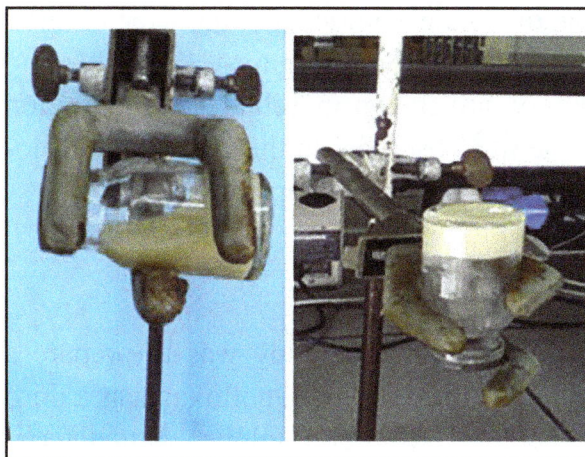

Figure 3. The chitosan/GP formulation at room temperature (left) and at 37°C (right).

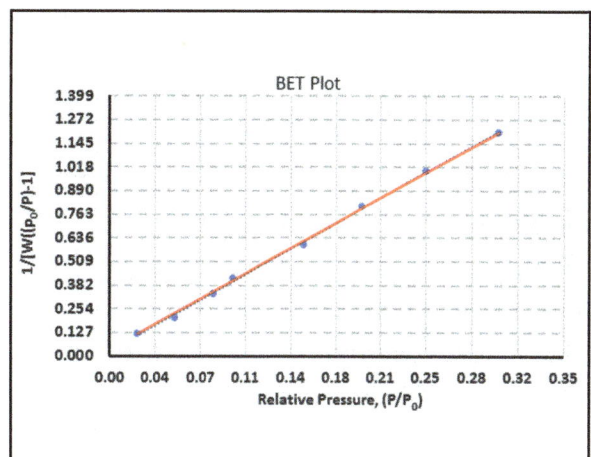

Figure 4. BET plot of the prepared MSNs.

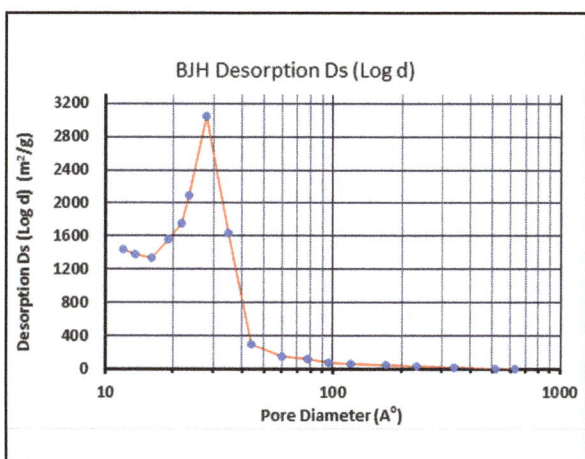

Figure 5. Pore size distribution of the prepared drug-free MSNs.

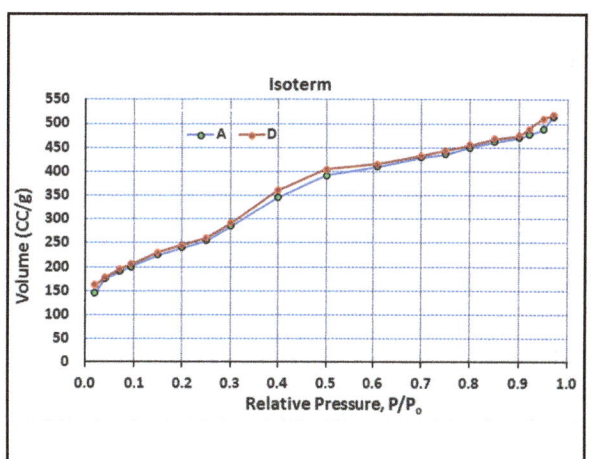

Figure 6. Nitrogen adsorption (A)/desorption (D) isotherm of the prepared MSNs.

1380 cm^{-1} represents the C-O stretching of the primary alcoholic group -CH2-OH.

In the wave length range of 800- 1200 cm^{-1}, the FTIR spectrum of chitosan showed three bands at 894,1030 and 1155 cm^{-1}. The wide band at 1030-1155 cm-1 represents the

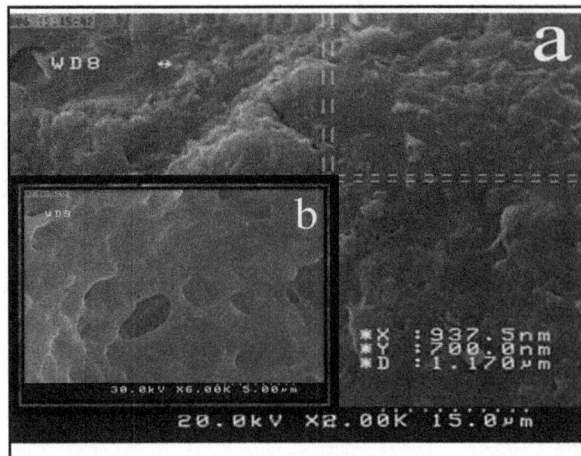

Figure 7. SEM of freeze-dried liposomal hydrogels (a) and swelled hydrogel in the phosphate buffer (b).

bridge C-O-C stretch of the glucosamine residues.

Two characteristic bands of GP appear at 976 cm^{-1} and 1069 cm^{-1}; the band at 976 cm^{-1} indicates aliphatic P-O-C stretching; the band at 1069 cm^{-1} is characteristic of the -PO42- group and the band at 920 cm^{-1} may indicate the presence of the -HPO42- group. The FTIR spectrum of the chitosan/β-GP system after the gelation indicates char acteristic bands for chitosan and glycerol phosphate disodium salt and there were no additional bands. For the chitosan/β-GP system, the bands of chitosan at 1380 and 1315 cm^{-1} were shifted to 1385 and 1319 cm^{-1}, respectively and the bands of GP at 1076 and 971cm^{-1} were shifted to 1069 and 976 cm^{-1}. No significant differences were seen on the FTIR spectra between the hydrogel and those of the danofloxacin, chitosan and β-GP.

Nanoparticle characterization: The Brunauer- Emmett- Teller (BET) surface areas and the BJH pore size distributions for NH2-MSN are shown in Fig. 4 and Fig. 5. The BET curve for MSN exhibited type-IV adsorption-desorption isotherm pattern according to IUPAC nomenclature for porous samples. The BET surface area for MSN

was found to be 890.54 m^2/g. The BJH pore size distributions for MSN showed 2.8 nm (Fig 5). The porous nature of the MSN was confirmed using nitrogen adsorption-desorption isotherms plot (Fig 6).

Morphology: The SEM photograph of the liposomal hydrogel shows that the formed gel had a rough and non-porous surface, while the swelled hydrogel in the phosphate buffer (pH=7) had a porous structure, as shown in Fig 7.

Antimicrobial activity: The antibacterial activities of the danofloxacin hydrogel and danofloxacin solution as diameter of their zones of inhibition against *S. aureus* and *E. coli* are shown in Table 1. No inhibition zone was observed for the gel without danofloxacin (the blank preparation).

Discussion

The aim of this study was to prepare a novel formulation of danofloxacin as a third generation fluoroquinolone antibacterial drug for sustained release drug delivery in veterinary medicine. In the present study on drug release, there was no prominent burst effect and the pattern of the release showed a smooth and sustained release with 27% and 53% of the cumulative in-vitro drug being released by the end of 24 and 48 h, respectively, although the release continued with a lower rate up to 168 h (85%). Regarding the kinetics of drug release and according to regression coefficient values, the drug release from the formulation was best fitted to Higuchi's kinetic model. This sustained release parenteral dosage form could be desirable for farm animals because it demonstrates minimized need for repeated injection, more compliance on drug therapy with promisingly better pharmacokinetic profile and antimicrobial efficacy in comparison to conventional dosage forms.

The injectable liposomal hydrogel has opened up a novel line of research in the field of minimally invasive and in situ forming gels as it can sustain the release of low-molecular weight hydrophilic drug-like danofloxacin for more than 96 h. Moreover, the system is biodegradable, biocompatible, and devoid of surfactants, and it shows minimal mechanical irritation upon in vivo implantation because of its soft and elastic nature. This type of formulation was prepared for cytarabine to reduce dosage frequency and sustain drug action (Mulik et al., 2009). It was capable of maintaining the therapeutic serum levels of cytarabine for more than 60 h. Thirumaleshwar et al. (2012) also designed a liposomal hydrogel as a wound dressing to provide an effective barrier to prevent the infection of the wound and further progression of infection to deeper tissues. Khaled et al. (2010) prepared an ocular prolonged-release liposomal hydrogel containing ciprofloxacin which effectively increased the ocular bioavailability of ciprofloxacin.

Drug release rate can also be controlled by functionalization of MSNs. For example, the release of vancomycin from cadmium sulfide (CdS) capped mobile crystalline material 41 (MCM-41) type MSNs was shown to be extended for up to 3 days and the loading and release mechanism of the MSN system was based on the capping and uncapping of the openings of the mesopores with CdS nanoparticles (Lai et al., 2003). A controlled release of captopril using MCM-41 showed enhanced release profile upon silylation and it is suggested that the drug release profile can be controlled by tailoring the surface properties and pore

size (Qu et al., 2006). Amine functionalized Santa Barbara-type mesoporous particle-15 (SBA-15) MSNs' release of tetracycline (TC) was shown to be extended up to 48 h and the TC-MCM-41 nanoparticles were more efficient than the free TC against *E. coli* in culture over a period of 24 h (Hashemikia et al., 2015). Thus, drug release could potentially be extended from our materials through surface functionalization.

In this study, the solidification of the liquid hydrogel was time- and temperature-dependent. All samples had the same gelation time above 37°C, lasting for about 15 min. By increasing the temperature from 32 to 37°C the gelation process was accelerated. It seems this process occurs via the creation of junction zones of the polymers mainly with changes in attractive versus repulsive forces like electrostatic repulsion between chitosan chains and strong chitosan-water interactions. These interactions were as a result of the polyol part of glycerophosphate which protects the chains against aggregation at low temperature. By increasing the temperature, chitosan chain polarity is reduced, protons from chitosan amine groups transfer to the phosphate moiety of glycerophosphate, sheets of water molecules around chitosan chains are removed and consequently attractive interchain hydrophobic and hydrogen bonding forces are strengthened to form hydrogel (Chenite et al., 2001).

Ruel Gariepy et al. (2002) reported that thermosensitive chitosan-beta-glycerophosphate (C-GP) solution containing loaded liposomes remained in sol state at 8-15°C and turned into a gel at body temperature after SC/IM injection. This system is reported to be able to sustain the drug release for more than 2 weeks. The major advantage of combining liposomes with the C-GP hydrogel system is the more sustained release of the drug along with overall stability compared with liposomal suspension. Moreover, this formulation offers some advantages over other systems. Zentner et al. (2001) reported that the onset of gelation of PLA- PEG-PLA was at 14°C and the transition to the solid-like gel state was complete around 18°C; this transition temperature which is very close to room temperature complicates handling of the preparation but our formulation remains liquid at room temperature for several hours and thus is easily injectable.

One of the main objectives of the current study was to prepare MSNs with an increased specific surface area and pore volume in order to achieve high loading of drug molecules. The chosen MSNs presented a high surface area and good pore volume, prior to the loading studies. Passive loading was chosen as the preferred method to load drug molecules and to increase the loading efficiency. In this study, the mean loading efficiency was about 45%. Hashemikia et al. (2015) reported TC loading in SBA-15 type MSNs as 42.3% w/w.

Among the factors affecting the loading process is the polarity of the organic solvent (Charnay et al., 2004). The chosen solvents were deionized water with a polarity index of 10.1. Since the interaction between water and silica nanoparticles prevents the loading process, a better choice may be methanol with a polarity index of 5.1. In addition, time and temperature also influence the loading process and should be further investigated.

The microbiological study showed an effective inhibitory property of this formulation on both Gram positive and Gram negative bacteria. The results showed that the inhibition zones of danofloxacin solution (positive control) were slightly greater than those of danofloxacin hydrogel. This may be due to the fact that the drug was not completely released within 24 hours and therefore produced lower danofloxacin concentrations in this in vitro test.

No drug delivery system is faultless, and this is the case with liposomal hydrogel as well. The cost of this drug delivery is high because of high costs associated with the raw materials as well as expensive equipment needed to increase manufacturing. Another issue is complication with sterilization of liposomes. As they are sensitive to high temperature, it is better for the initial solutions to be filtered through 0.45 μm and thereafter the entire production process to be performed under aseptic conditions (New, 1990).

Conclusion: In the present study, the liposomal hydrogel was solidified at body temperature with an appropriate gelation time. This promising formulation was capable of sustaining the release of danofloxacin for more than 96 h and showed suitable in vitro antibacterial effects. Although most novel antimicrobial drug delivery systems are currently in preclinical stages, with ongoing efforts in this field, nanoparticle-based drug delivery systems will improve the practice of antimicrobial therapy in veterinary medicine.

Acknowledgments

We would like to thank Tehran University of Medical Sciences and University of Tehran for supporting this work. Also, the authors are grateful for the support of Kimiafaam Pharmaceutical Co. (Tehran, Iran) for providing danofloxacin as a gift.

References

1. Beck-Broichsitter, M., Gauss, J., Packhaeuser, C.B., Lahnstein, K., Schmehl Seeger, W., Kissel, T., Gessler, T. (2009) Pulmonary drug delivery with aerosolizable nanoparticles in an ex-vivo lung model. Int J Pharm. 367: 169-178.

2. Chang, Y., Xiao, L., Tang, Q. (2009) Preparation and characterization of a novel thermosensitive hydrogel based on chitosan and gelatin blends. J Appl Polymer Sci. 113: 400-407.

3. Charnay, C., Begu, S., Tourne-Peteilh, C., Nicole, L., Lerner, D.A., Devoisselle, J.M. (2004) Inclusion of ibuprofen in mesoporous templated silica: drug loading and release property. Eur J Pharm Biopharm. 57: 533-540.

4. Chenite, A., buschmann, M., Wang, D., Chaput, C., Kandani, N. (2001) Rheological characterization of thermogelline chitosan/glycerol-phosphate solutions. Carbohydr Polym. 46: 39-47.

5. Hashemikia, S., Hemmatinejad, N., Ahmadi, E., Montazer, M. (2015) Optimization of tetracycline hydrochloride adsorption on amino modified SBA-15 using response surface methodology. J Colloid Interface Sci. 443: 105-114.

6. Jahangirian, H., Haron, M.J., Imail,M.H., Rafiee-Moghadam, R., Afsah-Hejri, L., Abdolahil, Y., Rezayi, M., Vafaei, N. (2013) Well diffusion method for evaluation of antibacterial activity of copper phenylL fatty hydroxamate synthesized from canola and palm kernel oils. Digest J Nanomater Biostruct. 8: 1263-1270.

7. Khaled, M.H. (2010) Ciprofloxacin as ocular liposomal hydrogel. AAPS Pharm Sci Tech. 11: 241-246.

8. Khodaverdi, E., Tafaghodi, M., Ganji, F., Abnoos, Kh., Naghizadeh, H. (2012) In vitro insulin release from thermosensitive chitosan hydrogel: AAPS Pharm Sci Tech. 13: 460-466.

9. Lai, C.Y., Trewyn, B.G., Jeftinija, D.M., Jeftinija, K., Xu, S., Jeftinija, S., Lin, V.S.A. (2003) Mesoporous silica nanosphere-based carrier system with chemically removable CdS nanoparticle caps for stimuli-responsive controlled release of neurotransmitters and drug molecules. J Am Chem Soc. 125: 4451-4459.

10. Liu, T., Li, L., Teng, X., Huang, X., Liu, H., Chen, D., Ren, J., He, J., Tang, F. (2011) Single and repeated dose toxicity of mesoporous hollow silica nanoparticles in intravenously exposed mice. 2011. J biomaterials. 32: 1657-1668.

11. Medlicott, N.J., Waldron, N.A., Todd, P.F. (2004) Sustained release veterinary parentral products. Adv Drug Deliv Rev. 56: 1345-65.

12. Mohseni, M., Gilani K., Mortazavi, S.A. (2015) Preparation and characterization of rifampin loaded mesoporous silica nanoparticles as a potential system for pulmonary drug delivery. Iran J Pharm Res. 14: 27-34.

13. Mulik, R., Kulkarni, V., Murthy, R.S. (2009) Chitosan-based thermosensitive hydrogel containing liposomes for sustained delivery of cytarabine. Drug Dev Ind Pharm. 35: 49-56.

14. New, R.R.C., Chance, S.M., Thomas, S.C., Peters, W. (1978) Antileishmanial activity of antimonials entrapped in liposomes. Nature. 272: 55-58.

15. Patois, E., Osorio-da Cruz., Tille, J.C., Walpoth, B., Gurny R., Jordan, O. (2009) Novel thermosensitive chitosan hydrogels: in vivo evaluation. J Biomed Mater Res A. 91: 324-30.

16. Prajapati, B.G., Patel, M.M. (2011) Cross-linked chitosan gel for local drug delivery of clotrimazole. E-J Sci Tech. 6: 43.

17. Qu, F., Zhu, G., Huang, S., Li, S., Qiu, S. (2006) Effective controlled release of captopril by silylation of mesoporous MCM-41. Chem Phys Chem 7: 400-406.

18. Ruel Gariépy, E., Leclair, G., Hildgen, P., Gupta, A., Leroux, J.C. (2002) Thermosensitive chitosan-based hydrogel containing liposomes for the delivery of hydrophilic molecules. J Control Release. 21: 373-83.

19. Sharma, A., Sharma, U.S. (1997) Liposomes in drug delivery: progress and limitations. Int J Pharm. 154: 123-140.

20. Shashi, K., Satinder, K., Bharat, P.A. (2012) complete review on: Liposomes. Int Res J Pharm. 3: 10-16.

21. Singhvi, G., Singh, M. (2011) Reviwe of in vitro drug release characterization models. Int J Pharm Studies Res. 2: 77-84.

22. Thirumaleshwar, S., Kulkarni, P.K., Gowda, D.V. (2012) Liposomal hydrogels: A novel drug delivery system for wound dressing. Curr Drug Therap. 7: 212-218.

23. Yang, F.,Sun, N., Liu, Y.M., Zeng, Z.L. (2014) Estimating danofloxacin withdrawal time in broiler chickens based on physiologically based pharmacokinetics modeling. Vet Pharm Ther. 38: 174-182.

24. Zentner, G.M., Rathi, R., Shih, C., McRea, J.C., Seo, M-H., Oh, H., Rhee, B.G., Mestecky, J., Moldoveanu, Z., Morgan, M., Weitman, S. (2001) Biodegradable block copolymers for delivery of proteins and waterinsolubledrugs. J Controll Release. 72: 203-215.

25. Zhou, H.Y., Zhang, Y.P., Zhang, W.F., Chen, X.G. (2011) Biocompatibility and characteristics of injectable chitosan-based thermosensitive hydrogel for drug delivery. Carbohydr Polym. 83: 1643-1651.

10

EPSA1 and VPF genes expression during embryonic and larval development period of Beluga, *Huso huso*

Taheri Mirghaed, A.[*]

Department of Aquatic Animal Health, Faculty of Veterinary Medicine, University of Tehran, Tehran, Iran

Key words:

Gene expression, larval development, sturgeon

Correspondence

Taheri Mirghaed, A.
Department of Aquatic Animal
Health, Faculty of Veterinary
Medicine, University of Tehran,
Tehran, Iran

Email: mirghaed@ut.ac.ir

Abstract:

BACKGROUND: The Endothelial PAS domain-containing protein 1 (EPSA1) is the key transcriptional regulator of hypoxic response and Vascular Permeability Factor (VPF) is an important growth factor for vascular development and angiogenesis. OBJECTIVES: In the present study, the levels of the EPSA1 coding gene and VPF transcripts were evaluated during Larval development of Beluga, *Huso huso*. METHODS: Samples at 12 developmental time-points including 1, 2, 4 days before hatch (eyed eggs), fresh hatched larvae (0), and larvae 1, 3, 6, 10, 15, 20, 25 and 50 days post-hatching were collected and stored in a −80 °C freezer until RNA extraction. Changes in EPSA1 and VPF mRNA expression were studied and differences in normalized mRNA expression levels among the different developmental stages of *H. huso* were analyzed by one-way analysis of variance (ANOVA). RESULTS: The transcripts of EPSA1 and VPF were detected in all developmental time-points of *H. huso* from embryos to fingerling fish. Our results revealed that the mRNA expression of EPSA1 and VPF was low during embryonic development and then upregulated significantly at the time of hatch and early larval time-points, whereas in the late larval development stages they started to decline. CONCLUSIONS: This study showed that there is an association between the EPSA1 and VPF mRNA expression during larval development of *H. huso*. The up regulation of EPSA1 and VPF transcripts at the time of hatch and during yolk sac fry development of *H. huso* is likely tied to the role of them in vasculogenesis and angiogenesis.

Introduction

The Endothelial PAS domain-containing protein 1 is encoded by the EPAS1 gene. This gene encodes a half of transcription factor involved in the induction of genes regulated by oxygen, which is induced as oxygen levels fall. Endothelial PAS domain-containing protein 1 is the key transcriptional regulator of hypoxic response in both adult and embryonic organisms (Bracken et al., 2003). The transcription factors hypoxia-inducible factor-1 (HIF-1 and EPSA1) is the key regulator responsible for the induction of genes that facilitate adaptation and survival of cells and the whole organism from normoxia to hypoxia (Ke and Costa, 2006). In mammals, expression of at least one hundred genes has been reported to be under the control of HIF-1a and EPSA1 (Rytkonen et al., 2007). A close related protein, EPSA1, shares 48% amino acid sequence identity with HIF-1. RNA expression patterns have indicated that both HIF-1 and EPSA1 are largely ubiquitously expressed in human and mouse tissues in an oxygen-independent manner (Ke and Costa, 2006). In normoxia, HIF and EPSA protein is transcriptionally inactive and rapidly degraded by the ubiquitin/proteasome pathway. Under hypoxia, however, HIF and EPSA becomes stabilized, translocates into the nucleus and heterodimerises with Aryl Hydrocarbon Nuclear Translocator (ARNT). This transcriptionally active complex then associates with hypoxia response elements (HREs) in the regulatory regions of target genes, binds transcriptional co-activators and induces target gene expression (Bracken et al., 2003).

Vascular Permeability Factor (VPF), a selective mitogen for endothelial cells, is an important growth factor for vascular development and angiogenesis (Liang et al., 2001). It is known that VPF is synthesized by different cell types, including aortic vascular smooth muscle cells, keratinocytes, macrophages and many tumor cells (Dvorak, 1995). VPFs have been found in all vertebrate species that have been examined so far and it has been stated that the sequence and genomic organization of the vertebrate VPF genes is highly conserved between teleost fish and mammals. VPF has been observed in teleost fish (zebrafish, Danio rerio and pufferfish, Fugu rubripes), frogs (Xenopuslaevis), birds (Gallus gallus), and mammals (Holmes and Zachary, 2005). It has also been noted that two isoforms of VPF that differ in the presence of exons 6 and 7, VPF165 and VPF121, are the dominant forms expressed in zebrafish embryo (Liang et al., 2001). In zebrafish, it has been suggested that Vascular Endothelial Growth Factor (VEGF) plays an important role in the vascular development and endoderm morphogenesis (Ober et al., 2004). Moreover, VPF is expressed throughout the zebrafish embryonic development (Liang et al., 1998) and it has been suggested that VPF can not only stimu-

late endothelial cell differentiation, but also, hematopoiesis in in zebrafish embryo (Liang et al., 2001).

Oxygen tension is a key physiological regulator of VPF-A gene expression. Transcriptional regulation of the VPF gene by hypoxia is mediated by the binding of the transcription factor HIF-1 to the hypoxia responsive enhancer elements (HREs) in its 5′ and 3′ UTRs (Holmes and Zachary, 2005). In mammals, HIF and EPSA signal an increase in VPF, which in turn stimulates the growth of blood vessels (Nikinmaa and Rees, 2005). According to a study on developmental defects in Baltic salmon (*Salmo salar*), it has been suggested that HIF regulates vascular development during normal development, presumably by modulating VPF levels, as in mammals (Vuori et al., 2004; Nikinmaa and Rees, 2005). In lake trout *Salvelinus namaycush*, the yolk sac fry has been shown to have an increasing expression pattern of HIF-1a protein and HIF-1 DNA binding after hatch, however, VPF protein expression was variable between different biological variations (Vouri et al., 2009).

Although the role of VPF in blood vessel formation is well known, it is presently not known how the VPF gene is transcribed during early development of any fish species, especially after hatching. It is also not known whether the transcription of HIFs is associated with VPF transcript during normal development of fish. We addressed these questions in early development of Beluga sturgeon, *Huso huso*, using quantitative real-time PCR (qPCR).

Materials and Methods

Animals and sampling protocol: All fertilized eggs were obtained from an artificially spawned sturgeon broodstock from Shahid Marjani Artificial Sturgeon Propagation and Rearing Center located in Aghalla, Iran. The Beluga Sturgeon larvae hatched seven days after fertilization (Water temperature 18°C), were reared in ferroconcrete and fiberglass tanks and fed with newly hatched Artemia. The Beluga Larvae started exogenous feeding at day 20. Samples were collected at 12 developmental time-points including 4 days before hatch, 2 days before hatch (eyed eggs), 1 day before hatch, newly hatched larvae (0), and larvae 1, 3, 6, 10, 15, 20, 25 and 50 days post-hatching. All individuals were killed by an overdose of tricaine methanesulfonate (MS-222) and deep-frozen in liquid nitrogen as soon as they were collected and stored in a −80°C freezer until RNA extraction.

Total RNA extraction and cDNA synthesis: The procedure of RNA extraction, control of RNA quality, measuring of RNA concentration and cDNA synthesis have been described by Akbarzadeh et al. (2011). Briefly, whole larvae or eggs were placed in the recommended proportions of Tri Reagent and homogenized using a Qiagen Tissue Lyser. Total RNA was isolated from six individuals at each stage described above (n = 6) using a Tri Reagent (Molecular Research Center, Inc., Cincinnati, OH, USA), treated with Invitrogen DNase I (Invitrogen, CA, USA) and cleaned up using the Nucleospin RNA II kit (Macherey-Nagel, Düren, Germany) in accordance with the manufacturer's instructions. The quality of RNA samples was evaluated by electrophoresis on a 1.5 % agarose gel and their concentration was determined by a NanoDrop ND-1000 Spectrophotometer (Thermo Scientific, Wilmington, DE, USA) reading at 260/280 nm. Every sample was measured in duplicate and a mean value was used. 1 µg of total RNA was used to synthesize First-strand cDNAs using a DyNAmoTM cDNA Synthesis Kit (Finnzyme, Espoo, Finland) for RT-PCR, following the manufacturer's instructions and a mixture of oligo-dT as primer.

Primer design: The qPCR primers for ESPA1 and VPF (Kolangi et al., 2013) were designed based on the conserved regions of the sequences in GenBank. Multiple qPCR primer combinations were designed for each gene using Primer3 and tested (Table 1). The specificity and size of the amplicons obtained with primer pairs were checked on a 1.5 % agarose gel. For each gene, qPCR efficiency was also taken into account for choosing the best qPCR primer pair with specific and correct size. Primers for ribosomal protein L6 (RPL6) (used as reference gene for standardization of expression levels) were referenced from Akbarzadeh et al. (2011). The method of PCR efficiency determination has been described in section 2.4.

Quantitative real-time PCR (qRT-PCR): Quantitative PCRs were run on a 7900 HT Fast Real-Time PCR System (Applied Biosystems) with Fermentas Maxima SYBR Green qPCR Master Mix (2×) (Fermentas) and all primers at [100 nM], using standard protocol [initial denaturation at 95°C for 10 min, 40 cycles of denaturation at 95°C for 15 s and annealing/extension at 60 °C for 1 min]. All reactions were run in triplicate. The mRNA expression levels of genes were recorded as Ct values that corresponded to the number of cycles at which the fluorescence signal can be detected above a threshold value. Baseline and threshold for Ct calculation were set manually using the SDS RQ manager v 1.2 (Applied Biosystems). Standard curves were constructed from dilution series of pooled cDNA (including seven dilutions from 1/10 to 1/2000), and the PCR efficiency was calculated using the equation $E\% = (10^{1/slope} - 1) \times 100$ (Radonic et al. 2004).

The fold change in relative mRNA expression of EPSA1 and VPF was calculated by the $2^{-\Delta\Delta Ct}$ method of Livak and Schmittgen (2001). The difference between Ct values of the reference genes and the target genes was calculated for each mRNA by taking the mean Ct of triplicate reactions and subtracting the mean Ct of triplicate reactions for the reference RNA measured on an aliquot from the same RT reaction ($\Delta Ct = Ct_{target\ gene} - Ct_{reference\ gene}$). All samples were then normalized to the ΔCt value of a calibrator sample to obtain a $\Delta\Delta Ct$ value ($\Delta Ct_{target} - \Delta Ct_{calibrator}$). Among the developmental time-points, the sample with the lowest Ct value was chosen as the calibrator sample in order to evaluate the putative differential mRNA expression of target gene.

Differences in normalized mRNA expression levels of EPSA1 and VPF among the different developmental stages of *H. huso* were analyzed by one-way analysis of variance (ANOVA), followed by a Tukey's HSD post hoc analysis for multiple comparisons. Differences were considered statistically significant at $p<0.05$. SPSS (version 18.0) software was used for statistical analysis.

Results

Relative transcription pattern of EPSA1: The transcript of EPSA1 was detected in all developmental time-points of *H. huso* from embryos to fingerling fish (Fig. 1 A&B). Changes in normalized EPSA1 transcription by using the RPL6 over development were statistically significant over time ($p<0.05$). Both EPSA1 (Fig. 1) relative mRNA levels were significantly upregulated from hatching time to late larval stages ($p<0.05$). The transcript levels of EPSA1 displayed a significant decrease from feeding time (20dph) to fingerling fish.

Relative transcription pattern of VPF: Figure 2 shows the result for the quantification of the developmental expression of VPF in *H. huso*. Similar to EPSA1, the mRNA of VPF could be detected as early as embryonic time (d-4). Changes in normalized VPF expression over embryonic and larval development of Beluga were statistically significant over time ($p<0.05$). After low expression during the embryonic stage (4, 2 and 1 days before hatch) the transcript levels of VPF displayed an increasing trend from hatching time (Fig. 2).

The relationship between the transcription patterns of EPSA1 and VPF: To show the relationship between the transcription of

EPSA1 and VEGF, maximal mRNA values were adjusted to 1, and other values were fractioned to indicate the proportion of the transcription levels compared to maximum. The results show a similar pattern was observed for EPSA1 and VPF transcripts in embryonic and larval development. The mRNA expression of both genes was low during embryonic development and then upregulated during hatching and early larval stages, whereas in the late larval and juvenile stages it remained fairly constant.

Discussion

In this study, we have found a direct relationship between the EPSA1 and VPF mRNA expression during normal development of *H. huso*. This is the first report of the association of HIFs and VPF mRNA expression during larval development of fish in a normal oxygen environment. The levels of EPSA1 and VPF transcripts were elevated significantly during and after hatching time and remained fairly constant in the late larval and juvenile stages.

The upregulation of EPSA 1 and VPF transcripts at the time of hatch and during yolk sac fry development of *H. huso* observed in the present study is likely to be tied to the role of EPSA1 and VPF in organogenesis, vasculogenesis and angiogenesis. It is well known that regulation of EPSA1, VPF and VPF receptor in the embryo is crucial to angiogenesis and, therefore, to organogenesis and survival (Bonventre et al., 2011). The role of EPSA on the regulation of the VPF gene and vascular development in hypoxia condition has been well studied (e.g. Levy et al., 1995; Forsythe et al. 1996; Miquerol et al., 2000; Holmes and Zachary, 2005; Kallergi et al., 2009). EPSA is an important regulator of hypoxia responses, including vascularization and erythropoiesis, and is required for normal development, including angiogenetic, hematopoietic, and neural development in mammalian embryos

Table 1. qPCR primer used in this study.

Primer name	Seq	Amplicon size	Accession number/Ref.
ESPA1 For	GAAGGTCCTGCACTGCACT		JQ027715.1
ESPA1 Rev	CTTGGTGCACAAGTTCTGGT		JQ027715.1
RPL6 For	GTGGTCAAACTCCGCAAGA		Akbarzadeh et al. (2011).
RPL6 Rev	GCCAGTAAGGAGGATGAGGA		Akbarzadeh et al. (2011).
VPF For	GCCTTCATGTGTACCACTCATG		Kolangi et al. (2013)
VPF Rev	GGTCTGCATTCACATGTACTGTG		Kolangi et al. (2013)

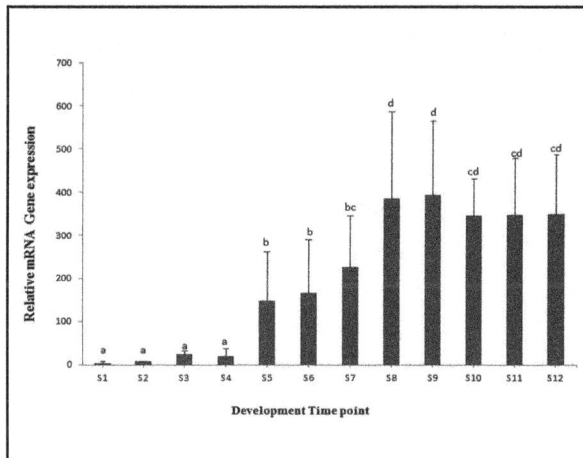

Figure 1. Relative expression levels of EPSA1 mRNA normalized using RPL6 during early development of Beluga. S1: 4 days before hatch; S2: 2 days before hatch; S3: 1 day before hatch; S4: newly hatched (day 0); S5: 1 day post-hatch (1 dph), S6:3 dph; S7: 6 dph; S8: 10 dph; S9:15 dph; S10: 20 dph; S11: 25 dph; S12: 50 dph. The values are represented as mean ± S.D. (n = 6). Statistical significance of differences of the normalized EPSA 1 data between groups was analyzed using one-way ANOVA and Tukey's multiple-comparison test. Bars with different letters are significantly different. p<0.05 was taken to show significant differences.

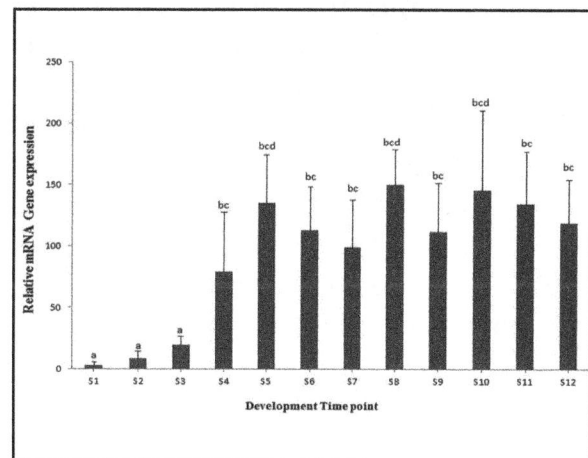

Figure 2. Relative expression levels of VPF mRNA normalized using RPL6 during early development of Beluga. S1: 4 days before hatch; S2: 2 days before hatch; S3: 1 day before hatch; S4: newly hatched (day 0); S5: 1 day post-hatch (1 dph), S6:3 dph; S7: 6 dph; S8: 10 dph; S9:15 dph; S10: 20 dph; S11: 25 dph; S12: 50 dph. The values are represented as mean ± S.D. (n = 6). Statistical significance of differences of the normalized VPF data between groups was analyzed using one-way ANOVA and Tukey's multiple-comparison test. Bars with different letters are significantly different. p<0.05 was taken to show significant differences.

(Vuori et al., 2004). In mammals, abnormal blood vessel development and vascularization are observed when embryos lacking a single VPF allele or HIFs are disturbed (Carmeliet et al., 1996; Ryan et al., 1998). In Baltic salmon, Vuori et al. (2004) found that both HIF-1 and VPF down-regulated in Baltic salmon suffer from abnormally high yolk-sac fry mortality (M74-syndrome). They suggested that HIF-1 regulates vascular development during normal development by modulating VPF levels. In lake trout, the expression of HIFs protein and HIF-1 DNA binding showed an increasing pattern after hatch and during yolk sac fry (Vuori et al., 2009).

Interestingly, the upregulation of VPF gene was observed at time of hatch and during yolk sac fry of *H. huso*. VPF has emerged as the single most important regulator of blood vessel formation (Holmes and Zachary, 2005). Various processes of early stage vascular development including vasculogenesis, large vessel formation (e.g. of the dorsal aorta), capillary sprouting, and the remodeling of the yolk sac vasculature are affected by VPF (Breier, 2000). Indeed, the expression of the VPF has been thoroughly studied during embryonic development. However, little is known about the role of VPF on vascular development at the time of hatching and during larval development of fish.

In zebrafish, overexpression of VPF in the embryo indicates a stimulation of both endothelial and hematopoietic lineages. It has also been demonstrated that VPF can stimulate hematopoiesis in zebrafish by promoting the formation of terminally differentiated red blood cells (Liang et al., 2001). Hendon et al. (2008) studied the effects of exposure to pyrene in the early life-stages of ship head minnow, *Cyprinodon variegatus*, and observed that the VPF gene is transcribed under conditions where the external environment is normoxic, and suggested that the oxygen tension in developing tissues is reduced to a level that prevents HIF degradation resulting in VPF transcription. In mouse, VPF was detected from embryonic day 7 in the extra-embryonic and embryonic endoderm, and by day 8 it is present at high levels in the trophoblast surrounding the embryo and in the embryonic myocardium, gut endoderm, embryonic mesenchyme and amniotic ectoderm. VPF expression declines in most tissues in the weeks after birth and is relatively low in most adult organs, except in a few vascular beds, including those of the brain choroid plexus, lung alveoli, kidney glomeruli and heart (Holmes and Zachary, 2005). VPF gene expression is also upregulated by a variety of growth factors and cytokines, including PDGF-BB, TGF-ß, basic fibroblast growth factor (FGF-2), interleukin-1ß and interleukin-6, some of which can act synergistically with hypoxia (Holmes and Zachary, 2005).

Our results indicate that VPF is involved in development of the vascular system of *H. huso* larvae in normoxic condition. It has been suggested that organogenesis is closely linked to vascular development and formation of the vertebrate closed circulatory system which involves both vasculogenesis and angiogenesis (Bonventre et al., 2011). During yolk sac fry development of fish, new capillaries are formed and larval-type red blood cells and hemoglobins are replaced by adult types (Iuchi and Yamamoto 1983; Wells and Pinder 1996).

The upregulation of VPF can therefore be considered a major factor by which the formation of blood vessels and cells is regulated.

The results of the present study also showed a marked upregulation of EPSA1 transcript at the time of hatch and larval development of *H. huso*. EPSA1 is a closely related protein complex which is regulated by cellular oxygen concentrations in a similar fashion. These hypoxia inducible factors activate transcription of target genes in response to hypoxia (Blancher et al., 2000; Losso and Bawadi, 2005). It has been demonstrated that EPSA1 is largely ubiquitously expressed in an oxygen-independent manner (Bracken et al., 2003). In normoxia, HIF protein is transcriptionally inactive and rapidly degraded by the ubiquitin/proteasome pathway (Bracken et al., 2003). However, Hypoxic conditions inhibit this degradation, which allows HIFs to accumulate in the cell (Kajimura et al., 2006). Interestingly, however, there are several reports of HIF protein expression at normoxia in which imply more diverse roles for HIF than solely regulating a hypoxic response (Bracken et al., 2003). EPSA1 is required for normal embryogenesis because it is central to oxygen homeostasis. HIF-1 and EPSA1 knockout mice died early or had syndromes of multiple organ pathology that included retinopathy, cardiac hypertrophy, mitochondrial abnormalities, hypoglycemia, altered Krebs cycle, and several biochemical abnormalities (Losso and Bawadi, 2005). The up-regulation of EPSA1 gene, especially at the time of hatch during development of *H. huso* in normoxic condition reveals the possible importance of HIF signaling during this period.

Conclusion: In conclusion, this is the first report of the association of EPSA1 and VPF mRNA expression during larval development of fish in a normal oxygen environment. Our data revealed that the levels of EPSA1 and VPF transcripts were elevated significantly during and after hatching time and remained fairly constant in the late larval and fingerling stages. The upregulation of EPSA1 and VPF transcripts at the time of hatch and during yolk sac fry development of *H. huso* observed in the present study is most likely tied to the role of EPSA1 and VPF in organogenesis, vasculogenesis and angiogenesis.

Acknowledgments

We would like to thank the staffs of Sturgeon Propagation and Rearing Center of Shahid Marjani (Gorgan, Iran) for their kind help. Special thanks are forwarded to Mr. Pasandi and Mr. Ghamsari for their guides and assistances.

References

1. Akbarzadeh, A., Farahmand, H., Mahjoubi, F., Nematollahi, M.A., Leskinen, P., Rytkonen, K., Nikinmaa, M. (2011) The transcription of L-gulono-gamma-lactone oxidase, a key enzyme for biosynthesis of ascorbic acid, during development of Persian sturgeon *Acipenser persicus*. Comp Biochem Physiol B. 158: 282-288.

2. Blancher, C., Moore, J.W., Talks, K.L., Houlbrook, S., Harris, A.L. (2000) Relationship of Hypoxia-Inducible Factor (HIF)-1a and HIF-2a expression to vascular endothelial growth factor induction and hypoxia survival in human breast cancer cell lines. Cancer Res. 60: 7106-7113

3. Bonventre, J.A., White, L.A., Cooper, K.R. (2011) Methyl tert butyl ether targets developing vasculature in zebrafish (*Danio rerio*) embryos. Aquat Toxicol. 105: 29-40.

4. Bracken, C.P., Whitelaw, M.L., Peet, D.J. (2003) The hypoxia-inducible factors: key transcriptional regulators of hypoxic responses. Cell Mol Life Sci. 60: 1376-1393.

5. Breier, G. (2000) Angiogenesis in embryonic development: A Review. Placenta. 14: 11-15.

6. Carmeliet, P., Ferreira, V., Breier, G., Pollefeyt, S., Kieckens, L., Gertsenstein, M., Fahrig, M., Vandenhoeck, A., Harpal, K., Eberhardt, C., Declercq, C., Pawling, J., Moons, L., Collen, D., Risau, W., Nagy, A. (1996) Abnormal blood vessel development and lethality in embryos lacking a single VEGF allele. Nature. 380: 435-439.

7. Dvorak, H.F., Brown, L.F., Detmar, M., Dvorak, A.M. (1995) Vascular permeability factor/vascular endothelial growth factor, microvascular hyperpermeability, and angiogenesis. Am J Pathol. 146: 1029-1039.

8. Forsythe, J.A., Jiang, B.H., Iyer, N.V., Agani, F., Leung, S.W., Koos, R.D., Semenza, G. (1996) Activation of vascular endothelial growth factor gene transcription by Hypoxia-Inducible Factor 1. Mol Cell Biol. 16: 4604-4613.

9. Hendon, L.A., Carlson, E.A., Manning, S., Brouwer, M. (2008) Molecular and developmental effects of exposure to pyrene in the early life-stages of *Cyprinodon variegatus*. Comp Biochem Physiol C. 147: 205-215.

10. Holmes, D.I., Zachary, I. (2005) The vascular endothelial growth factor (VEGF) family: angiogenic factors in health and disease. Genome Biol. 6: 209.

11. Kajimura, S., Aida, K., Duan, C. (2006) Understanding Hypoxia-Induced Gene Expression in Early Development: In Vitro and In Vivo analysis of hypoxia-inducible factor 1-regulated Zebra fish insulin-like growth factor binding protein 1gene expression. Mol Cell Biol. 26: 1142-1155.

12. Kallergi, G., Markomanolaki, H., Giannoukaraki, V., Papadaki, M.A., Strati, A., Lianidou, E.S., Georgoulias, V., Mavroudis, D., Agelaki, S. (2009) Hypoxia-inducible factor-1α and vascular endothelial growth factor expression in circulating tumor cells of breast cancer patients. Breast Cancer Res. 11: R84-12.

13. Ke, Q., Costa, M. (2006) Hypoxia-Inducible Factor-1 (HIF-1). Mol Pharmacol. 70: 1469-1480.

14. Kolangi Miandare, H., Farahmand, H., AKbarzaeh, A., Ramzanpour, S., Kaiya, H., Mi-

yazato, M., Rytkonen, K.T., Nikinmma, M. (2013) Developmental transcription of gene putatively associated with growth in two sturgeon species of different growth rate. Gen Comp Endocr. 182: 41-47.

15. Levy, A.P., Levy, N.S., Wegner, S., Goldberg, M.A. (1995) Transcriptional regulation of the rat vascular endothelial growth factor gene by hypoxia. J Biol Chem. 270: 13333-13340.

16. Liang, L., Xu X., Chin A.J., Balasubramaniyan, N.V., Teo, M.A.L., Lam, T.J., Weinberg, E.S., Ge, R. (1998) Cloning and characterization of vascular endothelial growth factor (VEGF) from zebrafish, *Danio rerio*. Biochim Biophys Acta. 1397: 14-20.

17. Liang, L., Chang, J.R., Chin, A.J., Smith, A., Kelly, C., Weinberg, E.S., Ge, R. (2001) The role of vascular endothelial growth factor (VEGF) in vasculogenesis, angiogenesis, and hematopoiesis in zebrafish development. Mech Dev. 108: 29-43.

18. Livak, K.J., Schmittgen, T.D. (2001) Analysis of relative gene expression data using real-time quantitative PCR and the $2^{-\Delta\Delta C_T}$ method. Methods. 25: 402-408.

19. Losso, J.N., Bawadi, H.A. (2005) Hypoxia Inducible factor pathways as targets for functional foods. J Agric Food Chem. 53: 3751-3768.

20. Iuchi, I., Yamamoto, M. (1983) Erythropoiesis in the developing rainbow trout, *Salmo gairdneri* irideus: histochemical and immunochemical detection of erythropoietic organs. J Exp Zool. 226: 409-417.

21. Miquerol, L., Langille, B.L., Nagy, A. (2000) Embryonic development is disrupted by modest increases in vascular endothelial growth factor gene expression. Development. 127: 3941-3946.

22. Nikinmaa, M., Rees, B.B. (2005) Oxygen-dependent gene expression in fishes. Am J Physiol Regul Integr Comp Physiol. 288: 1079-1090.

23. Ober, E.A., Olofsson, B., Makinen, T., Jin, S.W., Shoji, W., Koh, G.Y., Alitalo, K., Stainier, D.Y.R. (2004) VEGFc is required for vascular development and endoderm morphogenesis in zebrafish. EMBO Rep. 5: 78-84.

24 Radonic, A., Thulke, S., Mackay, I.M., Landt, O., Siegert, W., Nitsche, A. (2004) Guideline to reference gene selection for quantitative real-time PCR. Biochem Biophys Res Commun. 313: 856-862.

25. Ryan, H.E., Lo, J., Johnson, R.S. (1998) HIF-1 alpha is required for solid tumor formation and embryonic vascularization. EMBO J. 17: 3005-3015.

26. Rytkonen, K.T., Vuori, K.A.M., Primmer, C.R., Nikinmaa, M. (2007) Comparison of hypoxia-inducible factor-1 alpha in hypoxia-sensitive and hypoxia-tolerant fish species. Comp Biochem Physiol D. 2: 177-186.

27. Vuori, K.A., Soitamo, A., Vuorinen, P.J., Nikinmaa, M. (2004) Baltic salmon (*Salmo salar*) yolk sac fry mortality is associated with disturbances in the function of hypoxia-inducible transcription factor (HIF-1 alpha) and consecutive gene expression. Aquat Toxicol. 68: 301-313.

28. Vuori, K.A., Paavilainen, T., Nikinmaa, M. (2009) Molecular markers of yolk sac fry development in nine families of lake trout. J Aquat Anim Health. 21: 279-289.

29. Wells, P., Pinder, A. (1996) The respiratory development of Atlantic salmon, I. Morphometry of gills, yolk sac, and body surface. J Exp Biol. 199: 2725-2736.

11

Comparison of different tools for pain assessment following ovariohysterectomy in bitches

Saberi Afshar, F.[1*], Shekarian, M.[2], Baniadam, A.[2], Avizeh, R.[2], Najafzadeh, H.[3], Pourmehdi, M.[4]

[1]*Department of Surgery & Radiology, Faculty of Veterinary Medicine, University of Tehran, Tehran, Iran*

[2]*Department of Clinical Sciences, Faculty of Veterinary Medicin, Shahid Chamran University of Ahvaz, Ahvaz, Iran*

[3]*Department of Basic Sciences, Faculty of Veterinary Medicin, Shahid Chamran University of Ahvaz, Ahvaz, Iran*

[4]*Department of Food Hygiene, Faculty of Veterinary Medicine, Shahid Chamran University of Ahvaz, Ahvaz, Iran*

Key words:

bitches, ovariohysterectomy, pain, tramadol, VAS

Correspondence

Saberi Afshar, F.

Department of Surgery & Radiology, Faculty of Veterinary Medicine, University of Tehran, Tehran, Iran

Email: saberiafshar@ut.ac.ir

Abstract:

BACKGROUND: Accurate identifying and assessment of the degree of pain that the animal is suffering can be a challenge, and control of painful condition is becoming an increasingly important part of veterinary medicine. **OBJECTIVES:** This study was carried out to compare different tools for postoperative pain assessment in bitches. **METHODS:** Ten adult mixed breed bitches were selected and randomly divided into two equal treatment and control groups. Anaesthesia was premedicated with acepromazine (0.03 mg/kg, IM) and induced with Sodium thiopental (6-10 mg/kg, IV). Halothane was used for maintenance of the anesthesia. Ovariohysterectomy was performed in the two groups. Treatment group received 3 mg/kg of tramadol intramuscularly (i.m.) and control group received normal saline (equal volume with tramadol, i.m.) before the anesthetic induction. After operation the injections of tramadol and normal saline were repeated every 6 hours over a period of 7 days. The animals were monitored at hour 2, 3 and 4 after each injection and they were scored for signs of pain by two trained assessors who were blinded to the groups. The measured variables were pain assessment with different methods including Simple Descriptive Scale (SDS), Visual Analogue Scale (VAS), and University Melbourne Pain Scale (UMPS). Duration of anesthesia and duration of surgery, were also recorded. **RESULTS:** There were no significant differences between the two groups with regard to analgesia that were measured based on VAS and SDS methods, but in UMPS method, analgesia was significantly better in treatment group. Among simple clinical criteria body temperature and respiratory rate did not show any significant alterations, but heart rate had significant changes between the groups. **CONCLUSIONS:** The ability to quantify the degree of pain experienced by animals is an important aspect in the assessment of animal welfare; in addition, we concluded, that the great challenge for the veterinarians is the evaluation of postoperative pain in dogs.

Introduction

Definition of pain in human is an unpleasant sensory and emotional experience associated with actual or potential tissue damage (Wright and Aydede, 2017) and the definition of animal pain is an aversive, sensory experience representing awareness by the animal of damage or threat to the integrity of its tissues; (note that there might not be any damage) (Heuberger et al, 2016; Molony, 1997).

Postoperative pain is classified as acute and associated with actual or potential tissue damage (Duthie, 1998; Stessel et al., 2017; Yazbek and Fantoni, 2005;). Although accurate identification and assessment of the degree of pain being suffered by an animal can be a challenge (Landa, 2012; Sharkey, 2013), control of painful condition is becoming an increasingly important part of veterinary medicine (Jirkof, 2017; McMillan et al., 2008). Because of the lack of verbal communication, the level of postoperative pain in dogs is difficult to assess. Therefore, the assessment of pain in veterinary medicine relies on temperament, vocalization, posture, activity level, locomotion, reaction to palpation, and other behavioral changes and it should be considered that threshold and response to pain varies according to species, breed, healthy status and age (McMillan, 2016; Vedpathak et al., 2009). All those criteria are subjective and prone to numerous external factors. The objective indicators of pain are physiological and biochemical responses and pain threshold. The purpose of multimodal assessment of pain is to achieve objectiveness and credibility of results (Matičić et al., 2010). An important issue regarding pain management is familiarity with the personality of the animal subject to evaluation. In this instance the pet owner may be the best person to evaluate, for example, the level of anxiety or pain that the patient may be experiencing (Bufalari et al., 2007; Mathews, 2000). Pain assessment in animals is the mandatory step in the successful management of pain. For successful assessment, a number of scales have been used such as Simple Descriptive Scale (SDS), Visual Analogue Scale (VAS), and University of Melbourne Pain Scale (UMPS) (Bufalari et al., 2007; Hielm-Björkman et al 2011).

The SDS as the simplest of the three scales usually consists of four or five expressions used to describe various values of pain intensity, e.g. no pain, mild, moderate, or severe pain. Each expression is assigned a number, which becomes the pain score for that animal (Leonardi et al., 2006).

VAS is a measurement that tries to measure a characteristic or attitude that is believed to range across a continuum of values and cannot be directly measured. For example, the amount of pain that a patient feels ranges across a continuum from none to an extreme amount of pain (Elfving et al, 2016). VAS has been used by human patients to evaluate their own severity of pain, it includes the use of a line in which the left end of the line represents no pain and the right end of the line represents the most pain possible. Patients then indicate the intensity of the pain by placing a mark on the line (Elfving et al 2016; Lawrence et al., 1993). When a VAS is used for estimating pain in animals, the animals are observed, and the location at which the mark is placed is determined by an observer (Hielm-Björkman et al., 2011).

The University of Melbourne Pain Scale (UMPS) is one of the multiparametric scales used to assess postoperative pain in dogs which also considers interaction between the animal and the evaluator. UMPS is a scale based on specific behavioral and physiological responses and includes multiple descriptors in six categories of parameters or behaviors related to pain (Matičić et al., 2010).

Various agents can be used for pain relief, including centrally acting analgesics and non-steroidal anti-inflammatory agents (Yazbek and Fantoni, 2005). Some researchers showed that preoperatively administration of carprofen could alleviate pain in dogs (Welsh et al., 1997) and the same results were obtained with morphine and buprenorphine by the others (Brodbelt et al., 1997; Snyder et al, 2016). The analgesic properties of tramadol result from mixed opioid and nonopioid mechanisms (Manne and. Gondi, 2017; Monteiro et al., 2009). The nonopioid mechanism was shown to inhibit the reuptake of noreepinephrine and serotonine (Beakley et al 2015; Duthie, 1998) and possibly displacement of stored 5 hydroxytryptamine from nerve endings in spinal and supraspinal pathways (Driessen and Reimann,1992; Raffa et al., 1992), therefore preventing impulses reaching the brain (Beakley et al 2015; Duthie, 1998). Tramadol has low affinity for µ receptors and an analgesic potency of one-tenth that of morphine (Monteiro et al., 2009), however, tramadol produced similar analgesia to morphine in the early postoperative period following ovariohysterectomy in dogs (Mastrocinque and Fantoni, 2003). In human beings it has been reported that the incidence of nausea and vomiting of tramadol was lower than that of other opioids (Duthie, 1998). Human field investigations showed tramadol in comparison with morphine produces less respiratory depression,

does not release histamine and when used in therapeutic dosages does not have any effect on heart rate, ventricular function and blood pressure (Houmes et al., 1992). On the other hand, some side effects such as the decrease in prostacycline and prostaglandins synthesis which have been seen by non-steroidal anti-inflammatory drugs, do not occur with tramadol (Allegaert, 2016; Raffa et al., 1992).

The aim of this study was to compare different tools that would facilitate clinical evaluation of postoperative pain in dogs and to seek a simple and practical way to assess pain in this species.

Materials and Methods

This experimental study was carried out in ten adult mixed breed bitches weighing between 15 and 25 kg and aged between 1.5 and 3 years. Physical examination and complete blood count and biochemical serum analysis were performed in all dogs. Dogs were randomly divided into two equal treatment and control groups. Food and water was withheld from all dogs for 12 and two hours, respectively.

Ovariohysterectomy was performed under general anesthesia. Dogs were premedicated with intramuscular acepromazine 0.03mg/kg (Acepromazine 2%, Kela laboratoria NV., Belgium), administered 20 minutes before anaesthetic induction. Anesthesia was induced with Sodium thiopental (Biochemic GmbH, Vienna- Austria), 6-10 mg/kg intravenously. After endotracheal intubation, anesthesia was maintained using halothane (Pacegrove LTD., England)) at a concentration of 1 to 1.5% delivered in oxygen by using a closed circuit. Anesthetic was kept constant by the use of classi-

Table 1. Simple Descriptive Scale (SDS) for scoring of abdominal pain in dogs (according to Mastrocinque and Fantoni, 2003).

score	Criteria
0	Complete analgesia, with no overt signs of discomfort and no reaction to firm pressure applied to the injured region
1	Good analgesia, with no overt signs of discomfort but reaction to firm pressure
2	Moderate analgesia, with some overt signs of discomfort which were made worse by firm pressure
3	No analgesia, with obvious signs of persistent discomfort made worst by firm pressure

Table 2. Visual analogue scale, for assessment of abdominal pain in dogs.

score	Criteria
0	No pain: Dog is running, eating, jumping, and bouncy. Sitting or walking normally. Sleeping comfortably with dreaming. Normal affectionate response to caregiver. Appetite is normal
1	Probably no pain: Dog seems to be normal, but condition is not as clear-cut as previous category. Heart rate is normal or slightly increased because of excitement.
2	Mild discomfort: Dog will eat or sleep but may not dream. Dog may resist palpation of the surgical wound, but otherwise shows no sign of discomfort. Not depressed. There may be a slight increased in respiratory rate; heart rate may or may not be increased.
3	Mild pain or discomfort: Dog will guard incision, or the abdomen may be slightly tucked up. Dog looks a little depressed cannot get comfortable, may tremble or shake, seems to be interested in food and may still eat a little but somewhat picky. Respiratory rate may be increased and a little shallow. Heart rate may be increased or normal depending on weather on opioid was given previously
4	Mild to moderate pain: Dog resists touching of the operative site. Guarding or splinting of the abdomen or stretching all four legs. May look, lick, or chew at the painful area. The dog may sit or lie in an abnormal position and is not curled up or relaxed. May tremble or shake. May or may not seem interested in food. May start to eat and then stop after one or two bites. Respiratory rate may be increased or shallow. Heart rate may be increased or normal. Pupils may be dilated. May whimper occasionally, be slow to rise, and hang the tail down, and appear somewhat depressed
5	Moderate pain: Dog may be reluctant to move, depressed, or inappetent and may bite or attempt to bite when the caregiver approaches the painful area. Trembling or shaking with head down may be a feature, depressed. Dog may vocalize when caregiver attempts to move it or when it is approached. There is definite splinting of the abdomen and the dog may remain recumbent without moving for several hours. The ears may be pulled back. The heart and respiratory rates may be increased. Pupils may be dilated. The patient lies down but does not really sleep and may stand in the praying position
6	Increased moderate pain: Similar to previous category, but dog may vocalize or whine frequently without provocation and when attempting to move. Heart rate may be increased or within normal limits if an opioid was administered previously. Respiratory rate may be increased with an abdominal lift. Pupils may be dilated.
7	Moderate to severe pain: Similar to previous category, but in addition, the dog is quite depressed and is not concerned with its surroundings. The dog may urinate or defecate without attempting to move, cries out when moved, and will spontaneously or continually whimper. Occasionally, an animal does not vocalize. Heart and respiratory rates may be increased. Hypertension may also be present. Pupils may be dilated.
8	Severe pain: Signs same as previous category. Vocalizing may be more of a feature, or animal is so consumed with pain that it does not notice the caretaker's presence. The patient may thrash around in the cage intermittently. Tachycardia and tachypnea, with increased abdominal effort and hypertension are usually present, even if an opioid was given previously. These can be unreliable parameters if not present.
9	Severe to excruciating pain: Signs same as previous category, but the dog is hyperesthetic. The dog trembles involuntary when any part of the body in close proximity to wound or injury touched.
10	Excruciating pain: Signs same as previous category, but the dog is emitting piercing screams or almost comatose. The patient is hyperesthetic or hyperalgesic. The whole body is trembling, and pain is elicited wherever you touch the patient.

cal signs of anesthetic depth. All ovariohysterectomies were performed by a single trained surgeon. Duration of anesthesia and duration of surgery were recorded.

Table 3. University Melbourne Pain Scale (UMPS) for scoring of abdominal pain in dogs (according to Firth and Haldane, 1999). * Includes turning head toward affected area; biting, licking, or scratching at the wound; snapping at the handler; or tense muscles and a protective (guarding) posture. ** Does not include alert barking. Minimum total score=0, maximum total score=27.

Category	Descriptor	Score
Physiologic data	Physiologic data within reference range	0
a	Dilated pupils	2
b	Percentage increase in heart rate relative to preprocedural rate	
c Choose only one	>20%	1
	>50%	2
	>100%	3
d Choose only one	Percentage increase in respiratory rate relative to preprocedural rate	1
	>20%	2
	>50%	3
	>100%	
e	Rectal temperature exceeds reference range	1
f	Salivation	2
Response to palpation	No change from preprocedural behavior	0
Chose one only	Guards/reacts* when touched	2
	Guards/reacts* before touched	3
Activity	At rest, sleeping	0
Choose only one	Semiconscious	0
	Awake	1
	Eating	0
	Restless (pacing continuously, getting up and down)	2
	Rolling, thrashing	3
Mental status	Submissive	0
Choose only one	Overtly friendly	1
	Wary	2
	Aggressive	3
Posture	Guarding or protecting affected area (including fetal position)	2
a	Lateral recumbency	0
b. Choose only one	Sternal recumbency	1
	Sitting or standing, head up	1
	Standing, head hanging down	2
	Moving	1
	Abnormal posture (e.g., prayer position, hunched back)	2
Vocalization**	Not vocalizing	0
Choose only one	Vocalizing when touched	2
	Intermittent vocalization	2
	Continues vocalization	3

Table 4. Body weight, age, duration of anesthesia and duration of surgery in dogs undergoing ovariohysterectomy. (Mean ± SD)*. *No significant differences were seen between these criteria in two groups.

Group	Body weight (kg)	Age (year)	Duration of anesthesia (min)	Duration of surgery (min)
treatment	19.8±3.96	1.8±0.83	36.7±2.9	29.2±3.1
control	19.6±2.60	1.9±0.65	37.2±3.8	28.7±3.4

Table 5. Visual Analogue Scale (VAS) in both groups after ovariohysterectomy (Mean ± SD)*. *No statistically significant changes were seen between groups (p>0.05).

Time / Group	Day 1	Day 2	Day 3	Day 4	Day 5	Day 6	Day 7
Treatment	4.4±1.81	4.4±.89	3.8±1.09	3.6±.89	2.72±0.7	2.26±1.17	1.72±0.97
Control	3.52±1.56	3.18±1.64	2.4±1.34	1.6±1.51	1.4±1.34	0.86±0.86	0.8±0.83

Table 6. Simple Descriptive Scale (SDS) in both groups after ovariohysterectomy (Mean ± SD)*.*No statistically significant changes were seen between groups (p>0.05).

Time / Group	Day 1	Day 2	Day 3	Day 4	Day 5	Day 6	Day 7
Treatment	2.20±0.44	1.80±0.83	1.60±0.54	1.40±0.54	1.12±0.26	0.46±0.50	0.40±0.54
Control	1.86±0.77	1.40±0.54	0.92±0.91	0.92±0.91	0.80±0.83	0.60±0.54	0.40±0.54

Table 7. Heart rate (beat/minute) in both groups after ovariohysterectomy (Mean ± SD) (Mean±SD). *The changes were significant in compare with before surgery in each group (p<0.05).

Time / Group	Before surgery	Day 1	Day 2	Day 3	Day 4	Day 5	Day 6	Day 7
Treatment	130±16.20	117.6±13.64*	108.2±23.17	103.6±16.75*	93.2±25.22*	95.6±34.41*	98.2±32.47*	98.8±32.17*
Control	89±13.41	143.8±42.00*	90.4±18.88	100.2±46.90	106.8±49.08	108.6±50.00	115.2±45.00	110.2±41.69

Treatment group received 3 mg/kg of tramadol (MS Pharma, USA) intramuscularly and control group received normal saline (equal volume with tramadol, i.m.) before the anesthetic induction. The injections of tramadol or normal saline were repeated four times a day with 6 hour intervals in 7 days. The animals were monitored at hour 2, 3 and 4 after each injection. Dogs were scored for signs of pain by two trained assessors who were blinded to the groups. The assessors were a general veterinary practitioner with minimum 5 years' experience in the field of small animal practice. If a dog appeared uncomfortable at any time during the postoperative period, or if the total score of UMPS scale was higher than 8, tramadol was administered at 3mg/kg, i.m. as a rescue analgesic.

The variables measured were pain assessment with different methods including Simple Descriptive Scale (SDS) (Table 1), Visual Analogue Scale (VAS) (Table 2), and University Melbourne Pain Scale (UMPS) (Table 3). Statistical analysis of collected data was done using the SPSS 16 program. Parametric variables were analyzed using Student's t-test or repeated measures ANOVA as appropriate. Non-parametric variables were analyzed by chi-square test ($\chi 2$ test). The minimum level of significance was defined as p<0.05

Results

There were no significant differences among groups for body weight, age, duration of anesthesia and duration of surgery (p>0.05) (Table 4).

With regard to analgesia that was measured with VAS, SDS and UMPS methods, only UMPS showed highly significant an-

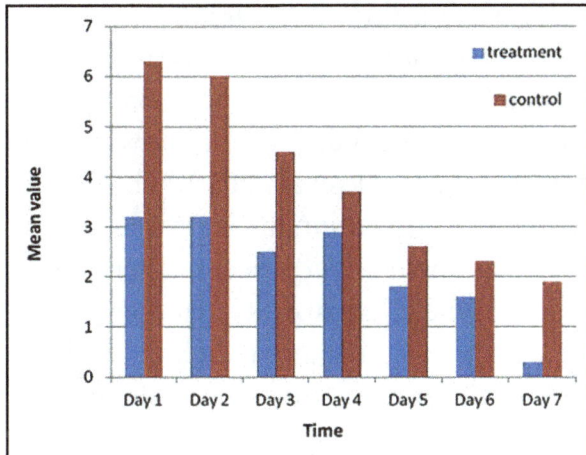

Figure 1. Comparative results of recorded UMPS scores between two groups.

algesia in treatment group (p<0.01) (Fig. 1) and VAS and SDS did not reveal any significant changes between groups (p>0.05) (Table 5 and 6). One dog in the control group was treated with supplemental tramadol.

In comparison with before surgery, heart rate decreased in treatment group significantly at day 1, 3, 4, 5, 6 and 7, and in control group significant increase of heart rate was seen on the first day after surgery (p<0.05) (Table 7).

Rectal temperature and respiratory rate did not show any significant changes in both groups.

Discussion

Pain is an individual experience and there is no objective method of measuring it today. In order to increase sensitivity and decrease bias while measuring the pain parameters, multiple objective and subjective pain assessment methods have been used (Matičić et al., 2010; Sharkey, 2013).

In the present study ovariohysterectomy was used as a model of surgical trauma for evaluation of three methods used for assessment of pain in dogs. Much of the animal pain research has focused on acute pain,

and the most common model used for this purpose is ovariohysterectomy of dogs. Ovariohysterectomy is a relatively standardized source of soft tissue pain which makes it suitable for clinical studies of analgesia (Hansen, 2003; Tsai et al., 2013). It is generally accepted that this surgical procedure causes some degree of moderate pain (Caulkett et al., 2003; Fox et al., 1994; Mastrocinque and Fantoni, 2003) while in the present study two subjective pain scales (VAS and SDS) did not show any significant changes between control and treatment groups.

Simple descriptive scales have initially been used for humans since 1975, but the application of these methods in animals is a relatively complex task to perform. This scale is easy to apply but its sensibility is weak (Holton et al., 2001). SDS is a scale based on observation of the animal and not the nature of the procedure performed. The main disadvantages of the SDS are that it is not a sensitive scale for assessment of pain because it consists of only four or five categories and observer bias may play a key role in determining the pain scale. On the one hand, some researchers believe that SDS in not adaptable to animals since it is not precise and specific (Bufalari etal., 2007). On the other hand, VAS like SDS is a scoring system that is used extensively for people and is generally completed by the patient experiencing the pain. The scale avoids the use of imprecise descriptive terms and provides many points from which to choose.

In veterinary medicine, VAS is used for the evaluation of acute (Holton et al., 1998), postoperative pain in dogs (Firth and Haldane, 1999) and cats (Cambridge et al, 2000). To avoid possible mistakes, it is necessary that the observer be well trained to recognize animal behavior during pain status and to discriminate species differences. Key disadvantages of the VAS in veterinary medicine occur primarily because the scale relies on an observer to identify and interpret pain behaviors. Observer bias may play a key role in assessment of pain, leading to the possibly of overdiagnosing or underdiagnosing pain. The most obvious limitation of VAS scale is that it simply places a numerical value on a subjective judgment, and indeed significant variability exists among observers with this device (Hansen, 2003; Holton et al., 1998).

There is no universal or self-sufficient pain assessment system. The comparison of clinical findings and behavioural parameters increase the objectivity of the results and help to explain their relationships, thus making the overall pain response clearer for the observer (Matičić et al., 2010). Some studies showed that UMPS is a reliable method of clinical pain assessment in dogs (Firth and Haldane, 1999; Matičić et al., 2010). The UMPS is regarded as more sensitive and more accurate than many descriptive and numerical rating scales (Firth and Haldane, 1999; Grant, 2006; Mich and Hellyer, 2008). The UMPS recognizes the importance of specific behavioural patterns, thereby eliminating the observers' bias. The behavioural and physiological parameters are taken into account and divided into six categories: physiologic data, response to palpation, activity, mental status, posture, and vocalization. The application of multiple parameters results in better accuracy and sensibility. The limitations of the system are the incapability of detecting subtle behavioural changes, the exclusive use for postoperative patients and the requirement of broad knowledge of manifestations of pain in animals (Matičić et al.,

2010; Mich and Hellyer, 2008).

Clinical parameters used for the assessment of acute pain are heart rate, respiratory rate, temperature, arterial pressure and mydriasis (Matičić et al., 2010). The first reaction to painful stimulus is the increase of these parameters, but it seems after stabilization of the circulatory system these criteria lose their significance (Mich and Hellyer, 2008). Clinical parameters by themselves are not specific enough to differentiate pain from anxiety or fear, but these conditions can influence the circulation. The analgesic agents, like opioids, can decrease the clinical response, even in the case of insufficient analgesia (Hansen, 2000).

In our study significant increase in heart rate in control group was only seen on the first day after operation and surgical trauma and probably pain might be a logical reason for this change, although some researchers showed low correlation between clinical and behavioral parameters of pain in animals (Conzemius et al., 1997). Opioid-like effect of tramadol can explain the decrease inheart rate in most of the days after surgery in treatment group and this phenomenon may happen even in the case of insufficient analgesia (Hansen, 2000).

Comparison of the clinical and behavioral indices increases the objectivity of the results and helps to explain their relationships, thus making the overall pain response clearer for the assessors. Although our study did not demonstrate concordance of the dynamics of pain measured by the SDS, VAS and UMPS, indicate the greater reliability of UMPS method of pain assessment in dogs.

Acknowledgements

The authors would like to sincerely thank

Shahid Chamran University of Ahvaz for the use of their facilities and the financial support.

References

Allegaert, K. (2016) Comment on: pharmacokinetics of tramadol and O-Desmethyltramadol Enantiomers following administration of extended-release tablets to elderly and young subjects. Drugs Aging. 33: 159-60.

Beakley, BD., Kaye, AM., Kaye, AD. (2015) Tramadol, pharmacology, side Effects, and serotonin syndrome: A review. Pain Physician. 18: 395-400.

Brodbelt, DC., Taylor, PM., Stanway, GW. (1997) A comparison of preoperative morphine and buprenorphine for postoperative analgesia for arthrotomy in dogs. J Vet Pharmacol Ther. 20: 284-289.

Bufalari, A., Adami, C., Angeli, G., Short, CE. (2007) Pain assessment in animals. Vet Res Commun. 31: 55-58.

Cambridge, AJ., Tobias, KM., Newberry, RC., Sarkar, DK. (2000) Subjective and objective measurements of post-operative pain in cats. J Am Vet Med Assoc. 217: 685-690.

Caulkett, N., Read, M., Fowler, D., Waldner, C. (2003) A comparison of the analgesic effects of butorphanol with those of meloxicam after elective ovariohysterectomy in dogs. Can Vet J. 44: 565-570.

Conzemius, MG., Hill, CM., Sammarco, JL., Perkowski, SZ. (1997) Correlation between subjective and objective measures used to determine severity of postoperative pain in dogs. J Am Vet Med Assoc. 210: 1619-1622.

Driessen, B., Reimann, W. (1992) Interaction of central analgesic, tramadol, with the uptake and release of 5-hydroxytryptamine in the rat brain in vitro. Br J Pharmacol. 105: 147-151.

Duthie, DJR. (1998) Remifentanil and tramadol. Br J Anaesth. 81: 51-57.

Elfving, B., Lund, I.C.LB., Boström, C. (2016) Ratings of pain and activity limitation on the visual analogue scale and global impression of change in multimodal rehabilitation of back pain - analyses at group and individual level. Disabil Rehabil. 38: 2206-16.

Firth, AM., Haldane, SL. (1999) Development of a scale to evaluate postoperative pain in dogs. J Am Vet Med Assoc. 214: 651-659.

Fox, SM., Mellor, DJ., Firth, EC., Hodge, H., Lawoko, CR. (1994) Changes in plasma cortisol concentrations before, during and after analgesia, anaesthesia and anaesthesia plus ovariohysterectomy in bitches. Res Vet Sci. 57: 110-118.

Grant, D. (2006) Pain Management in Small Animals: A Manual for Veterinary Nurses and Technicians. Butterworth-Heinemann. Edinburgh, London, New York, Oxford, Philadelphia, St. Louis, Sydney, Toronto. p. 74-75.

Hansen, B. (2000) Acute pain management. Vet Clin North Am Small Anim Pract. 30: 899-916.

Hansen, BD. (2003) Assessment of Pain in Dogs: Veterinary Clinical Studies. ILAR J. 44: 197-205.

Heuberger, R., Petty, M., Huntingford, J. (2016) Companion animal owner perceptions, knowledge, and beliefs regarding pain management in end-of-life care. Top Companion Anim Med. 31: 152-159.

Hielm-Björkman, AK., Kapatkin, AS, Rita HJ. (2011) Reliability and validity of a visual analogue scale used by owners to measure chronic pain attributable to osteoarthritis in their dogs. Am J Vet Res. 72: 601-7.

Holton, L., Reid, J., Scott, EM., Pawson, P., Nolan, A. (2001) Development of a behaviour-based scale to measure acute pain in dogs. Vet Rec. 148: 525-531.

Holton, LL., Scott, EM., Nolan, AM., Reid, J., Welsh, E., Flaherty, D. (1998) Comparison of three methods used for assessment of pain in dogs. J Am Vet Med Assoc. 212: 61-66.

Houmes, RJM., Voets, MA., Verkaaik, A., Erdmann, W., Lachmann, B. (1992) Efficacy and safety of tramadol versus morphine for moderate and severe postoperative pain with special regard to respiratory depression. Anesth Analg. 74: 510-514.

Jirkof, P. (2017) Side effects of pain and analgesia in animal experimentation. Lab Anim. 22; 46: 123-128.

Landa, L. (2012) Pain in domestic animals and how to assess it: a review. Vet Med. 57: 185-192.

Lawrence, J., Alcock, D., McGrath, P., Kay, J., MacMurray, SB., Dulberg, C. (1993) The development of a tool to assess neonatal pain. Neonatal Netw. 12: 59-66.

Leonardi, F., Zanichelli, S., Botti, P. (2006) Pain in the animals: diagnosis, treatment and prevention. annali della facoltà di medicina veterinaria di parma (Vol. XXVI). 45-66.

Manne, VS., Gondi, SR. (2017) Comparative Study of the Effect of Intravenous Paracetamol and Tramadol in Relieving of Postoperative Pain after General Anesthesia in Nephrectomy Patients. Anesth Essays Res. 11: 117-120.

Mastrocinque, S., Fantoni, DT. (2003) A comparison of preoperative tramadol and morphine for the control of early postoperative pain in canine ovariohysterectomy. Vet Anaesth Analg. 30: 220-228.

Mathews, KA. (2000) Pain assessment and general approach to management. Vet Clin North Am Small Anim Pract. 30: 729-755.

Matičić, D., Stejskal, M., Pećin, M., Kreszinger, M., Pirkić, B., Vnuk, D., Smolec, O., Rumenjak, V. (2010) Correlation of pain assessment parameters in dogs with cranial cruciate surgery. Vet Arh. 80: 597-609.

McMillan, CJ., Livingston, A., Clark, CR., Dowling, PM., Taylor, SM., Duke, T., Terlinden, R. (2008) Pharmacokinetics of intravenous tramadol in dogs. Can J Vet Res. 72: 325-331.

McMillan, FD. (2016) The psychobiology of social pain: Evidence for a neurocognitive overlap with physical pain and welfare implications for social animals with special attention to the domestic dog (Canis familiaris). Physiol Behav.1. 167: 154-171.

Mich, PM., Hellyer, PW. (2008) Objective, categorical methods for assessing pain and analgesia. In: Handbook of Veterinary Pain Management. Gaynorm J.S., Muirm W.W, (eds.). (2nd ed.). St. Louis, Mosby, USA. p. 78-109.

Molony, V. (1997) Comments on Anand and Craig (Letters to the Editor). Pain. 70: 293.

Monteiro, ER., Junior, AR., Assis, HM., Campagnol, D., Quitzan, JG. (2009) Comparative study on the sedative effects of morphine, methadone, butorphanol or tramadol, in combination with acepromazine, in dogs. Vet Anaesth Analg. 36: 25-33.

Raffa, RB., Friderichs, E., Reimann, W., Shank, RP., Codd, EE., Vaught, JL. (1992) Opioid and nonopioid components independently contribute to the mechanism of action of tramadol, an "atypical" opioid analgesic. J Pharmacol Exp Ther. 260: 275-285.

Sharkey, M. (2013) The challenges of assessing osteoarthritis and postoperative pain in dogs. AAPS J. 15: 598-607.

Snyder, LB., Snyder, CJ., Hetzel, S. (2016) Effects of buprenorphine added to bupivacaine infraorbital nerve blocks on isoflurane minimum alveolar concentration using a model for acute dental/oral surgical pain in dogs. J Vet Dent. 33: 90-96.

Stessel, B., Fiddelers, AA., Marcus, MA., van Kuijk, SM., Joosten, EA., Peters, ML., Buhre, WF., Gramke, HF. (2017) External validation and modification of a predictive model for acute postsurgical pain at home after day surgery. Clin J Pain. 33: 405-413.

Tsai, TY., Chang, SK., Chou, PY., Yeh, LS. (2013) Comparison of postoperative effects between lidocaine infusion, meloxicam, and their combination in dogs undergoing ovariohysterectomy. Vet Anaesth Analg. 40: 615-22.

Vedpathak, HS., Tank, PH., Karle, AS., Mahida, HK., Joshi, DO., Dhami, MA. (2009) Pain management in veterinary patients. Vet World. 2: 360-363.

Welsh, EM., Nolan, AM., Reid, J. (1997) Beneficial effects of administering carprofen before surgery in dogs. Vet Rec. 141: 251-253.

Wright, A., Aydede, M. (2017) Critical comments on Williams and Craig's recent proposal for revising the definition of pain. Pain. 158: 362-363.

Yazbek, KVB., Fantoni, DT. (2005) Evaluation of tramadol, an "atypical" opioid analgesic in the control of immediate postoperative pain in dogs submitted to orthopedic surgical procedures. Braz J Vet Res Anim Sci. [online]. 42: 250-258.

12

Acute toxicity evaluation of five herbicides: paraquat, 2,4-dichlorophenoxy acetic acid (2,4-D), trifluralin, glyphosite and atrazine in *Luciobarbus esocinus* fingerlings

Alishahi, M.*, **Tulaby Dezfuly, Z., Mohammadian, T.**

Department of Clinical Sciences, Faculty of Veterinary Medicine, Shahid Chamran University of Ahvaz, Ahvaz, Iran

Key words:

acute toxicity, echo-pollutant, *Luciobarbus esocinus,* herbicide, LC50

Correspondence

Alishahi, M.
Department of Clinical Sciences, Faculty of Veterinary Medicine, Shahid Chamran University of Ahvaz, Ahvaz, Iran

Email: alishahim@scu.ac.ir

Abstract:

BACKGROUND: Evaluation of herbicide pollution in aquatic environments needs the great concern and the most important echo-pollutant effects of herbicides are related to their effects on non target aquatic organisms. Native fish can serve as a proper bio-indicator for evaluation of pollution on aquatic ecosystems. OBJECTIVES: To find environmentally friendly herbicides, in this study the acute toxicity of five widely used herbicides in Iran as aquatic ecosystems pollutants on *Luciobarbus esocinus* were investigated. METHODS: Acute toxicity (96 h LC50) of five herbicides (Paraquat, 2,4-dichlorophenoxy acetic acid, Trifluralin, Glyphosite and Atrazine) were determined via OECD standard method. *L.esocinus* exposed to Serial concentrations (more than 6 in triplicates) of each herbicide. Mortalities at 24, 48, 72 and 96 hours after exposure were recorded and the LC50 were calculated using Probit software. RESULTS: Results showed that acute toxicity of these herbicides are significantly different in *L. esocinus*. The 96 h LC50 of Paraquat, 2,4-D, Trifluralin, Glyphosite and Atarzine in *L.esocinus* were 54.66, 138.8, 1.09, 716.83 and 44.30 mg/l respectively. Glyphosite showed lowest toxicity in *Luciobarbus esocinus* among the five herbicids. The highest toxicity of herbicides in *L. esocinus* belongs to Trifluralin. The mortality rate of exposed fish to herbicides enhanced either by increasing herbicides concentration or duration of exposure. Mortality patterns during 96 hours of toxicity evaluation were similar in all five herbicides. CONCLUSIONS: Regarding the high application and similar efficacy of herbicides in most of the cane farms of Khouzestan province, and based on different toxicities of these five herbicides for fish as a non targeting organism, Glyphosite is highly recommendable as a proper alternative to Trifluralin, Atrazine, Paraquat and 2,4-dichlorophenoxy acetic acid.

Introduction

Unfortunately, most cyprinid ponds in Iran are located close to agricultural areas. Because of modern pest management practices, large amounts of herbicides are used in these areas for crop protection. Herbicides are actively used in terrestrial and aquatic ecosystems to control unwanted weeds, and their use has generated serious concerns about the potential adverse effects of these chemicals on the environment and human health (Oleh et al., 2009).

Herbicides may reduce environmental quality and influence essential ecosystem functioning by reducing species diversity and community structures, modifying food chains, changing patterns of energy flow and nutrient cycling and changing the stability and resilience of ecosystems.

In aquatic toxicology, laboratory experiments are normally used to estimate the potential hazard of chemicals and to establish "safe" levels of pollutants (Cattaneo et al., 2011).

Paraquat dichloride is a non-selective contact herbicide, used in controlling pests of cultivated farmlands of sugar cane, rice, fruit, and vegetable. It quickly kills a wide range of annual grasses, broad leaves, weeds and some perennial grasses when sprayed directly onto leaves. More so, the active ingredient is rapidly absorbed by clay and silt particles in the soil and does not leave any effective soil residue. It has a long half life in the environment and poses a threat to aquatic organisms and human health because of its bioavailability, resistance to microbial degradation, and resistance to decomposition in the presence of light (Yao et al., 2013). 2,4-dichlorophenoxyacetic acid (2,4-D) is a common and worldwide herbicide that is employed for post-emergence foliar spray and is also used for weed control of sugar cane, wheat, rice, maize and aquatic weeds (Farah et al., 2004). As a phenoxyherbicide, 2,4-D may cause an array of adverse effects to the nervous system such

as myotonia, disruption of nervous system activity and behavioral changes (Bortolozzi et al., 2004).

Trifluralin is a dinitroaniline-type preemergence herbicide for control of grass and broadleaf weeds. Trifluralin has also been used to control larval mycosis in penaeid shrimp culture. It is extensively accumulated in the environment and slowly eliminated. (Schultz and Hayton, 1993). Its adverse effects on biotic components of a freshwater ecosystem were reported in chronic concentrations (Poleksic and Karan, 1999).

Glyphosate is one of the widely used herbicides that could be persistent and mobile in soil and water, and it is known to be one of the most common terrestrial and aquatic contaminants. It is used as a non-selective herbicide and for control of a great variety of annual, biennial, and perennial grasses, sedges, broad-leaved weeds, and woody shrubs. They are also used in fruits orchards, vineyards, conifer plantations and many plantation crops. It is perhaps the most important herbicide ever developed (Ayoola, 2008).

Atrazine (2-Chloro-4-ethylamino-6-Isopropylamino-s-triazine) is one of the most commonly used herbicides found in the rural environments. It is extensively used for corn, sugar cane, sorghum, and to some extent in landscape vegetation. Rated as moderately toxic to aquatic species, atrazine is mobile in the environment and is among the most detected pesticides in streams, rivers, ponds, reservoirs and ground water (Battaglin et al., 2008).

One of the largest sugar cane farms (over 100,000 hectares) of Asia is located in Khouzestan Province, Iran, in which large amounts of herbicides (hundreds of tonnes) are being used annually. More than 30% of Iran's running water flows in the rivers of Khuzestan province (Haji Sharafi and Shokuhfar, 2009).

The toxicity of a chemical is totally dependent on the concentration of the chemical in organisms or even the concentration at the target receptor in the organism. Herbicides at high concentration are known to reduce the survival, growth and reproduction of fish, and produce many visible effects on fish (Ladipo and Dohetry, 2011). There are few works on comparison of different herbicide toxicity in aquatic animals (Deivasigamani, 2015).

Besides, toxicity testing of chemicals on animals has been used for a long time to detect the potential hazards posed by chemicals to environment and human. Bioassay technique has been the cornerstone of programs on environmental health and chemical safety (Moraes et al., 2007). Aquatic bioassays are necessary in water pollution control to determine whether a potential toxicant is dangerous to aquatic life and if so, to find the relationship between the toxicant concentration and its effect on aquatic animals (Olaifa et al., 2003). The application of environmental toxicology studies on non-mammalian vertebrates is rapidly expanding (Ayoola, 2008), thus in this study the toxicity of five common herbicides in Iranian agriculture were compared in *Luciobarbus esocinus* to find which herbicides induce less impact on aquatic animals and environment.

Materials and Methods

Fish: 1200 fingerlings *Luciobarbus esocinus* were purchased from Native Fish Breeding and Cultivation Center in Hami-

dieh, Khouzestan. Fish were transferred to aquarium room of Veterinary Faculty, Shahid Chamran University of Ahvaz, Iran. Fish were acclimatized for 2 weeks in 300 L indoor fiberglass tanks and were fed with standard diet.

Fish were kept in continuously aerated water in a static system and with a natural photoperiod (12 h light - 12 h dark). During acclimation, fish were fed once a day with commercial fish pellets. For the LC determinations, 528 fingerlings were uniformly distributed in 21 40-L plastic aquaria. Each herbicide was tested using 6 to 9 different concentrations, with 2 repetitions. Two aquaria were kept as control (without herbicide). Fingerlings were observed at 24 h intervals, for 96h (acute toxicity) when the test was concluded. During the experimental period, fingerlings were not fed and water exchange was stopped. Later (after adaptation) they were transferred into 20 liter aquaria (10 fish weighing about 3-5 g in each aquarium. All products used were purchased from local stores. The generic, commercial, and chemical names, and pesticide group of each product tested are shown in Table 1, and the concentrations used are shown in Table 2. Before addition, each product was mixed in a small volume of water from each aquarium and then added to the water using a glass pipette. Fingerlings were then observed for 96h and the mortality recorded; swimming behavior (normal, erratic swimming, lethargy) was checked and compared to the control group.

Feeding was terminated 48 h prior to the initiation of the experiment. All experiments were carried out for a period of 96 h and the number of dead fish were counted every 24 h. During the acute toxicity test of experiment, water in each aquarium was aerated

Table 1. Specifications of the test herbicides.

Herbicide	Chemical Name	Supplier	Purity Rate	Acute Oral LD50 For Rat	Statue
Paraquat	1,1-dimethyl-4,4'-bipyridinium	Aria Shimi Co, Iran	20%	129-157 MG/KG	water soluble green liquid.
2, 4 - D	2-(2,4-dichlorophenoxy)-acetic acid	Shimagro Co, Iran	67.5%	2100 MG/KG	water soluble brown liquid
Trifluralin	α-trifluoro-2,6-dinitro-N,N-dipropyl-p-toluidine),	Aria Shimi Co, Iran	48%	5000 MG/KG	water soluble orange liquid
Glyphosate or Roundup	N- phosphonomethyl glycine	Sinochem Co, China	41%	5600 MG/KG	water soluble yellow liquid
Atrazine	Chloro-4-ethylamino-6-isopropylamino-1-3-5-triazinre	Moshkfam Co, Iran	80%	1350 MG/KG	water soluble white powder

Table 2. The selected herbicides concentrations to determine their acute toxicity for *L. esocinus*.

Herbicide	Number of treatments	Number of replicates	Total exposed fish	Concentrations (mg/l)
Paraquat	7	3	210	0, 16, 32, 64, 100, 128, 256
2,4-D	7	3	210	0, 25, 50, 100, 200, 400, 800
Trifluralin	9	3	270	0, 0.32, 0.65, 1.25, 2.5, 5, 7.5, 10, 15
Glyphosite	8	3	240	0, 80, 160, 320, 640, 1280, 2560, 5120
Atrazine	6	3	180	0, 10, 20, 40, 80, 160

and had the same conditions as follow: dissolved oxygen 8.1±0.5 mg/l, temperature 25±1°C,

pH 7.8± 0.2, water total hardness 640 mg/l as CaCO3, NH3 and NO2 <0.01 mg ml^{-1}.

The lethal concentration (LC50) was tested by exposing 10 fish per group according to Table 2 herbicides per liter of water for 96 hours. The control group was kept in experimental water without herbicides with all of the other conditions kept constant. The movement and the behavior of the fish were examined during the study. Motionless fish and those without any opercula movement were considered dead and were removed from the tanks.

Then fish were exposed to 6-9 sequential concentrations of each herbicide in a way that zero and 100% mortality yield after 96 hours. The mortality rate was recorded after 24, 48, 72, and finally 96 hours. The concentration of herbicides to induce 10, 15, 50, 85, 95 and 100 percent mortality (LC10, LC15, LC50, LC85, LC95, LC100) was estimated after 24, 48, 72, and 96 hours using Probit software verion 1.5 designed by U.S. EPA. This software estimates LC concentration based on regression between mortality rate and log of toxin concentration. Estimation was presented with lower and upper range with 95% confidence level (Aydin and Kuprucu, 2005). The selected herbicides concentrations for estimating their acute toxici-

Table 3. Lethal concentrations of herbicides (mg/l) (95% confidence intervals) depending on exposure time for *L. esocinus*.

Type of Toxicant	Lethal concentra-(tion (mg/l	Exposure time (h)			
		h 24	h 48	h 72	h 96
Paraquat	LC10	68.78	61.47	41.3	31.44
	LC15	73.33	65.51	45.4	34.95
	LC50	96.17	85.74	67.72	54.66
	LC85	126.12	112.22	101.02	85.5
	LC95	147.88	131.43	127.76	111.17
	LC100	176.73	156.87	166.2	149.18
2,4-D	LC10	226.22	173.09	121.52	60.44
	LC15	245.48	190.14	134.68	70.86
	LC50	346.83	282.9	208.02	138.82
	LC85	490.02	420.90	321.32	271.95
	LC95	600.23	531.45	414.75	403.57
	LC100	753.38	690.11	552	627.1
Trifluralin	LC10	0.413	0.46	0.36	0.39
	LC15	0.56	0.6	0.47	0.47
	LC50	2.17	1.76	1.45	1.09
	LC85	8.3	5.15	4.43	2.52
	LC95	18.26	9.68	8.5	4.12
	LC100	44.13	19.61	17.72	7.13
Glyphosite	LC10	846.43	532.9	410.04	226.3
	LC15	988.06	637.012	487.25	282.14
	LC50	1900.54	1354.44	1010.62	716.83
	LC85	3655.72	2879.87	2096.14	1821.22
	LC95	5367.18	4484.29	3216.71	3148.33
	LC100	8251.8	7363.97	5196.85	5812.30
Atrazine	LC10	86.81	38.54	28.65	25.58
	LC15	90.91	41.48	31.61	28.41
	LC50	110.53	56.56	47.93	44.30
	LC85	134.39	77.14	72.67	69.06
	LC95	150.72	92.55	92.77	89.62
	LC100	171.39	113.50	121.97	120.01

ty in *L. esocinus* are brought in Table 2.

Results

None of the herbicides, even at the highest concentration, altered the water quality parameters. Lethargy, swimming at the water surface and erratic swimming (mainly vertical swimming) were the main behavioral changes observed throughout the experiment, in the presence of herbicides. The behavioral changes were observed with different herbicides, usually at the high concentrations tested.

The fish mortality rate following the exposure to increasing concentrations of herbicides after 24, 48, 72, and 96 hours showed that the higher the herbicide concentration, the greater the mortality rate. The mortality rate increased along with increasing the exposure time. Acute toxicity of Paraquat, 2,4-D, Trifluralin, Glyphosite and Atarzine was determined in *L. esocinus* after 24, 48,

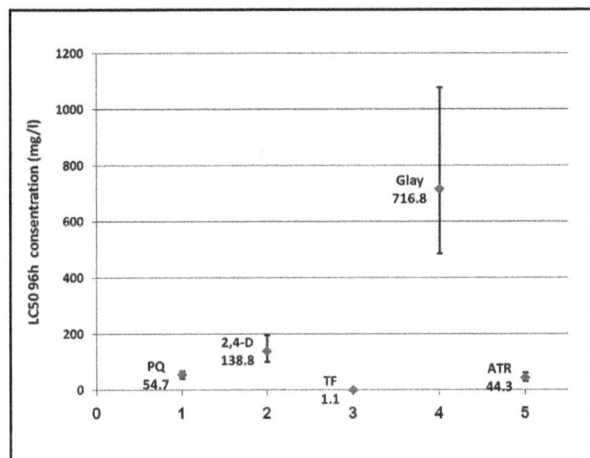

Figure. 1. Comparison of LC50 96h concentrations of selected herbicides in *L. esocinus*.

72 and 96 hours of exposure. 96 hours LC50 value (Median lethal concentration) was calculated at 54.66, 138.82, 1.09, 716.83 and 44.30 mg/l in *L. esocinus*, (Table 3) and MAC of these herbicides was 5.46, 13.88, 0.1, 71.68 and 4.43 mg/l respectively. The greatest LC50 was 716.83 mg/l for Glyphosate and the least was 1.09 mg/l for Trifluralin. Therefore, the most toxic herbicides for *L. esocinus* were Trifluralin, Atrazine, and Paraquat, respectively.

The glyphosate showed significantly lesser lethality (higher LC50 concentration) than other tested herbicides. Trifluralin and Atrazine showed the highest lethality (lower LC50 concentration) in *L.esocinus* among the examined herbicides. (Fig 1).

Discussion

In Khouzestan province of Iran, most cyprinid fish ponds are built close to agricultural areas with shared water sources. Water contamination by agricultural herbicides is a potential threat to productivity and a major cause of fish mortality. However, water contamination with herbicides at non-lethal concentrations might pass unnoticed including loss in growth, health and resistance to

diseases which, in most cases, might be difficult to assess (Nwani et al., 2010). From an ecotoxicological point, contamination of water sources poses a potential threat to aquatic organisms including fish. Since fishes are the last chain of the food web in aquatic ecosystems there may be bioaccumulation problems in addition to acute effects (World Health Organization, 1984). The toxicity of different echotoxicants such as herbicides and their adverse effects on aquatic animals was mostly assayed by 96h LC50 (median lethal concentration) in native fish. The 96-h LC50 of several commonly used agricultural herbicides were determined in this study. *Luciobarbus esocinus* fingerlings were used because this fish species is an ubiquitous native species in rivers, wetlands and ponds in southwest Iran and has been newly cultivated in polyculture system of cyprinid farms.

In this study all tested herbicides were toxic for *Luciobarbus esocinus*, such that Median lethal concentration after 96 h exposure (96 h LC50) of five herbicides: Paraquat, 2,4-D, Trifluralin, Glyphosite and Atrazine in *Luciobarbus esocinus* was 54.66, 138.82, 1.09, 716.83 and 44.30 mg/l respectively. The results showed although toxicity of five tested herbicides was different for *L. esocinus*, their toxicity revealed positive correlation not only to herbicide concentration, but also to exposure duration. The most toxic herbicide tested was Trifluralin, which is used in cane farms for controlling the unwanted plant growth. Among the evaluated herbicides Trifluralin and Atrazine were more toxic than the others, and Trifluralin, which was used in large scale in cane (over one hundred thousand hectares farms) for controlling weed growth was the most toxic. All environmental parameters, herbicides concentration and examined fish source were quite similar in this study based on OECD regulation, then the differences in herbicides toxicity just refer to each herbicide toxicity mechanism in fish. The results of this work, like other toxicity assessment studies, showed somehow different results compared to a similar report in other fish, but it is worth considering that toxicity of chemicals to aquatic organisms has been shown to be affected by age, size and health of the species. Physiological parameters like quality, temperature, pH, dissolved oxygen and turbidity of water, concentration and formulation of chemical and its exposure also greatly influence such studies.

The data obtained for acute toxicity of trifuralin in this study were in the range of LC50 concentrations established for juvenile rainbow trout and bluegill sunfish 0.01-0.04 and 0.02- 0.09 mg/l, respectively. Poleksic and Karan (1999) showed that Median lethal concentration (LC50) on Carp, after 24h and 48h exposure was 0.185 mg/l and 0.066 mg/l, and 0.045 mg/l after 96 h (Poleksic and Karan, 1999). The herbicide trifrluralin has been classified in the group of highly toxic substances, according to its LC50 values to fish (OECD, Chemical Group and Management Committee, 1992). Trifrluralin affects fish health, making them more sensitive to environmental changes and less resistant to diseases.

Water contamination with trifluralin may occur via agricultural farms leaching after raining or irrigation. Nevertheless, only 0.5% of the quantity applied to the soil in field conditions is leached and may consequently contaminate water sources. This percentage means rather low water contamination, representing smaller concentrations than 1.0 µg l[-1]. (Grover et al., 1997).

LC50 (48h) of trifluralin was reported 19 µg l[-1] in bluegill fish (Lepomis macrochirus), 19 µg l[-1] in Mola mola, 1 mg/l in Cyprinus carpio and 0.56 mg/l in pollutant biomarker, Daphnia magma , respectively. Also, the amount of LC50 after 96 hours in *Oncorhynchus mykiss* was 0.21 mg/l and 10-90µg l[-1] in *Lepomis macrochirus* (Gangolli ,1999).

Toxicity mechanisms of trifluralin include genotoxicity effects which cause DNA breaks, loss of genetic material, immunotoxicity and mutations which lead to cell death. Besides, trifluralin causes hemoglobin oxidation (by forming metahemoglobin), red blood cell destruction, damage to kidney and the liver.

Existing reports characterize trifluralin as a highly acute toxic substance to fish, but there are not enough descriptions of its chronic toxicity and cytotoxic effect. Studies mainly related to its genotoxic, mutagenic and carcinogenic potential are mostly inconclusive or even contradictory.

Paraquat is a chlorinated herbicide which is mainly used to control weeds in agriculture, however, once it enters surface waters it may affect other organisms such as fish as a non-target organism either in natural or culture conditions. In the present study the 96 h LC50 of paraquat was estimated to be 54.66 ppm in *Lusiobarbus esocinus* fingerling. Yeo (1967) reported that paraquat at 1.0 and 3.0 ppm was toxic to small mouth bass (Micropterus dolomieui) and to mosquito fish (Gambusia affinis) in 180-gallon plastic pools that had an average pH of 9.4. The 96-hour LC50's for the blue gill and channel catfish were 13 ppm and greater than 100 ppm, respectively. Besides, the acute toxicity (96 h LC50) of the herbicide paraquat for *Oreochromis niloticus* was

12.25 mg l^{-1} (Babatunde and Oladimeji, 2014). Deivasigamani et al. (2015) reported that common carp weighing 300-400 g died within 15 min after exposure to paraquat at the concentration of 100 ppm, but they did not describe the source of the test chemical (Deivasigamani et al., 2015).

Paraquat-induced endothelial cell toxicity occurs by NO synthase which causes NADPH oxidation, moreover, Paraquat-induced cytotoxicity is potentiated in cytokine-activated macrophages in a manner that correlates with its ability to block NO formation.

The difference in toxicity between pure chemical and formulated commercial products may be attributable to the other ingredients supplemented into the formulated products. The difference in toxicity rate of paraquat in various fish species can be ascribed to species sensitivity, age and weight of fish as well as environmental parameters.

Based on the findings, the amount of lethal concentration of 2,4-D for 50 percent of fish was determined to be 138.82mg/l after 96 hours. The maximum value equals 13.89 mg/l which is also called NOEC (or ineffective concentration). The minimum concentration level (LOEC) which is also called LC10 96h was 60.44 mg/l (Table 3).The lethal concentration allowing 50 percent of the fish to perish was determined to be 346.83, 282.9, 208.02, and 138.82 after 24, 48, 72, and 96 hours respectively (Table 3). It reveals an increase in the herbicide toxicity following an increase in exposure time.

2-4-D herbicides toxicity in fish mostly induced by chromosomal damage including chromosome breakage, sister chromatid exchange and micronuclei anisocytosis as well as altered nuclear morphology. Disrupted chromosome material and erythrocytes with several micronuclei present is a conventional effect of 2-4-D in fish. There are some bacteria and fungi that use 2-4-D as a source of carbon and energy (Daugherty and Karei, 1995). The widespread use of chlorophenoxy acetic acid as a herbicide and a growth regulator in agriculture, forestry, and households has compounded the damage incurred by these toxic compounds on the environment and human health.

Abdelghani et al. (1997) found 96 h LC values of 2,4D as 181.2 for catfish, 266.3 for bluegill, and 750.1 mg/l for crawfish, respectively. Farah et al. (2004) found the LC50 values of 2,4-D as 81 ppm for *Heteropneustes fossilis*, 122 ppm for Clarias batrachus, 107 ppm for Channa punctatus and 302 ppm for Culex pipiens fatigans. Sarikaya et al. (2002), found LC50 value of 2,4-D on tench (Tinea tinea) as 48 mg/l. Sarikaya and Yilmaz (2003) reported 96 h LC50 value for Cyprinus carpio as 63.24 mg/l. In the current study, we found that acute toxicity of 2,4D (LC50) significantly increased in accordance with the exposure time from 346.83 mg/l at 24 h to 138.82mg/l at 96 h.

In the present study the 96-h LC50 determined for the glyphosate in *Luciobarbus esocinus* was 716.83 mg l^{-1}. It is much higher than that reported by other authors in other fish species as 17.8 mg/l in Gambusia yucatana (Rendsn-Van-Osten et al., 2005) and 120 mg/l in *Oncorhynchus mykiss* (GIESY et al., 2000). Glyphosate (Roundup®) exhibited very slight toxicity in *Luciobarbus esocinus* which was the lowest toxicity among 5 highly used herbicides in Iran. In other works different results reported about the toxicity of glyphosate in various fish species, 96-h LC50 of glyphosate for *Huso huso, Acipenser stellatus, A. persicus* and *Oncorhynchus mykiss* were reported 26.4,

23.2 ,27.5 and 86 mg l^{-1} respectively. Sturgeon fries exposed to concentrations of 60 to 100 mg l^{-1} showed an increase in mortality. Glyphosate exhibited a slight to moderate toxicity in sturgeon species (Filizadeh and Rajabi Islami, 2011). Most of the studies indicated a slight or moderate toxicity for fish species. Fish exposed to 10 mg/l of glyphosate for two weeks were found to have gill and liver damage. For commercial formulations, the LC 50 found varied from 13 to 33mg/l in coho salmon. Even et al., report that the toxicity of glyphosate-based herbicides might be attributed to the presence of the surfactant (POEA), which is more toxic than glyphosate itself, however Rodeo® has no surfactant, and is registered for aquatic use (Fryer, 1977).

Glyphosite toxicity causes some oxidative stress in high concentration in fish Hence, after exposure, an increase in antioxidative stress enzymes was seen.

Despite the toxicity levels of glyphosate in mentioned works, Hildebrand et al. (1980) found that Roundup® treatments at concentrations up to 220 kg/ha did not significantly affect the survival of Daphnia magna or its food base of diatoms under laboratory conditions. It appears that under most conditions, rapid dissipation from aquatic environments of even the most toxic glyphosate formulations prevents build-up of herbicide concentrations that would be lethal to most aquatic species.

The results of the LC50 (median lethal concentration) of the present study at 96 h was 44.30 mg/l for atrazine. This result indicated moderate toxicity of atrazine among the tested herbicides. In other works different results reported about the toxicity of atrazine in various fish species. In tilapia (*Oreochromis mossambicus* and *Oreochro-*

mis niloticus) the LC50 in 96 h was 8.8 and 5.02 mg/l, respectively. This indicates , that the species used in this study are less sensitive to atrazine than those used in other studies.

Although the 96 h LC50 of 44.30 mg/l reported for *L. esocinus* exposed to atrazine in the present study differed from the report of Bathe et al. (1973), Neskovic et al. (1993) and Hussein et al. (1996) who reported LC50 of 16.0, 18.8 and 9.37 mg/l for *Lepomis macrochirus* (Bluegill sunfish), *Cyprinus carpio* and *Oreochromis niloticus* respectively exposed to atrazine, the present findings seem to be consistent with other research which found 37 mg/l (LC50 96h) for grass carp fingerlings. On the other hand, we can showthat fingerlings are less sensitive to some chemicals and toxins than adult or juvenile fishes.

In toxicity studies, the sensitivity of organisms can be different, even using the same product (Botelho et al., 2012).

It has been reported that atrazine-induced apoptosis, defined by both morphological and biochemical criteria, in carp cells occurred in a dose- and time-dependent manner. Intracellular free Ca2+ is thought to act as an important messenger in a variety of cellular signaling pathways and metabolic processes and has a crucial role in the apoptotic process. Recent evidence suggests that intracellular Ca2+ involved in atrazine-induced apoptosis in fish cells (Mizuhashi et al., 2000).

In conclusion, there is evidence that trifluralin and Atrazine tend to be more toxic to *L. esocinus* than other herbicides. Respective industries should be encouraged to look into the possibility of reducing the rate of these herbicides because of their potency to harm non target aquatic organisms. Also, for sustainable agricultural activity, especially in areas that fish ponds and agriculture farms use the same water sources, it is highly recommended to use glyphosate as an alternative to Trifluralin and Atrazine. To the best of our knowledge, this work is the first study to compare the toxicity of different common herbicides on a high risk native fish.

Acknowledgments

This work was financially supported by the Research Council of Shahid Chamran University, Ahvaz, Iran.

References

1. Ayoola, S.O. (2008) Toxicity of glyphosate herbicideon Nile tilapia (*Oreochromis niloticus*) juvenile. Afr J Agric Res. 3: 825-834.

2. Abdelghani, A.A., Tchounwou, P.B., Anderson, A.C., Sujono, H., Heyer, L.R., Monkiedje, A. (1997) Toxicity evaluation of single and chemical mixtures of roundup, Garlon-3A, 2,4-D, and syndets surfactant to channel catfish (*Ictalurus punctatus*), bluegill sunfish (*Lepomis microchirus*), and crawfish (*Procambarus* spp.). Environ. Toxicol Water Qual. 12: 237-243.

3. Aydin, R., kuprucu, K. (2005) acute toxicocity of diazinon the common carp (embryos and larvae, Pest Biochem Physiol. 82: 220-225.

4. Babatunde, M.M, Oladimeji, A.A. (2014) Comparative study of Acute toxicity of Paraquat and Galex to *Oreochromis niloticus*. IJAST. 3: 437-444.

5. Bathe, R., Ullmann, L., Sachsse, K. (1973) Determination of pesticide toxicity to fish. In: Berlin Dahlem publication. Wasser-Boden Luft, Ver (eds.). Germany, Section. 37: 241-246.

6. Battaglin, W.A., Rice, C.K., Foazio, M.J., Salmon, S., Barry, R.X. (2008) The occurrence of glyphosate, atrazine, and other pesticides in vernal pools and adjacent streams in Washington, DC, Maryland, Iowa and Wyoming 2005-2006. Environ Monit Assess. 155: 281-307.

7. Botelho, R.G., Santos, J.B., Fernandes, K.M., Neves, C.A. (2012) Effects of atrazine and picloram on grass carp: acute toxicity and histological assessment, Toxicol Environ Chem. 94: 121-127.

8. Bortolozzi, A., Evangelista, A., De Duffard, R. Duffard, M. Antonelli (2004) Effects of 2,4 dichlorophenoxyacetic acid exposure on dopamine D2-like Receptors in rat brain, Neurotoxicol Teratol. 26: 599-605.

9. Deivasigamani, S. (2015) Effect of herbicides on fish and histological evaluationof common carp (*Cyprinus carpio*). Int J Appl Res. 1: 437-440

10. Daugherty D.D., Karei. S.F. (1995) Degradation of 2,4-di Chlorophenoxyacetic acid by *Pseudomonas capacia* DBo1 (pR01D1) in a Dual-substrate Chemostat. Appl Environ Microbiol. 60: 3261.

11. Farah, M.A., Ateeg, B., Ali, M.N., Sabir, R., Ahmad, W. (2004) Studies on lethal concentrations and toxicity stress of some xenobiotics on aquatic organisms. Chemosphere. 55: 257-265.

12. Fernandes, Thaís C. C., (2013) Characterization, Modes of action and effects of trifluralin: in Herbicides-current research and case Studies in use, Merlin pub, Online Access via InTech Open Access Books, Chapter 19: 490-515. Missouri, USA.

13. Filizadeh, Y., Rajabi Islami, H. (2011) Toxicity determination of three sturgeon species exposed to Glyphosate, Iran J Fish Sci. 10: 383-392.

14. Fryer, J.D. (1977) Weed control handbook

edited by make peace. Group of Experts on the Scientific Aspects of Marine Pollution (GESAMP). 1: 118-121, 384-389.

15. Gangolli, S. (1999) The dictionary of substances and their effects. Cambridge publication: Royal Socety Chemistry. UK. 7: 998p.

16. Grover, R., Wolt, J.D., Cessna, A.J., Schiefer, H.B. (1997) Environmental fate of trifluralin. Rev Environ Contam Toxicol. 153: 1-64.

17. Haji Sharafi, GH.H., Shokouhfar, A.R. (2009) Replace herbicide sugarcanes to reduce consumption and optimal use of pesticide in agro industrial Sugarcane Khuzestan. J Crop physiol. (in Persian). 1: 49- 57.

18. Hussein, S.Y., El-Nasser, M.A., Ahmed, S.M. (1996) Comparative studies on the effects of herbicide atrazine on freshwater fish *Oreochromis niloticus* and *Chrysichthys auratus at* Assiut Egypt. Bull Environ Cont Toxicol. 57: 503-510.

19. Hildebrand, L.D., Sullivan, D.S., Sullivan, T.P. (1980) Effects of RoundupR herbicide on populations of *Daphnia magna* in a forest pond. Bull Enviorn Contam Toxicol. 25: 353-357.

20. Ladipo, M.K., Doherty, V.F. (2011) Acute toxicity, behavioural changes and histopathological effect of paraquat dichloride on tissues of catfish (*Clarias gariepinus*). Int J Biol Sci. 3: 67-74.

21. Moraes, B.S., Loro, V.L., Glusczak, L., Pretto, A. (2007) Effects of four rice herbicides on some metabolic and toxicology parameters of teleost fish (*Leporinus obtusidens*). Chemosphere. 68: 1597-1601.

22. Mizuhashi, S., Ikegaya, Y., Matsuki, N. (2000) Cytotoxicity of tributyltin in rat hippocampal slice cultures. Neurosci Res. 38: 35-42.

23. Neskovic, N., Elezonic, K., Karan, I., Poleksic, V., Budimir. V. (1993) Acute and sub acute toxicity of atrazine to Carp (*Cyprinus carpio*). Ecotoxicol Environ Saf. 25: 173-182.

24. Nwani, C.D., Nagpure, N.S., Kumar, R., Kushwaha, B., Kumar, P., Lakra, W.S. (2010) Lethal concentration and toxicity stress of Carbosulfan, Glyphosate and Atrazine to freshwater air breathing fish *Channa punctatus* (Bloch) Int Aquat Res. 2: 105-111.

25. Lushchak, O.V., Kubrak, O.I., Storey, J.M., Storey, K.B., Lushchak, V.I. (2009) Low toxic herbicide Roundup induces mild oxidative stress in goldfish tissues Chemosphere. 76: 932-937.

26. Olaifa, F.E., Olaifa, A.K., Lewis, O.O. (2003) Toxic Stress of Lead on Clariasgariepinus (African catfish) Fingerlings. AJBR. 6: 101-104.

27. Poleksic, H.V., Karan, V. (1999) Effects of Trifluralin on Carp: Biochemical and Histological Evaluation, Ecotoxicol Environ Saf. 43: 213-221.

28. Roberta Cattaneo, R., Clasen, B., Menezes, C.C., Baldisserotto, B., Loro, V.L., Pretto, A., Santi, A., Avila, L.A. (2011) Toxicological responses of *Cyprinus carpio* exposed to a commercial formulation containing glyphosate. Bull Environ Contam Toxicol. 87: 597-602.

29. Sarikaya, R., Yilmaz, M., Gul, A. (2002) The acute toxic effect of 2,4-D upon tench (*Tinea tinea* L., 1758). J Inst Sci Technol Gazi Uni. 15: 289-296.

30. Schultz, I.R., Hayton, W.L. (1993) Toxicokinetics of trifluralin in Rainbow trout, Aquat Toxicol. 26: 287-306.

31. Sarikaya, R., Yilmaz, M. (2003) Investigation of acute toxicity and the effect of 2,4-D (2,4-dichlorophenoxyacetic acid) herbicide on the behavior of the common carp (*Cyprinus carpio* L., 1758; Pisces, Cyprinidae).

Chemosphere. 52: 195-201.

32. Shakil, A.S., Grantley, D.C., Michael, J.B., Lynn, H.L.K. (2008) Mechanism of trifluralin-induced thyroid tumors in rats, Toxicol Lett. 180: 38-45.

33. Vesna, P., Vesela, K. (1999) Effects of trifluralin on carp: Biochemical and histological evaluation, Ecotoxicol Environ Saf. 43: 213-221.

34. Ward, G.S., Parrish, P.R. (1982) Manual of Methods in Aquatic environmental research. Part 6. Toxicity Tests. FAO Fisheries Technical Paper, No 185 FIRI/T185.

35. Yao, F., Liu, H., Wang, G., Du, L., Yin, X., Fu, Y. (2013) Determination of paraquat in water samples using a sensitive fluorescent probe titration method. J Environ Sci. 25: 1245e51.

36. Yeo, R.R. (1967) Dissipation of diquat and paraquat, and effects on aquatic weeds and fish. Weeds. 15: 42-46.

13

The effect of rice husk as an insoluble dietary fiber source on intestinal morphology and Lactobacilli and *Escherichia coli* populations in broilers

Abazari, A.[1], Navidshad, B.[2*], Mirzaei Aghjehgheshlagh, F.[2], Nikbin, S.[2]

[1]*Graduated from Department of Animal Sciences, University of Mohaghegh Ardabili, Ardabil, Iran*
[2]*Department of Animal Sciences, University of Mohaghegh Ardabili, Ardabil, Iran*

Key words:
broilers, gut bacteria population, intestine morphology, particle size, rice husk

Correspondence
Navidshad, B.
Department of Animal Sciences, University of Mohaghegh Ardabili, Ardabil, Iran

Email: bnavidshad@uma.ac.ir

Abstract:

BACKGROUND: There are some reports on the positive effects of dietary insoluble fiber on the performance of broilers. **OBJECTIVES:** This study was carried out to determine the effect of inclusion rate and particle size of rice husk in the diet of broilers on the ileal and cecal bacteria populations and small intestine morphology. **METHODS:** The experimental diets consisted of a control husk-free diet and four diets containing 7.5 or 15 g/kg rice husk with particle sizes of less than 1 mm or between 1-2 mm. **RESULTS:** The dietary insoluble fiber did not affect feed intake of the experimental groups. The best body weight gain and feed conversion ratio was recorded in the broiler chickens fed the diet containing 15g/kg rice hulls with particle size of less than 1 mm (p<0.05). In the duodenum and jejunum, the crypt depth to villi height ratio in the control group was significantly lower than other groups (p<0.05). In the ileum, all the birds fed rice husk except the group fed the diet that contained 15g/kg rice husk with particle size of 1-2 mm, had higher *Lactobacilli* and lower *E. coli* and coliforms populations than the control group (p<0.05). **CONCLUSIONS:** The results of the present study suggest that the 7.5g/kg dietary inclusion and more coarse particles size of rice husk (1-2 mm) were more effective to promote broiler growth performance. The positive effects of dietary insoluble fiber on the growth performance of broilers in this study are probably a result of favorable changes in the bacteria populations of the gastrointestinal tract and not any improvement in small intestine absorptive capacity.

Introduction

To date, most attention has focused on fermentable carbohydrate components such as fructooligosaccharides and mannan oligosaccharides which have beneficial effects on intestinal microflora of broilers (Navidshad et al., 2015). However, the research conducted in recent years has shown that incorporation of low levels of different sources of insoluble fiber in diet improves development of digestive organs (Hetland and Svihus, 2007; Rezaei et al., 2011a,b, 2014) and increased secretion of bile acids, HCl and digestive enzymes (Hetland et al., 2003). These changes may improve the digestibility of nutrients, the health of the digestive tract (Montagne et al., 2003) and ultimately improve animal welfare (Van Krimpen et al., 2009). The crypt depth to villi height ratio is an indicator of digestion potential in the small intestine and a smaller ratio suggests an improvement on the intestinal mucosa (Hampson, 1986).

Lactic acid bacteria which are included *Lactobacilli* are the most commonly used probiotics (Brashears et al., 2003). Some strains of *E. coli* cause illness that can be fatal in domestic birds (Sackey et al., 2001).

Previous studies have shown that cellulose as an active component of the diet may increase the number of intestinal beneficial bacteria, particularly bifidobacteria and *Lactobacilli* and also affect potential pathogenic bacteria (Cao et al., 2003). It is generally accepted that the phenolic components of pure lignin have antimicrobial properties (Baurhoo et al., 2008). It has been shown that cellulose has an abrasive effect on the intestine and causes increased secretion of mucous (Montagne et al., 2004). Mucous layer has a dynamic nature (continually under construction and destruction) and is involved in protection, creating fluidity and nutrients absorption in small intestine. After creating friction by dietary cellulose, the secretion of mucin in the gastrointestinal tract by goblet cells is increased (Montagne et al., 2004).

Based on the literature review, there is a lack of information on the effect of the level and particle size of the dietary fiber on the microbial population of small intestine of broilers. This study was carried out to determine the effect of inclusion rate and particle size of rice husk in the diet of broilers on the ileal and cecal bacteria populations and small intestine morphology.

Materials and Methods

The rice husk (Hashemi cultivar) required in the trial was obtained from a commercial rice processing factory, Astara, Iran. After grinding with hammer mill with sieve sizes of 1 and 2 mm the husk was divided in two parts with particle sizes less than 1 mm and 1-2 mm, respectively. The dry matter, crude protein, fat, fiber and ash of the rice husk and experimental diets were determined (AOAC, 2000). The concentration of neutral detergent fiber (NDF), acid detergent fiber was determined based on Van Soest (1963). The lignin content of rice husk was considered 22.34% (Senthil Kumar et al., 2010).

Animal care guidelines were followed for animal use for experimental and other scientific purposes. The study lasted for 42 days, 200 broilers (Ross 308) of both sexes were used in a completely randomized design with 5 treatments, 4 replicates and 10 birds per replication. In this study, the experimental diets were isonitrogenous and isocaloric and were formulated based on Ross (308) broilers nutritional requirements tables (Table 1). The environmental conditions (temperature, humidity and light) were controlled based on the recommendation of the strain catalog. Access to water and feed was free from day 1 to the end of the experiment. The chicks with similar weights received one of the following experimental diets from 11 d of age:

1. The control diet without rice husk (C).
2. Diet containing 7.5 g/kg rice husk with particle sizes less than 1 mm (RSL).
3. Diet containing 15 g/kg rice husk with particle sizes less than 1 mm (RSH).
4. Diet containing 7.5 g/kg rice husk with particle size between 1 to 2 mm (RBL).
5. Diet containing 15 g/kg rice husk with particle size between 1 to 2 mm (RBH).

Feed intake and weight gain were measured periodically and the feed conversion ratio was calculated. Before the weighting, the birds were fasted for 7 hours to empty the gut contents. Mortality was recorded daily. European efficiency index (EEI) for each replication was calculated as follows,

EEI = (livability × live weight in kg/length of fattening period in days × FCR) × 100

At 42 d of age, two birds of each replication were randomly selected and slaughtered. Digestive tract was removed immediately. Digesta samples of the ileum (the boundary between Meckel's diverticulum and the branching point of the ceca) and ceca were immediately collected and transferred to sterile tubes containing 20% glycerol phosphate buffer saline and stored in -20°C until the tests.

Ileal and cecal bacterial populations were quantified using 'standard Koch's plate method (Merck Microbiology Manual, 2007). Samples were placed in buffer peptone 1% (w/v 1:9) and then the serial dilutions were prepared. The following bacterial species were quantified using specific culture media (Merck, Germany), lactic acid bacteria in MRS agar, *E. coli* on Chromocult TBX agar and coliforms on coliform Agar ES. All samples were plated in triplicate and incubated at 37°C for 4 h (Merck Microbiology Manual, 2007). All the collected data were analyzed using general linear model (GLM) of SAS statistical software14 and the comparison of means was done by Duncan procedure at 0.05 probability level.

Results

The chemical composition obtained for rice husks was as follows, 93% dry matter, apparent metabolizable energy of 834 kcal / kg, ash 16.8%, ether extract 3.49%, crude protein 3.23%, crude fiber 37.5% , NDF 76.0%, ADF 56.1%, calcium 0.8% and total P 0.27%.

The effect of dietary inclusion of rice husk on the production traits and EEI of broilers is shown in Table 2. The experimental diets had no effect on feed intake of birds. During the grower phase, the live weight gain of broilers fed diets containing 15g/kg rice husk (RSH and RBH treatments) was higher than the groups fed the lower level (7.5g/kg) rice husk (RSL and RBL) treatments (p<0.05). In the finisher phase, the differences observed in live weight gains were not significant, but numerically the

diets with lower level of rice husk (RSL and RBL treatments) had higher weight gain. This effect resulted in an improved weight gain in the RBL group compared to the control group in the whole experiment period (p<0.05). During the experimental period, the best feed conversion ratio was also observed in RBL group such that the difference with the RSL group was significant (p<0.05).

European efficiency index in the experimental period was affected by the diets, such that as in all the rice husk fed birds except for RSL, EEI was higher than the control group (p<0.05). Table 3 shows the effect of rice husk on the intestinal morphology of broilers. Unexpectedly, dietary rice husk reduced the villi height compared to the control group in all parts of the small intestine (p<0.05), although this difference was not significant in the ileum. The small intestine epithelial thickness was not affected by the diets. In duodenum, the highest number goblet cells were observed in the control group and the lowest was in the RBH treatment (p<0.05). In the jejunum and ileum rice husk consumption resulted in increased numbers of goblet cells compared to the control group, such that in the jejunum the differences with RSL and RBH groups, and in ileum, the difference with the RSL group were significant (p<0.05). In duodenum, a dipper crypt was observed in RBH group rather than in the control and RSH groups (p<0.05). In the jejunum and ileum, crypt depth was not affected by diet. In the duodenum and jejunum, the crypt depth to villi height ratio in the control group was significantly lower than other groups (p<0.05), but this parameter was not affected in the ileum.

The bacterial flora of the gastrointestinal tract was also under the influence of rice husk in diets (Table 4). In the ileum, all the birds fed rice husk except RBH, had a higher lactic acid bacteria and lower *E. coli* and coliforms populations than the control group (p<0.05). Fewer numbers of *E. coli* were observed in the ileal

Table 1. Composition of experimental diets. 1Vitamin premix provided the following per kilogram of diet, vitamin A (retinyl acetate), 9,000 IU; vitamin D (cholecalciferol), 5,500 IU; vitamin E (dl-α-tocopheryl acetate), 68 IU; menadione, 9.0 mg; pyridoxine, 7.0 mg; riboflavin, 26.0 mg; Ca-pantothenate, 26.3 mg; biotin, 0.41 mg; thiamine, 3.66 mg; niacin, 75 mg; cobalamin, 0.03 mg; and folic acid, 3.70 mg. 2Mineral premix provided the following per kilogram of diet, Fe, 82 mg; Mn, 60 mg; Zn, 115 mg; Cu, 15 mg; I, 0.85 mg; and Se, 0.4 mg.

| | Starter | Grower | | | Finisher | | |
| | | Control | Rice hulls | | Control | Rice hulls | |
Ingredient, %			7.5 g/kg	15 g/kg		7.5 g/kg	15 g/kg
Rice hulls	0	0	0.75	1.5	0	0.75	1.5
Corn	45.92	48.55	47.19	46.11	51.96	50.59	49.23
Soybean meal	43.83	40.29	40.44	40.53	37.34	37.49	37.63
soybean oil	5.88	7.19	7.67	7.91	6.96	7.44	7.91
DCP	2.09	1.72	1.72	1.72	1.6	1.6	1.6
Calcium Carbonate	1.19	1.07	1.05	1.04	1.02	1.01	1.02
Common salt	0.23	0.44	0.44	0.44	0.44	0.44	0.44
Vitamin premix1	0.25	0.25	0.25	0.25	0.25	0.25	0.25
Mineral premix2	0.25	0.25	0.25	0.25	0.25	0.25	0.25
DL-Methionin	0.32	0.25	0.25	0.25	0.18	0.18	0.19
HCl-Lysin	0.04	0	0	0	0	0	0
Chemical analysis							
Metabolisabld energy (Kcal/kg)	2980	3100	3100	3090	3130	3130	3130
Crude protein	23.27	22	22	22	21	21	21
Ca	1.033	0.9	0.9	0.9	0.85	0.85	0.85
AvP	0.52	0.45	0.45	0.45	0.42	0.42	0.42
Na	0.198	0.2	0.2	0.2	0.2	0.2	0.2
Lys	1.41	1.297	1.297	1.304	1.223	1.223	1.223
Met	0.69	0.5992	0.5992	0.599	0.524	0.524	0.524
Met+Cys	1.06	0.95	0.95	0.95	0.86	0.86	0.86
CF	4.7	4.49	11.45	11.86	4.39	11.54	11.92
NDF	11.61	11.44	11.87	12.31	11.45	11.88	12.30
ADF	5.01	4.80	5.19	5.59	4.6	5.05	5.44
Lignin	0.67	0.61	0.80	0.99	0.61	0.80	0.97

Table 2. Performance characteristics of broilers fed experimental diets contained rice husk. 1C=Control. RSL= The diet contained 7.5g/kg rice husk with particle size of less than 1 mm, RSH= The diet contained 15 g/kg rice husk with particle size of less than 1 mm, RBL= The diet contained 7.5g/kg rice husk with particle size of 1-2 mm, RBH= The diet contained 15g/kg rice husk with particle size of 1-2 mm. EEI= European efficiency index. Within a column not sharing a common superscript differ significantly at p<0.05.

| | Daily feed intake (gram/bird/day) | | | Daily weight gain (gram/bird/day) | | | Feed conversion ratio | | | EEI |
	11-24 d	25-42 d	11-42 d	11-24 d	25-42 d	11-42 d	11-24 d	25-42 d	11-42 d	
C1	81. 7	166.8	126.5	54.5ab	87.9	72.2b	1.50	1.89	1.75ab	292.5b
RSL	81.0	175.0	134.2	52.3b	92.5	74.0ab	1.54	1.90	1.79a	307.4b
RSH	85.6	169.9	131.7	56.3a	93.6	76.6ab	1.52	1.82	1.72ab	342.7a
RBL	82.9	174.3	131.6	55.0ab	101.3	79.6a	1.51	1.72	1.65b	345.8a
RBH	84.4	172.7	133.0	56.8a	96.1	78.4ab	1.49	1.80	1.69ab	346.0a
MSE	1.64	4.86	2.53	1.13	4.06	2.19	0.043	0.051	0.045	5.12
p value	0.34	0.51	0.82	0.04	0.32	0.03	0.19	0.33	0.02	0.03

Table 3. Small intestinal morphology of broilers fed experimental diets that contained rice husk. 1C=Control. RSL= The diet contained 7.5g/kg rice husk with particle size of less than 1 mm, RSH= The diet contained 15g/kg rice husk with particle size of less than 1 mm, RBL= The diet contained 7.5g/kg rice husk with particle size of 1-2 mm, RBH= The diet contained 15g/kg rice husk with particle size of 1-2 mm. Within a column, not sharing a common superscript differs significantly at p<0.05.

	Duodenum					Jejunum					Ileum				
	VH2	CD	CD:VH	ET	G	VH	CD	CD:VH	ET	G	VH	CD	CD:VH	ET	G
C1	1738[a]	141.8[c]	0.081[b]	41.8	10.4[a]	843[a]	143.0	0.169[b]	40.2	9.8[c]	778	101.6	0.130	39.4	9.2[b]
RSL	1713[bc]	157.6[ab]	0.092[a]	42.0	7.2[cd]	825[b]	145.2	0.176[ab]	39.0	12.4[a]	769	101.0	0.131	38.8	10.8[a]
RSH	1711[bc]	152.0[b]	0.089a	39.4	9.2[bc]	823[b]	143.6	0.174[ab]	36.4	11.2[abc]	767	102.1	0.131	38.7	10.0[ab]
RBL	1706[c]	155.8[ab]	0.091a	39.6	8.4[bc]	824[b]	145.6	0.177[a]	37.2	10.8[bc]	766	103.2	0.135	40.4	10.4[ab]
RBH	1717[b]	158.2[a]	0.092a	42.4	6.2[d]	825[b]	146.8	0.178[a]	39.6	11.8[ab]	868	102.6	0.133	38.6	11.8[ab]
MSE	2.89	1.95	0.001	1.42	0.43	3.01	1.92	0.002	1.42	0.43	3.93	2.22	0.003	0.43	0.42
p value	0.02	0.02	0.01	0.66	0.03	0.01	0.12	0.04	0.15	0.02	0.42	0.36	0.61	0.59	0.03

Table 4. Ileum and cecum bacteria population of broilers fed experimental diets that contained rice husk. 1C=Control. RSL= The diet contained 7.5g/kg rice husk with particle size of less than 1 mm, RSH= The diet contained 15 g/kg rice husk with particle size of less than 1 mm, RBL= The diet contained 7.5g/kg rice husk with particle size of 1-2 mm, RBH= The diet contained 15g/kg rice husk with particle size of 1-2 mm. Within a column, not sharing a common superscript differs significantly at p< 0.05.

	Ileum (log 10 cfu/g)			Cecum (log 10 cfu/g)		
	Lactobacillus. sp	*E. coli*	Coliforms	*Lactobacillus*. sp	*E. coli*	Coliforms
C1	7.56b	9.95a	9.99a	9.60	8.60a	8.94a
RSL	8.25a	6.52c	6.55c	8.79	8.51ab	8.74a
RSH	8.54a	8.12b	8.53b	8.63	6.85c	7.55b
RBL	8.44a	6.64c	7.09bc	8.73	7.62bc	8.05ab
RBH	7.36b	7.74bc	7.94bc	9.44	8.30ab	8.62ab
MSE	0.22	0.46	0.48	0.52	0.34	0.42
p value	0.02	0.02	0.04	0.23	0.02	0.03

digesta of RBL and RSH groups (p<0.05) and the coliforms were also reduced in the BCL group. The total number of treatments in BCL (p<0.05). In ceca, the only significant difference was lower populations of coliforms and *E. coli* in RSH group compared with the control group (p<0.05).

Discussion

In this study, the use of the rice husk at 15 g/kg of the diet as a source of lignocellulose led to improved body weight gain of broilers at grower phase. However, this situation was changed at the finisher phase such that during the experimental period the birds fed the diet containing 7.5 g/kg rice husk with particle size of 1-2 mm showed better weight gain. This finding suggests that the dietary fiber effect on chick's performance will change with gastro-intestinal development and a coarse and higher level of fiber may accelerate this development. These findings confirm the results of previous reports that the moderate levels of an insoluble fiber could improve the growth performance of broilers (Sarikhan et al., 2010; González-Alvarado et al., 2010; Mateos et al., 2012).

The insoluble dietary fiber speeds up the passage rate of digesta in the intestinal tract, which in turn may increase the feed intake (Hetland et al., 2003; Montagne et al., 2003). Such observations in broilers have also been reported using pure cellulose (Cao et al., 2003) and lignin (Mateos et al., 2012).

Increased goblet cell numbers in the jejunum and ileum of broilers in this study were reported in previous studies because of its abrasive effect that resulted in a change in mucin secretion (Montagne et al., 2003; Rezaei et al., 2011a,b, 2014). The mucus layer overlying the epithelium secreted by the goblet cells improves the elimination of gut contents and provides the first line of defense against physical and chemical injury caused by ingested food, microbes and the microbial products (Kim and Ho, 2010).

Increased crypt depth in the duodenum of chicks fed rice husk is in agreement with a report on chicks fed cellulose (Wils-Plotz and Dilger, 2013). Unexpectedly, in the present study, dietary rice husk decreased small intestine villi height compared to the control group. The crypt depth to villi height ratio in this study was reduced in all the experimental groups fed the diets that contained rice husk compared to the control group, which is not compatible with the more superior growth performance observed in the rice husk fed groups.

The results of the present study showed that adding rice husk as a lignocellulose source could promote the growth of beneficial Lactobacillus bacteria and reduce the population of pathogenic bacteria such as some *E. coli* in the ileum and cecum of broilers at 42 d of age. In the same report, it was shown that 4% alfalfa meal in the broiler diet increased *Lactobacilli* bacteria population and reduced the number of *E. coli* compared with the control group (Hampson, 1986).

The mechanism of lignocellulose action on bacterial populations in the gastrointestinal tract is not entirely clear. It can be assumed that this effect is due to different actions of cellulose and lignin in the intestinal environment. It has been found that the decomposition of insoluble dietary fiber (NDF) by chicken's bacterial enzymes is about 35% (Jamroz et al., 2001) but the effect on the microbial population is mainly due to fiber physicochemical properties. The friction effect of dietary insoluble fiber on the surface of gut, facilitates removal of pathogen bacteria from mucous layer (Mateos et al., 2012). This effect in turn is able to boost the growth of beneficial micro-

flora. The positive effect of lignocellulose on gut Bifidobacterium and *lactobacilli* population has been confirmed in the previous reports (Cao et al., 2003). Some bacteria release bacteriocins which prevent further proliferation of pathogens in the gut (O'Shea et al., 2012). It has been reported that lignin Alcell decreased the growth of aerobic bacteria in mice in both in vivo and in vitro situations (Nelson et al., 1994).

The results of the present study suggest that a minimum amount of dietary insoluble fiber is needed to achieve the best growth performance of broiler chickens. So, diets of broilers should be formulated to provide enough insoluble fiber. The 7.5g/kg dietary inclusion and more coarse particles size of rice husk (1-2 mm) were more effective to promote broiler growth performance. The positive effects of dietary insoluble fiber on the growth performance of broilers in this study is probably a result of favorite changes in the bacteria populations of the gastrointestinal tract and not any improvement in small intestine absorptive capacity.

Acknowledgments

This work was supported by the Vice-Chancellor for Research and Technology of University of Mohaghegh Ardabili.

References

1. AOAC International. (2000) Official Methods of Analysis. (18th ed.) AOAC International, Gaithersburg, MD, USA.
2. Baurhoo, B., Ruiz-Feria, C.A., Zhao, X. (2008) Purified lignin, nutritional and health impacts on farm animals - a review. Anim Feed Sci Technol. 144: 175-184.
3. Brashears, M.M., Jaroni, D., Trimble, J. (2003) Isolation, selection, and characterization of lactic acid bacteria for a competitive exclusion product to reduce shedding of *Escherichia coli* O157, H7 in cattle. J Food Prot. 66: 355-363.
4. Cao, B.H., Zhang, X.P., Guo, Y.M., Karasawa,

Y., Kumao, T. (2003) Effects of dietary cellulose levels on growth, nitrogen utilization, retention time of diets in digestive tract and caecal microflora of chickens. Asian-Australas. J Anim Sci. 16: 863-866.

5. González-Alvarado, J.M., Jiménez-Moreno, E., González-Sánchez, D., Lázaro, R., Mateos, G.G. (2010) Effect of inclusion of oat hulls and sugar beet pulp in the diet on productive performance and digestive traits of broilers from 1 to 42 days of age. Anim Feed Sci Technol. 162: 37-46.

6. Hampson, D.J. (1986) Alteration in piglet small intestine structure at weaning. Res Vet Sci. 40: 32-40.

7. Hetland, H., Svihus, B., Krögdahl, Å. (2003) Effects of oat hulls and wood shavings on digestion in broilers and layers fed diets based on whole or ground wheat. Br Poult Sci. 44: 275-282.

8. Hetland, H., Svihus, B. (2007) Inclusion of dust bathing materials affects nutrient digestion and gut physiology of layers. J Appl Poult Res. 16: 22-26.

9. Jamroz, D., Jacobsen, K., Orda, J., Skorupinska, J., Wiliczkiewicz, A. (2001) Development of the gastrointestinal tract and digestibility of dietary fibre and amino acids in young chickens, ducks and geese fed diets with high amounts of barley. Comp Biochem Physiol A. 130: 643-652.

10. Kim, Y.S., Ho, S.B (2010) Intestinal Goblet Cells and Mucins in Health and Disease: Recent Insights and Progress. Curr Gastroenterol Rep. 12: 319-330.

11. Mateos, G.G., Jiménez-Moreno, E., Serrano, M.P., Lázaro, R.P. (2012) Poultry response to high levels of dietary fiber sources varying in physical and chemical characteristics. J Appl Poult Res. 21: 156-174.

12. Merck Microbiology Manual. (2012) 12th. Merck, Darmstadt, Germany.

13. Montagne, L., Pluske, J.R., Hampson, D.J. (2003) A review of interactions between dietary fibre and the intestinal mucosa, and their consequences on digestive health in young non-ruminant animals. Anim Feed Sci Technol. 108: 95-117.

14. Montagne, L., Piel, C., Lalles, J.P. (2004) Effect of diet on mucin kinetics and composition, nutrition and health implications. Nutr Rev. 62: 105-114.

15. Navidshad, B., Liang, J.B., Faseleh Jahromi, M., Akhlaghi, A., Abdullah, N. (2015) A comparison between a yeast cell wall extract (Bio-Mos®) and palm kernel expeller as mannan-oligosaccharides sources on the performance and ileal microbial population of broiler chickens. Ital J Anim Sci. 14: 3452.

16. Nelson, J.L., Alexander, J.W., Gianotti, L., Chalk, C.L., Pyles, T. (1994) Influence of dietary fiber on microbial growth in vitro and bacterial translocation after burn injury in mice. Nutrition. 10: 32-36.

17. O'Shea, E.F., Cotter, P.D., Stanton, C., Ross, R.P., Hil, C. (2012) Production of bioactive substances by intestinal bacteria as a basis for explaining probiotic mechanisms, bacteriocins and conjugated linoleic acid. Int J Food Microbiol. 152: 189-205.

18. Rezaei, M., Karimi Torshizi, M.A., Rouzbehan, Y. (2011a) Effect of dietary fiber on intestinal morphology and performance of broiler chickens. Anim Sci J Pajouhesh Sazandegi. (In Persian). 90: 52-60.

19. Rezaei, M., Karimi Torshizi, M.A., Rouzbehan, Y. (2011b) The influence of different levels of micronized insoluble fiber on broiler performance and litter moisture. Poult Sci. 90: 2008-2012.

20. Rezaei, M., Karimi Torshizi, M.A., Shariatmadari, F. (2014) Inclusion of processed rice hulls as insoluble fiber in the diet on performance and digestive traits of Japanese quails. J Anim Sci Adv. 4: 962-972.

21. Sackey, B.A., Mensah, P., Collison, E., Sakyi-Dawson, E. (2001) Campylobacter, Salmonella, Shigella and *Escherichia coli* in live and dressed poultry from metropolitan Accra. Int J Food Microbiol. 71: 21-28.

22. Sarikhan, M., Shahryar, H.A., Gholizadeh, B., Hosseinzadeh, M.H., Beheshti, B., Mahmood-nejad, A. (2010) Effects of insoluble fiber on growth performance, carcass traits and ileum morphological parameters on broiler chick males. Int J Agric Biol. 12: 531-536.

23. Senthil Kumar, P., Ramakrishnan, K., Dinesh Kirupha, S., Sivanesan, S. (2010) Thermodynamic and kinetic studies of cadmium adsorption from aqueous solution onto rice husk. Brazil J Chem Eng. 27: 347-355 .

24. Van Krimpen, M.M., Kwakkel, R.P., Van Peet-Schwering, C.M.C., Den Hartog, L.A. Verstegen, M.W.A. (2009) Effects of nutrient dilution and nonstarch polysaccharide concentration in rearing and laying diets on eating behavior and feather damage of rearing and laying hens. Poult Sci. 88: 759-773.

25. Van Soest, P.J. (1963) Use of detergents in the analysis of fibrous feeds. II. A rapid method for the determination of fiber and lignin. J Assoc Offic Agric Chem. 46: 829-835.

26. Wils-Plotz, E.L., Dilger, R.N. (2013) Combined dietary effects of supplemental threonine and purified fiber on growth performance and intestinal health of young chicks. Poult Sci. 92: 726-734.

14

Serum biochemical and hematological parameters in dogs with benign prostatic hyperplasia (BPH)

Khaki, Z.[1*], Masoudifard, M.[2], Khadivar, F.[3], Shirani, D.[4], Fathipour, V.[1], Taheri, M.[5]

[1]Department of Clinical Pathology, Faculty of Veterinary Medicine, University of Tehran, Tehran, Iran

[2]Department of Radiology and Sonography, Faculty of Veterinary Medicine, University of Tehran, Tehran, Iran

[3]Graduated student, Faculty of Veterinary Medicine, University of Tehran, Tehran, Iran

[4]Department of Small Animal Internal Medicine, Faculty of Veterinary Medicine, University of Tehran, Tehran, Iran

[5]Dr. Rastegar Laboratories, Faculty of Veterinary Medicine, University of Tehran, Tehran, Iran

Key words:

acid phosphatase, benign prostatic hyperplasia, CRP, dog, prostate

Correspondence

Khaki, Z.

Department of Clinical Pathology, Faculty of Veterinary Medicine, University of Tehran, Tehran, Iran

Email: zkhaki@ut.ac.ir

Abstract:

BACKGROUND: Clinical prostatic diseases occur in 80% of dogs over 5 and 95% over 9 years of age. It seems that benign prostatic hyperplasia (BPH) affects Scottish terriers more severely than the other breeds. **OBJECTIVES:** This study aimed to evaluate the changes of biochemical and hematological parameters in BPH dogs. **METHODS:** Blood samples were collected from 10 male dogs (mostly terrier or mix) older than five years with weight 8.91 ± 2.5 kg.suffering from BPH which referred to Small Animal Hospital of the Veterinary Faculty of Tehran University. The diagnosis of BPH was based on clinical, laboratory surveys and ultrasonography. 10 normal male dogs with same age, breed and weight were selected as control group. Then serum acid phosphatase (TAP and PAP), CRP, urea, creatinine, total protein, albumin, globulins and hematological parameters were assayed and the results were analyzed by Independent student T-test. Also, Pearson's linear correlation test was used to determine the correlation between TAP, PAP, CRP and ESR with length and width of prostate. **RESULTS:** The length (p=0.008), width (p= 0.01) of prostates was significantly higher in dogs suffering from BPH compared to the healthy dogs. TAP and PAP levels significantly increased in all dogs in BPH group (approximately 6 times) compared to the controls (p=0.001). Moreover, serumic CRP concentration was elevated in some BPH dogs (approximately 6 times) (p=0.001). While there was significant ESR elevation in some of the dogs in disease group compared to the normal dogs, no significant difference was observed in other biochemical and hematological parameters between two groups (p>0.05). There was a highly significant correlation between serum TAP and PAP (p≤ 0.01) with prostate's length and width which was more than CRP. **CONCLUSIONS:** The serum acid phosphatase, CRP and ESR were elevated in BPH dogs but the increase in serum acid phosphatase was more important than the others. It is recommended that each laboratory should use its own values of acid phosphatase in dogs.

Introduction

The prostate gland is a bi-lobed structure that lies within the pelvis just behind the bladder and directly below the rectum (Francey, 2010). Clinical prostatic diseases occur only in humans, chimpanzee, dogs (Steiner et al., 1999) and, rarely, in cats (Francey, 2010). It has been reported that it may occur in 80% of intact dogs over 5 and 95% over 9 years of age. BPH seems to affect Scottish terriers more severely than other breeds. Prostatic tumors are rather uncommon in dogs (Francey, 2010) and prostatic adenocarcinoma is the main prostatic neoplasia in humans and dogs (Swinney, 1998).

Due to the high frequency of prostatic lesions in dogs, "in vivo" diagnostic methods should be established in order to determine the specific lesion, treatment and prognosis. The human prostate gland secretes many glycoproteins. Prostatic Acid Phosphatase (PAP) and Prostatic Specific Antigen (PSA) levels are high in human patients with BPH (Corrazza et al., 1994; Wadstrom et al., 1984). PAP and PSA have been used for the identification of human prostate cancer (McEntee et al., 1987). Although PSA has been identified in normal, hyperplasic and neoplastic canine prostatic cells, it was not detected in serum or seminal from healthy dogs or those with prostatic disease (Francey, 2010). However, Amorim et al 2004 tried to evaluate PSA in serum and urine of normal dogs with human detector. Their methodology was monoclonal antibodies raised against human, thus, the sensitivity of the test for dogs was weaker (Amorim et al., 2004).

Similar to human, PAP level is hormone dependent, and its levels are variable with age (Aumüller et al., 1987; Corrazza et al., 1994); however, Gadelha et al (2013) reported that PAP levels did not correlate with age (Gadelha et al 2013). Quantitative changes in canine PAP are less remarkable than in human, nevertheless, they are important in the evaluation of the prostatic epithelial cells secretory activity (Aumüller et al., 1987; Corrazza et al., 1994),

C-reactive protein (CRP) is an Acute Phase Protein (APP) which participates in the acute phase response. This response is a nonspecific inflammatory reaction of the host that occurs shortly after any tissue injury. Therefore, it can be considered as one of the earliest markers for any pathologic process or disease (Ceron et al., 2005; Kaneko, 2010). CRP is thought to possess high diagnostic specificity, as it is only induced by proinflammatory hypercytokinaemia. These properties should facilitate the use of canine CRP as a marker of systemic inflammatory activity for routine diagnostic, monitoring and screening purposes (Kjelgaard-Hansen et al., 2013; Kaneko, 2010). Production and response of APPs varies depending on the species. For example, a strong response occurs with CRP in dogs; however, in cats, significant increases of CRP have not been detected after an inflammatory stimulus. (Ceron et al., 2005).

The results of different experiments on whether the measurement of acid phosphatase could be used as a diagnostic test for prostatic disease (Gadelha et al., 2013) are not reliable. However, for veterinary pa¬tients (BPH dogs), the activity of acid phosphatase is not routinely used for screening purposes in Iran and there are no data about blood serum biochemical and hematological parameters in BPH dogs. Therefore, the aim of current study was to evaluate related blood serum biochemical (TAP, PAP, CRP, urea, creatinine, total protein, albumin and globulin) and hematological parameters in dogs suffering from BPH.

Materials and Methods

Thesurvey was conducted on dogs which referred to Small Animal Hospital of the Veterinary Faculty of Tehran University. Blood and urine samples were collected from 10 male dogs older than five years old suffering from Benign Prostatic Hypertrophy (BPH). The breeds of dogs were mostly Terrier or mix with Spitz, Shih Tzu, and Pekingese and one German shepherd. The average weight and age were 8.91 ± 2.5 kg and 113.9 ± 14.19 months, respectively. The diagnosis of benign prostatic hypertrophy was based on prostatic enlargement (judged by rectal digital palpation and ultrasonography) accompanied by one or more of the following signs: dysuria, difficulty in defecating, hematuria and sanguineous discharge from the tip of the penis unrelated to urinating. Moreover, cytology of the urine sediment was performed for diagnosis of prostatic adenocarcinoma (Corrazza et al., 1994).

Ten normal male dogs with same age, breed and weight were selected as control group. The control animals were examined according to the clinical, hematological and ultrasonography evaluation.

In all dogs, volume of each prostate was estimated by using the following formula (Francey, 2010):

Volume [cm3] = (0.867 X BW [kg]) + (1.885 X age [year]) + 15.88.

Blood samples were collected into EDTA (for hematologic), citrate tubes (for ESR) and without anticoagulant for serum separation and biochemical assessment. For mea-

suring biochemical parameters, the blood tubes were inserted in water and ice flask. The whole blood was allowed to clot for 30 minutes at 25° C and then centrifuged at 2000 rpm for 15 minutes at 4 C°. The serum layer was pipetted off and then stored on ice and assayed the same day. Colorimetric methods (Commercial Iranian kit-Zeist Chimi) were used for measurement of serum Total Acid Phosphatase (TAP) and Prostatic Acid Phosphatase (PAP).

CRP concentration was measured by using a commercial canine CRP ELISA kit (Tridelta Development Ltd, Kildare, UK). The serum samples were kept at -20 C° until assayed.

In addition, other serum biochemical analysis such as urea, creatinine, total protein, and albumin were determined by using an Elitech automated analyzer (SELECTRA prom, France) and commercial kits (Pars Azmoon, Tehran, Iran). Globulin concentration was calculated by subtracting the serum albumin from the total protein concentration (Thrall et al., 2012).

ESR was measured by Westergren method. It was done by transferring 1.8 mL of blood into a vial containing a defined amount of 3.8% sodium citrate (0.2 mL) solution. The blood was mixed thoroughly and sucked into the Westergren ESR tube to the top mark (0 mark).The tube was then stood vertically for 1 hour and the level of the red cells was read as the ESR (Thrall et al., 2012).

Hematological parameters including total erythrocyte count (RBC), hematocrit value (HcT), hemoglobin concentration (Hb), mean corpuscular volume (MCV), mean corpuscular hemoglobin concentration (MCHC), and total white blood cells (WBC) were determined by the NIHONKOHDEN hematology analyzer (Italy). Differential leukocyte counts were also estimated manually as described by Meyer and Harvey (2004).

For statistical analysis, Independent t-Test (SPSS version16) was used to compare and determine statistical differences in laboratory-obtained values between two groups. All values were expressed as mean and Standard Error (SE). Also, Pearson's linear correlation test was used to determine the correlation between TAP, PAP, CRP, and ESR with length and width of prostate. A p value <0.05 was considered significant.

Results

In dogs suffering from BPH compared to healthy dogs, the prostates were higher, wider and larger (p<0.05) (Table 1).

Mean serum TAP and PAP activities were increased in BPH group significantly (71.02±2.91 and 32.19±2.83 U/L respectively) compared to control (12.14±1.63 and5.38±1.11 U/L respectively) (p=0.001). Statistical analysis revealed that there were significant differences in serum CRP between two groups. Mean serum CRP concentration was increased in BPH group (5.5±1.4 mg/l)compared to the control (0.9±0.2 mg/l) (p=0.001) (Table2). Although serum total protein, globulin and urea were increased in BPH group, it was not significant (p>0.05). Moreover, there was no significant difference in other biochemical parameters between control and BPH dogs (p>0.05) (Table3).

There were significant rises in ESR of BPH group compared to normal dogs. Mean ±SE of ESR in BPH and control dogs was 8.8±0.57 and 6±0.47 mm/h respectively. Additionally, as it can be seen in Table 3, there were no significant differences in

Table 1. The mean±SE of length, width and volume of prostrates in sonography of BPH and control groups. *-Significant.

	group BPH mean±SE (min-max)	Control group mean±SE (min-max)	p value
Length of prostate (mm)	45.78±4.78 (31.11-71.57)	28.51±2.93 (12.8-36.47)	0.008*
Width of prostate (mm)	45.78±4.78 (19.9-66.1)	26.05±2.18 (14.8-35.04)	0.01*
Volume of prostate (cm3)	41.5±3.05 (29-62)	28.5±2.93 (12.8-36.47)	0.056

Table 2. Serum acid phosphatase (TAP and PAP) activities and CRP in BPH and control groups. *-Significant.

p value	Control group mean±SE (min-max)	BPH group mean±SE (min-max)	
Serum TAP (U/L)	12.14±1.63 (3.8-19.7)	71.02±2.91 (56.3-85)	0.001*
Serum PAP (U/L)	5.38±1.11 (0.9 - 13.1)	32.19±2.83 (21.2-52)	0.001*
CRP (mg/l)	0. 9±0. 2 (0. 2 -2. 3)	5.5±1. 4 (1. 6-10.3)	0.001*

Table 3. Serum total protein, albumin, globulin, urea and creatinine in BPH and control groups.

	Control group mean±SE (min-max)	BPH group mean±SE (min-max)	p value
total protein (g/dl)	6.86±0.2 (5.96-8.4)	7.08±0.34 (5.73-9.4)	0.59
albumin (g/dl)	3.86±0.18 (2.71-4.43)	3.6±0.18 (2.56-4.18)	0.33
globulin (g/dl)	3±0.28 (1.59-4.32)	3.48±0.35 (1.84-5.4)	0.3
urea (mg/dl)	31.6±3.89 (20-52)	35.35±3.88 (19-57)	0.5
creatinine (mg/dl)	0.97±0.14 (0.5-1.7)	0.88±0.09 (0.4-1.3)	0.6

RBC indices, WBC counts, and differential leukocyte count.

There was a severe significant correlation between serum TAP and PAP (p≤ 0.01) with prostate's length and width which was more than CRP. Only correlation between CRP and width of prostate was significant (p=

Table 4. Hematological parameters in BPH and control groups. *-Significant.

	Control group mean±SE (min-max)	group BPH mean±SE (min-max)	p value
ESR mm/h	6±0.47 (4-9)	8.8±0.57 (6-12)	*0.001
HcT (%)	45.17±2.32 (33.8 -59.1)	41.29±2.34 (26.8-52.8)	0.25
RBC (106μl)	6.92±0.34 (5.5-8.9)	6.52±0.38 (4.7-8.6)	0.45
Hb (g/dl)	15.06±0.73 (-19 11.7)	15.55±0.55 (11.9-18)	0.6
WBC (103μl)	9.12±0.81 (5.82-14)	9.32±1.54 (4.4-18.9)	0.9
Neut.seg (%)	6377.3±812.8 (3621- 11900)	6276±1271.2 (2412-15050)	0.94
Neut.band (%)	70.9±33.09 (0-280)	65.8±30.27 (0-237)	0.91
Monocyte (%)	218±51.95 (0-473)	415.4±180.41 (0-1890)	0.3
Lymphocyte (%)	2175.6±269.9 (729- 3708)	2163.3±410.5 (616-5292)	0.98
Eosinophil (%)	269±127.18 (0-1235)	392.8±101.12 (0-957)	0.45
Basophil (%)	13.2±13.2 (0-132)	12.7±12.7 (0-127)	0.97

Table 5. Correlation between TAP,PAP,CRPand ESR with length and width of prostate. *-Significant.

	length	width
TAP	r=0.593 p=0.007*	r=0.562 p=0.012*
PAP	r=0.617 p=0.005*	r=0.582 p=0.000*
CRP	r=0.460 p=0.085	r=0.547 p=0.035*
ESR	r=0.322 p=0.179	r=0.415 p=0.077

0.03). There was no correlation between ESR and prostate's size (Table 5).

Discussion

The dog's prostatic glands are the best natural models for the study of human prostatic diseases (Amorim et al., 2004) because they are the animal models that spontaneously develop prostatic hyperplasia (Gadelha et al., 2013).

Benign Prostatic Hyperplasia is best treated by the administration of estrogens or by castration(Noakes et al., 2001), because they remove the source of androgens responsible for maintaining prostatic size (Feldman and Nelson, 2004).We used castration for dogs suffering from BPH. Our experience showed that maximum atrophy of prostate was noted after 6 to 9 weeks of therapy. After castration in the dog, retained prostate exhibited a similarly high incidence of neoplasia.Thus, all of the BPH dogs in current study were treated by castration and their clinical signs improved.

Quantitative changes in canine PAP are less remarkable than in human, nevertheless, they are important in the evaluation of the prostatic epithelial cells secretary activity (Aumüller et al., 1987). In our study, serum TAP and PAP levels were particularly elevated (approximately 6 times) in all dogs with benign prostatic hypertrophy. Corrazza et al (1994) found that PAP serum concentrations were particularly elevated in dogs with benign prostatic hypertrophy, which had the same result as the current experiment. However, they showed that serum concentration of TAP and PAP increased 0.5 and 3 times respectively in some dogs suffering from BPH. In addition, they mentioned that elevated TAP and PAP is probably due to a degeneration of the prostatic secretary epithelial cells induced by an increased dihydrotestosterone concentration within the gland (Corrazza et al., 1994). Salo et al (1990) have concluded that intracapsular cancer does not elevate serum acid phosphatase levels as it was determined by radioimmunoassay or an enzymatic method.

BPH alone leads to significant rises in PAP concentration. The degree of BPH correlates with PAP level (Salo et al., 1990); however, Corrazza et al (1994) described that dogs with prostatic adenocarcinoma had significantly higher TAP, PAP serum concentrations than dogs with benign prostatic hypertrophy, normal dogs and dogs with nonprostatic disease (Corrazza et al., 1994).

In the present study, the activity of acid phosphatase was higher than the values obtained in other studies. The results of Gadelha et al. (2013) showed that the PAP values in the serum were lower than Corazza et al. (1994) and Amorim et al. (2004). As Gadelha et al (2013) described previously, this could be explained by the difference in the reagent used by the different laboratories. Also, the difference in dog's breed may be important, and it is recommended that each laboratory should establish and use its own values (Gadelha et al., 2013;Thrall et al., 2012) .

C-reactive protein (CRP) is a major acute phase protein in dogs characterized by low physiological level, a marked and fast increase shortly after a systemic inflammatory stimulus (Kjelgaard-Hansen et al., 2013). Although the acute phase response, which by definition only lasts a few days, seems to play a positive role in the innate host defense mechanisms, increases in APPs have also been described in chronic inflammation (Ceron et al., 2005). Moreover, CRP can be used as a monitor and quantitative marker of the inflammatory stimulus of aseptic elective soft tissue surgery (Kjelgaard-Hansen et al., 2013).

APPs concentration in adult dogs should be interpreted with caution, as they can be influenced greatly by analytic condition. This is particularly important for APPs due to the lack of reference materials for international harmonization of assays in small animals (Eckersall et al., 1999).

In this study, the result showed that dogs with BPH had significantly higher mean serum CRP concentration (5.5 ± 1.4 mg/l) than normal dogs (0.9 ± 0.2 mg/l) ($p<0.001$) an increase of approximately 6-fold. Although CRP is a major APP (Francey, 2010) in BPH dogs, CRP rose moderately in current study. As our observation, relatively increased levels of CRP have been found in inflammatory bowel disease (Jergens et al., 2003) and in hematological and neoplastic diseases of the dog (Tecles et al., 2005). Increases of 95-fold were found in CRP concentration after surgical trauma compared with 40- to 50-fold increases after turpentine oil injection (Ceron et al., 2005). In our study, increase of CRP was not shown in all BPH dogs. Only 66.6% of them showed high concentration of CRP in serum which indicated that normal serum concentration of CRP does not rule out BPH in the dog.

The result showed that there was a greater correlation between serum acid phosphatase ($p\leq0.01$) and prostate's length and width than CRP. Only correlation between CRP and width of prostate was significant ($p= 0.03$).

Although the mean of total protein and globulins in BPH groups was more than healthy dogs and albumin levels in patients was less than the others, there were no significant changes in the above parameters. If the repeated sampling was done, presumably the levels of protein parameters would increase or decrease. Albumin is a negative acute phase protein and its concentration falls gradually during infectious and inflammatory disease (Kaneko et al.,2010), also elevated levels of globulin are reported in acute and chronic period of disease.(Kaneko et al., 2010). Although the measurement of albumin is easier and cheaper, currently it seems to have a lower clinical value in diagnosing and monitoring inflammation (Ceron et al., 2005).

From 10 patients, in one out of two with prostatic cyst, actual elevation of protein (9.4 g/dl) was seen due to increasing globulin (5.4 g/dl).

In this study, there was no significant change in serum urea of BPH dogs. In measurement of GFR, the accuracy of serum creatinine was higher than urea because of the lack of tubular reabsorption and minimal tubular secretion (Thrall et al., 2012). In current study, dogs suffering from BPH did not show any elevation of serum creatinine concentration. It seems that kidneys were not significantly affected by BPH. As in our investigation, Rule et al (2005) mentioned that Prostatic enlargement in human was not associated with chronic kidney disease (Rule et al., 2005); however, Sataria and Staskin (2000) described that there was a relationship between BPH and chronic kidney disease due to abnormalities of the lower urinary tract and uretrovesical junction (Sataria and Staskin ,2000).

Erythrocytes sedimentation rate (ESR) is known as acute phase response as CRP. ESR is an indirect measure of the acute phase reaction. Its value lies in the fact that it is a simple and inexpensive laboratory test for assessing inflammation. In human, the researchers believe that it has even been used for the prognosis of noninflammatory condition, such as prostatic cancer, coronary artery disease and stroke(Husain and Kim, 2002).It seems that increased ESR could be important in BHP dogs because in our study, mean of ESR was elevated sig-

nificantly in them (not in all cases). There was no significant change in means of other hematological parameters. Although Corazza et al (1994) mentioned that mild leukocytosis was seen in dogs suffering from BPH (Corazza et al., 1994) our survey showed that only in 2 dogs was WBC increased. They showed neutrophilia without left shift and lymphopenia which was presumably caused by stress.

In conclusion, the serum acid phosphatase, CRP and ESR were elevated in BPH dogs; however, the increase in serum acid phosphatase was more significant than the others. It is recommended that each laboratory should establish and use its own values of acid phosphatase in dogs.

Acknowledgments

This research was supported by the research fund of University of Tehran, Tehran, Iran.

References

Amorim, R.L., Moura, V.M.B.D., Di Santis, G.W., Bandarra, E.P., Padovani C. (2004) Serum and urinary measurements of prostatic acid phosphatase (PAP) and prostatic specific antigen (PSA) in dogs. Arq Bras Med Vet Zootec. 56: 320-324.

Aumuller, G., Vedder, H., Enderle-SchmitT,U. (1987) Cytochemistry and Biochemistry of Acid Phosphatases VII: Immunohistochemistry of canine prostatic acid phosphatase. Prostate. 11: 1-15.

Ceron, J.J., Eckersall, P.D., Martınez-Subiela, S. (2005) Acute phase proteins in dogs and cats: current knowledge and future perspectives. Vet Clin Pathol. 34: 85-99.

Corrazza, M., Guidi, G., Romagnoli, S., Tognetti, R. , Buonaccorsi A. (1994) Serum total prostatic and non-prostatic acid phosphatase in healthy dogs and in dogs with prostatic diseases. J Small Anim Pract. 35: 307-310.

Eckersall, P.D., Duthie, S., Toussaint, M.j., Gruys, E., Heegaard, P., Alava, M., Lipperheide, C., Madec, F. (1999) Standardization of diagnostic assays for animal acute phase proteins. Adv Vet Med. 41: 643-655.

Felman, E.C., Nelson, R.W. (2004) Canine and Feline Endocrinology and Reproduction. (3rd ed.) WB. Saunders. Missouri, USA.

Francey, T. (2010) Prostatic Diseases. In: Textbook of Veterinary Internal Medicine. Ettinger, S.J., Feldman, E.C. (eds.). (7th ed.) vol 2, WB. Saunders, Philadelphia, USA. p. 1926-1930.

Gadelha, C.R.F., Vicente, W.R.R., Ribeiro, A.P.C., Apparicio, M., Covizzi, G.j., Campos, A.C.N. (2013) Prostatic acid phosphatase in serum and semen of dogs. Arch Med Vet. 45: 321-325.

Husain, T.M., Kim, H.D. (2002) C - reactive protein and erythrocyte sedimentation rate in orthopaedics. University of Pennsylvania. Orthopaedic Journal. 15: 13-16.

Jergens, A.E., Schreiner, C., Frank, D.E., Niyo, Y., Ahrens, F.E., Eckersall, P.D., Benson, T.J., Evans, R. (2003) A scoring index for disease activity in canine inflammatory bowel disease. J Vet Int Med. 17: 291 -297.

Kjelgaard-Hansen, M., Strom, H., Mikkelsen, L., Eriksen, T., Jensen, A.L., Luntang-Jensen, M. (2013) Canine serum C-reactive protein as a quantitative marker of the inflammatory stimulus of aseptic elective soft tissue surgery. Vet Clin Pathol. 42: 342-345.

Kaneko, J.J., Harvey, J.W., Bruss, M.L. (2008) Clinical Biochemistry of Domestic Animals. (6th ed.) Elsevier, Academic Press, London, UK.

McEntee, M., Issaacs, I., Smith, C. (1987) Adenocarcinoma of the canine prostate: immunohistochemically examination for secretory antigens. Prostate. 11: 163-170.

Meyer, D.J., Harvey, J.W. (2004) Veterinary Laboratory Medicine. (3rd ed.) WB Saunders, London, UK.

Noakes, D.E., Parkinson, T,J., England, G.C.W. (2001) Arthur's Veterinary Reproduction and Obstetrics. (8th ed.) WB Saunders, London, UK.

Rule, A.D., Jacobson, D.J., Roberts, R.O.,Girman, C.J., McGree, M.E., Lieber, M.M., Jacobson, S.J. (2005) The association between benign prostatic hyperplasia and chronic kidney disease in community-dwelling men. Kidney Int. 67: 2376-2382.

Salo, J.O., Rannikko, S., Haapiainen, R. (1990) Serum acid phosphatase in patients with localized prostatic cancer, benign prostatic hyperplasia or normal prostates. Br J Urol. 66: 188-192.

Sataria, P.M., Staskin, D.R. (2000) Hydronephrosis and renal deterioration in the elderly due to abnormalities of the lower urinary tract and ureterovesical junction. Int Urol Nephrol. 32: 119-126.

Steiner, M.S., Couch, R.C., Raghow, S., Stauffer D. (1999) the chim panzee as a model of human benign prostate hyperplasia. J Urol. 162: 1454-1461.

Swinney, G.R. (1998) Prostatic neoplasia in five dogs. Aust Vet J. 76: 669-674.

Tecles, F., Spiranelli, E., Bonfanti, U., Ceron, J.J., Paltrinieri, S. (2005) Preliminary studies of serum acute-phase protein concentrations in hematologic and neoplastic diseases of the dog. J Vet Int Med. 19: 865-870.

Thrall, M.A., Weiser, G., Allison ,R., Campbell, T.W. (2012) Veterinary Hematology and Clinical Chemistry. (2th ed.) Wiley-Blackwell, Iowa, USA.

Wadström, J., Huber, P., Rutishauser, G. (1984) Elevation of serum prostatic acid phosphatase levels after prostatic massage. Urology. 24: 550-551.

15

Effects of camphor on histomorphometric and histochemical parameters of testicular tissue in mice

Morovvati, H.[1], Adibmoradi, M.[1*], Kalantari Hesari, A.[1], Mazaheri Nezhad Fard, R.[2], Moradi, H.R.[1]

[1]*Department of Basic Sciences, Faculty of Veterinary Medicine, University of Tehran, Tehran, Iran*
[2]*Division of Food Microbiology, Department of Pathobiology, School of Public Health, Tehran University of Medical Sciences, Tehran, Iran*

Key words:

camphor, histochemistry, mice, testis, vitamin E

Correspondence

Adibmoradi, M.
Department of Basic Sciences,
Faculty of Veterinary Medicine,
University of Tehran, Tehran,
Iran

Email: adibmoradi@ut.ac.ir

Abstract:

BACKGROUND: In traditional medicine of some Asian countries it is believed that camphor could act as a sexual depressant. However, limited studies have been published on this issue. **OBJECTIVES:** In the current study, effects of camphor on testes, sperm and serum factors, and roles of vitamin E as antioxidant in treatment of toxicity of camphor for testes were studied. **METHODS:** Fifty adult male mice (20-25 g) were categorized into five groups. Control group, two control sham groups received olive oil and combined vitamin E and olive oil respectively, and two treatment groups received camphor and combined camphor and vitamin E, respectively. Camphor with doses of 30 mg/kg/day and vitamin E with doses of 100 mg/kg/day were prepared. All substances were administered using gavage. After 35 days, blood was collected from the animal heart for serology and testosterone assessment. Sperms were collected and tissue samples were removed and fixed in Bouin and liquid nitrogen. Paraffin embedded and freezing sections were stained with H&E and specific stain and studied. **RESULTS:** Results showed a significant decrease in sperm count, average proportions of live and mature sperms and major testicular morphometric parameters (p>0.05). Although histochemical changes were seen, no changes were observed in serum testosterone in groups that received camphor. Vitamin E moderated toxicity of camphor in immature sperms, diameter of lumen and TDI index. **CONCLUSIONS:** It can be concluded that camphor includes adverse effects on parameters of testes and sperm quality. Furthermore, vitamin E, as an antioxidant, can moderate toxicity of camphor.

Introduction

Camphor is a solid, greasy and clear white crystal with sharp odor. It is well known in Asian nations. Camphor is derived from Cinnamonom camphor. Nowadays, the industrial type of camphor is synthesized and extensively used in medicine, health and various industries (Yu et al., 2003; Anczewski et al., 2003; Lattanzi et al., 2003). This substance is used as anticipative, odorant, cosmetics, stimulator of blood circulation and respiration, psychological stimulant, libido modulator, anti-conceptive and abortive (Libelt and Shannon, 1993; Reynolds, 1996; Gerald et al., 2002; Liu et al., 2006). Camphor is synthesized from turpentine oil in ointment, lotion and gel forms and used as antibacterial, anti-itching, local analgesic and anti-sunlight (Yu et al., 2003; Anczewski et al., 2003; Lattanzi et al., 2003). Furthermore, it is used in UV-filter oils, sanitation materials, gums, cigarettes, prevention of insect biting and mummification (Chatterjie and Alexander, 1986; Liu et al., 2006).

Evidence indicates adverse effects of camphor on the body. However, there is limited information on effects of camphor on body organs such as the genital system. Camphor can be absorbed through skin, digestive system (5-90 min after consumption) and respiratory system. Overdose of camphor causes toxicity with signs of vision obscurity, vomiting, colitis, vertigo, delirium, heart muscle spasm, hard breathing, paroxysm and death. In one of the recent investigations on the role of camphor in the reproductive system of male mice, camphor (30 mg/kg/day) was shown to make histological changes in testes and induce immature seminiferous tubules (Nikravesh and Jalali, 2004). Studies indicate that organic compounds such as camphor may decrease P450 B1 cytochrome activity. This enzyme interferes with one of the key enzymes in testosterone synthesis, hydroxilase-17 (Barzegari and Mirhosseini, 2012; Mokhtari et al., 2007). Studies have shown that camphor content of UV-filter oil affects gonadotropines and sex hormones and causes impotency in teenagers and atrophy of copulatory organs in both sexes (Durrer et al., 2007; Schlumpf et al., 2004). In one study, researchers have shown that use of camphor ointment includes no effects on gonadotropines (LH and FSH) and testosterone (Janjua et al., 2004). Furthermore, they have reported that camphor content of UV-filter oil causes inhibition of 17b-hydroxysteroid dehydrogenase Type 3 which catalyses the last step of testosterone synthesis (Nashev et al., 2010). Effects of camphor on gene expression of estrogen and estrogen receptor activity have been studied (Maerkel et al., 2007; Heneweer et al.,

2005). In contrast, compounds have been studied with protective effects on genital system. One of these compounds, vitamin E (tocopherol), is a powerful non-enzymatic antioxidant that is involved in lipid peroxidation in cell membrane by limiting action of free radicals; thereby, inhibiting protected cell membranes from induced damage. Vitamin E protects testes and sperms via antioxidant defense system (Ganesh et al., 2012). In traditional medicine in Iran, camphor is used as libido suppressor. A small study has been carried out on the effects of camphor on sperm and testis parameters. Therefore, the aim of the current study was to investigate these effects of camphor on reproductive parameters and the role of vitamin E in treatment of sexual disorders caused by camphor.

Materials and Methods

Fifty adult male mice (balb/c) weighing 20-25 g were randomly selected and equally divided into five groups including one control group, two control sham groups and two treatment groups. They were housed under standard conditions with proper food and water available. Before the trial, animals were accustomed to the environment with 12-h day/night illuminating cycles at 23-25 °C. Since olive oil is reported as the most appropriate solvent for camphor, doses of 30 mg/kg/day of camphor (Henan Xingfa, China) were dissolved in olive oil and prescribed using gavage for 35 days (Budavari et al., 1996). Vitamin E (α-tocopherol) (Zahravi, Iran) was prescribed daily with doses of 100 mg/kg/day via gavage one hour after receiving camphor (Ganesh et al., 2012). Animal groups were categorized as follows: Control group received normal saline (0.3 ml); sham Group 1 received equal volume of olive oil (0.3 ml); sham Group 2 received olive oil (0.3 ml) with vitamin E (100 mg/kg/day); treatment Group 1 received camphor (30 mg/kg/day) dissolved in olive oil (0.3 ml); and treatment Group 2 received camphor (30 mg/kg/day) dissolved in olive oil (0.3 ml) with vitamin E (100 mg/kg/day) (Nikravesh and Jalali M., 2004; Ganesh et al., 2012).

After 35 days of experiment, animals were weighed and then sacrificed using chloroform. Blood samples were collected from the heart and centrifuged at 4,000 rpm for 10 min to separate serum. Serum samples were assessed for antioxidant activity (AOA) using ferric reducing ability of plasma (FRAP) method, and lipid malonaldehyde (MAD) peroxidation using reaction with thiobarbituric acid method (Kheradmand et al., 2013; Koracevic et al., 2001). Serum testosterone level was assessed using testosterone measurement kit (DRG Instruments, Germany). Volume of testes was quantified using graduated tubule containing water. Left testes were used for histochemical study including alkaline phosphatase (ALP), lipid and periodic acid Schiff (PAS) staining. Right testes were used for histological and morphometric studies. Assessment of sperms included sperm count and motility using hemocytometer slide and sperm viability using eosin-nigrosin staining. Rate of DNA fracture was calculated using acridine-orange staining and nucleus maturation using aniline-blue staining (Rezvanfar et al., 2008; Rezvanfar et al., 2013). Testes were fixed for histological studies using dehydration, clearing, paraffin embedding, blocking, sectioning to 5-7 µm thickness, mounting on slides, and staining processes. Histological studies included capsule, interstitial tissue and seminiferous tubules for appearance, attachment and abnormal features. Histometrical studies of testes included thickness of capsule, height of germinal epithelium of seminiferous tubules, number of Sertoli cells (in each seminiferous tubule), number of Leydig cells, and seminiferous tubule and lumen diameters. Spermatogenesis and spermiogenesis studies included tubular differentiation indices (TDI), spermiogenesis indices (SI) and repopulation indices

(RI) (Kalantari Hesari et al., 2015). Histomorphometrical studies were carried out using Dino-Lite lens digital camera and Dino-capture 2 Software. Frozen specimens in liquid nitrogen were sectioned to 15-20 µm using cryostat at -45 °C. SPSS V.19 Software was used for data analysis. Distribution of data was controlled by K-S test and since distribution of all data was normal, parametric tests were used for data analyses. One way ANOVA test was used to compare two groups and t-test to compare several groups with each other. When necessary, Tukey test was used followed by ANOVA test. Results were shown as average ±SD (standard deviation) with a minimum significance $p > 0.05$.

Results

Body weight and testes volume: No significant difference was observed in average body weight between control, control sham and treatment groups (p=0.61). The maximum body weight (34.75 ±2.46 g) was seen in olive oil receiving group while the minimum body weight was seen in group receiving a combination of camphor and vitamin E (29.25 ±2.84 g). No significant difference was observed in average testis volume between groups (p= 0.66) (Table 1).

Quality of sperm: The average percentage of motile sperms and sperms with intact (normal) DNA included no significant difference (p= 0.22 and p= 0.84, respectively). However, changes were seen in other parameters as follows: total number of sperms showed a significant decline in camphor group (7,250,000 ±11.64) compared to that in control, control sham and treatment groups. A significant difference was observed in control, olive oil and combined camphor and vitamin E groups. No significant difference was seen in combined camphor and vitamin E group (p= 0.6). Other groups showed no significant difference (Table 2). Camphor group showed a significant

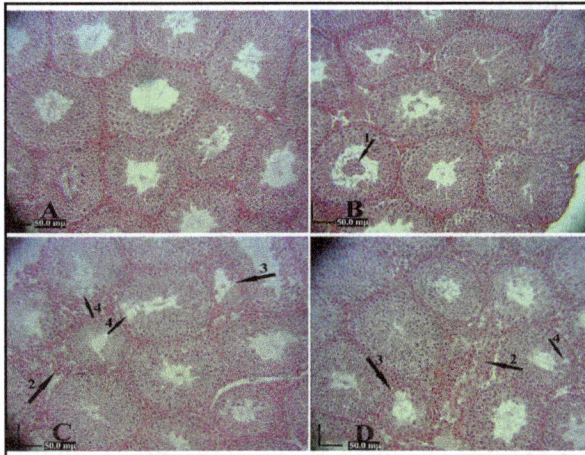

Figure 1. Histology of testes stained by H&E (100×). A, control group; B, olive oil group; C, Camphor group; D, Camphor + Vitamin E group. No. 1, indicates spermatogenesis line cells were separated and poured into the lumen of seminiferous; No. 2, increased of Leydig cells; No. 3, degenerative tubules; No. 4, Vacuoles appearing on spermatogenesis cell lines.

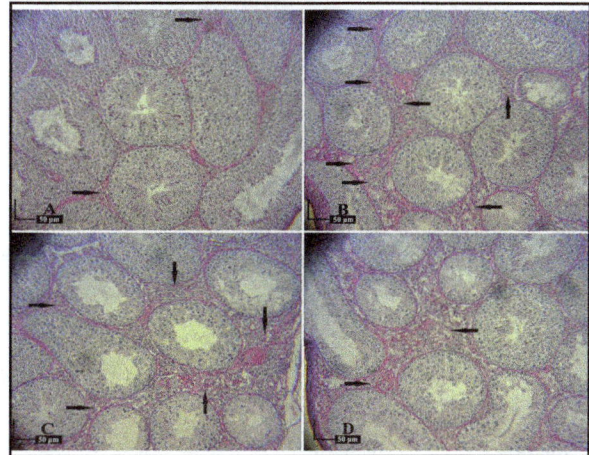

Figure 2. Excessive increase the number of Leydig cells in the groups receiving olive oil (PAS staining) (100×). A: In control group, Leydig cells are normal; B: olive oil group; C and D: Respectively group that received of camphor solution in olive oil and group that received of camphor solution in olive oil + vitamin E, increased the number of Leyding cells, especially near the capsule, in both groups was observed.

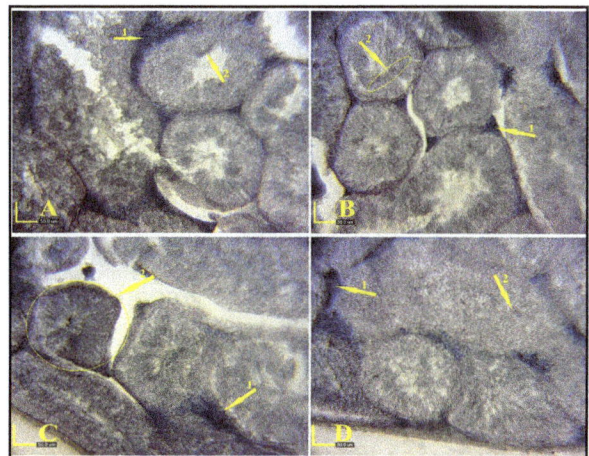

Figure 3. Alkaline phosphatase staining in control, control sham and treatment mice (400×). A, control group slightly reacted with ALP stain; B, olive oil group with a significant increase in the intensity of stain compared to control group; C, camphor group with maximum reaction with ALP stain compared to other groups; D, combined camphor and vitamin E group. Arrows no. 1 indicate ALP particles in Leydig cells; arrows no. 2 indicate ALP particles in spermatogenesis cells.

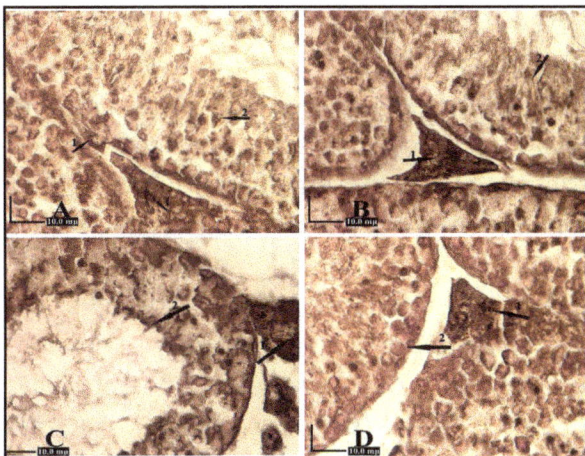

Figure 4. Sudan-black staining in control, control sham and treatment mice (100×). A, control group; B, olive oil group; C, camphor group (the highest accumulation of lipids was observed in cells of seminiferous tubules. Leydig cells were similar to those in sham groups); D, combined camphor and vitamin E group. Arrows no. 1 indicate Sudan black stain in Leydig cells; arrows no. 2 indicate Sudan black stain in spermatogenesis cells.

decrease in motile sperms (34.75% ±2.81). A significant difference was seen in control and olive oil groups. No significant difference was observed in the other groups. (Table 2). A majority of immature sperms were reported in camphor group (28.25% ±2.50), compared to that in control, olive oil, and combined olive oil and vitamin E groups (p<0.05). However, immature sperms showed an insignifi-

cant increase in camphor group, compared to that in combined camphor and vitamin E (p≥ 0.05). Immature sperms showed a significant increase in combined camphor and vitamin E group, compared to that in control, and combined olive oil and vitamin E groups (p< 0.05) (Table 2).

Histological results: Histological study of testes showed normal structures in control

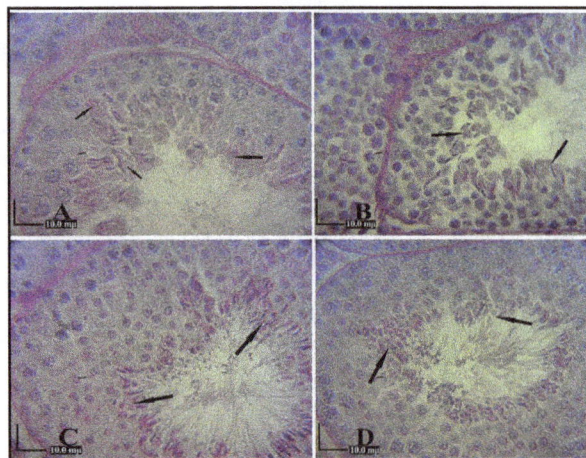

Figure 5. PAS staining in control, control sham and treatment mice (400×). A, control group; B, olive oil group; C, camphor group; D, combined camphor and vitamin E group.

group, including normal capsule and lack of congestion edema. No degenerated tubules or detached spermatogenic cells were observed (Fig. 1.A). Histological study in olive oil group demonstrated abnormal features including detached spermatogenic cells (spermatocytes and spermatids) inside lumen of seminiferous tubules and significantly increased Leydig cells in interstitial tissue. This increased number of Leydig cells was more obvious near the capsule in all groups, except control group (Fig. 2). Testis capsule was normal; however, degrees of edema and congestion were seen (Fig. 1.B). Furthermore, numerous degenerated tubules were seen in testis tissue sections. In group receiving combined olive oil and vitamin E, tissue sections showed that capsule and other histological structures including spermatogenic cells were normal (Fig. 1.C). Histological study in camphor group showed changes including increased number of degenerated tubules, wider epithelium and therefore a smaller lumen of seminiferous tubules, excessively increased number of Leydig cells in interstitial tissue, and presence of vacuoles in spermatogenic cells. No changes, edema and congestion were observed in tissue of testes (Fig. 1.D). Histological study in combined camphor and vitamin E group showed similar findings but with a lower rate. However, cap-

sule was normal and no edema or congestion was observed (Fig. 1.E).

Morphometric results: In morphometric study, capsule thickness of testes showed a significant increase in combined camphor and vitamin E group, compared to that in control group ($p < 0.05$). Minimum and maximum thicknesses were seen in control group (8.82 ±1.05 μm) and combined camphor and vitamin E (12.7 ±1.21 μm), respectively. No significant difference was seen in capsule thickness of testes in other groups ($p \geq 0.05$) (Table 3). Diameter of seminiferous tubules revealed a significant decrease in olive oil group, compared to that in other groups except control group ($p < 0.05$). The smallest diameter of seminiferous tubules was seen in olive oil group (161.65 ±9.29 μm). No significant difference was observed in diameter of seminiferous tubules in other groups ($p \geq 0.05$) (Table 3). Germinal epithelium thickness showed a significant increase in camphor group, compared to that in olive oil group ($p < 0.05$). No significant difference was seen in germinal epithelium thickness in other groups ($p \geq 0.05$) (Table 3). Internal lumen diameter of seminiferous tubules showed a significant decrease in camphor group, compared to that in olive oil, and combined camphor and vitamin E groups ($p < 0.05$). Maximum internal lumen diameter of seminiferous tubules was seen in control group (12.24 ±7.32 μm) (Table 3). No significant difference was seen in internal lumen diameter of seminiferous tubules in other groups ($p \geq 0.05$) (Table 3). No significant difference was seen in number of Sertoli cells in study groups ($p = 0.06$) (Table 3). Minimum and maximum numbers of Leydig cells were observed in control (14.375 ±1.51 μm), and combined camphor and vitamin E groups (25 ±3.55 μm), respectively, ($p = 0.064$) (Table 3). TDI index showed a significant decrease in camphor group, compared to that in combined olive oil and vitamin E, and combined camphor and vitamin E groups ($p < 0.05$). The lowest TDI index was seen in camphor group

Table 1. Average weight of body and testis volume in control and treatment mice. No significant difference was seen between the groups.

	Control	Olive oil	Olive oil + vitamin E	Camphor	Camphor + vitamin E
Body weight (g)	31 ±2.61	34.75 ±2.46	32 ±0.85	32 ±2.94	29.25 ±2.84
Testis volume	0.07 ±0.01	0.09 ±0.01	0.09 ±0.01	0.08 ±0.01	0.10 ±0.03

Table 2. Sperm parameters in control and treatment groups. Dissimilar letters indicate significant differences between the groups (p< 0.05).

	Control	Olive oil	Olive oil + vitamin E	Camphor	Camphor + vitamin E
Total count of sperm	54375000 ±117.26[a]	52750000 ±151.90[a]	60375000 ±14.77[a]	7250000 ±11.64[b]	20375000 ±10.08[ab]
Sperm viability (%)	53 ±2.74[a]	39.75 ±3.71[a]	51.25 ±4.42[ab]	34.75 ±2.81[b]	47.25 ±6.44[ab]
Sperm motility (%)	84.5 ±3.62	82.25 ±2.25	76.50 ±1.76	67.25 ±5.50	77.75 ±7.61
Sperm with intact DNA (%)	99.25 ±0.48	99 ±0.58	98.50 ±0.65	99 ±0.71	99.5 ±0.29
Immature sperm (%)	9.5 ±1.55[a]	13.5 ±1.19[ac]	11.75 ±1.80[a]	28.25 ±2.50[b]	19.50 ±1.32[c]

(79% ±071), compared to that in other groups (Table 3). RI index showed a significant decrease in olive oil group (64% ±1.25), compared to that in other groups except control group (p< 0.05). No significant difference was seen in RI index in other groups (p≥ 0.05) (Table 3). SI index showed a significant decrease in olive oil group, compared to that in camphor group (p< 0.05). Maximum SI index was seen in camphor group (89.25% ±0.73). No significant difference was observed in SI index in other groups (p≥ 0.05) (Table 3). Assessment of degenerated tubules showed a significant increase in camphor, and combined camphor and vitamin E groups, compared to that in control group (p< 0.05). Minimum and maximum numbers of degenerated tubules were seen in control group (1% ±0.27), and combined camphor and vitamin E (15.5% ±3.51), respectively. No significant difference was seen in number of degenerated tubules in other groups (p≥ 0.05) (Table 3).

Histochemical results: Results of testicular tissue section staining using ALP have revealed the highest rate of small brown particles in cytoplasm of Leydig and spermatogenic cells in camphor group, compared to

that in other groups. Furthermore, ALP staining results showed a similar finding in olive oil group but with a lower rate. A higher density was seen in combined camphor and vitamin E group than control group (Fig. 3, Table 4). Cytoplasm of testicular cells included black particles with lipid contents using Sudan-black staining. These black particles were mostly detected in cells closed to lumen. Furthermore, Sudan-black staining showed a significant increase in lipids in olive oil, combined olive oil and vitamin E, combined camphor and vitamin E, and camphor groups, compared to that in control group. A majority of black particles was seen in spermatogenic cells in camphor group and then in combined olive oil and camphor, and vitamin E groups, respectively (Fig. 4, Table 4). PAS staining findings have revealed normal in all groups capsule. PAS positive particles were mostly detected in cytoplasm of spermatogenic cells, specifically in spermatids. PAS positive particles were mostly observed in groups with the thickest epithelium, compared to other groups. No other significant differences were reported (Fig. 5, Table 4).

Serum tests: In the present study, antiox-

Table 3. histomorphometrical and serum parameters in control and treatment groups. Dissimilar letters indicate significant differences between the groups (p< 0.05).

	Control	Olive oil	Olive oil + vitamin E	Camphor	Camphor + vitamin E
Testicular capsule thickness (μ)	8.82 ±1.04[a]	12.70 ±1.20[ab]	18.37 ±3.51[ab]	14.14 ±2.16[ab]	21.22 ±11.00[b]
Diameter of Seminiferous tubules (μ)	194.92 ±4.86[ab]	161.65 ±9.28[b]	219.81 ±9.07[a]	221.08 ±7.93[a]	215.93 ±10.19[a]
Thickness of the seminiferous tubular epithelium (μ)	65.77 ±4.55[ab]	64.19 ±4.32a	66.67 ±4.06[ab]	75.73 ±3.35[b]	72.09 ±3.48[ab]
Diameter of seminiferous tubules lumen (μ)	112.24 ±7.30[ab]	84.09 ±6.51[a]	98.54 ±5.26[ab]	115.85 ±11.13[b]	83.69 ±4.17[a]
Number of Sertoli (n)	18.12 ±1.09	15.25 ±0.67	15.00 ±1.10	15.50 ±1.22	18.87 ±1.46
Number of Leydig cells (n)	14.37 ±1.51	16.12 ±3.02	15.25 ±1.38	20.37 ±3.76	25.00 ±3.54
TDI (%)	82.50 ±1.61[ab]	81.25 ±1.39[a]	86.00 ±1.03[a]	79.00 ±0.70[b]	84.00 ±1.16[a]
RI (%)	69.50 ±0.82[ab]	64.00 ±1.25[b]	74.50 ±1.89[a]	73.75 ±1.39[a]	73.25 ±3.03[a]
SI (%)	79.50 ±1.93[ab]	80.50 ±1.61[a]	86.00 ±1.10[ab]	89.25 ±0.73[b]	82.00 ±3.02[ab]
Degenerative tubules (%)	1.00 ±0.26[a]	12.05 ±4.01[ab]	6.00 ±0.88[ab]	13.25 ±3.34[b]	15.50 ±3.51[b]
Antioxidant activity of serum or AOA (μmol/l)	0.813 ±0.018[a]	0.809 ±0.027[a]	0.931 ±0.013[b]	0.791 ±0.005[a]	0.837 ±0.014[a]
Malondialdehyde concentration of serum or MDA (TBARS μmol/ml)	0.295 ±0.003	0.275 ±0.007	0.299 ±0.002	0.318 ±0.004	0.314 ±0.010
Testosterone level of serum (ng/ml)	4.52 ±1.14	7.62 ±3.61	5.87 ±0.31	3.01 ±0.99	2.75 ±1.10

Table 4. Qualitative assessment of alkaline phosphatase and Sudan-black stained testicular tissues in control, control sham and treatment mice. Nos. 1-5 were used to show minimum and maximum levels of staining for alkaline phosphatase and Sudan-black staining, respectively. Other groups are shown by the stain levels 1-5.

	Control	Olive oil	Olive oil + vitamin E	Camphor	Camphor + vitamin E
Alkaline phosphatase staining	1+	3+	2+	5+	4+
Sudan-black staining	1+	4+	2+	5+	3+

idant activity of plasma was assessed using AOA method. The highest antioxidant activity was seen in combined olive oil and vitamin E group (0.931 ±0.01 mmol/l). AOA showed a significant increase in combined olive oil and vitamin E group, compared to that in other groups (p< 0.05). No significant difference was seen in other groups (p≥ 0.05) (Table 3). No significant difference was seen in lipid peroxidation in groups (p= 0.06). Minimum and maximum values of MDA were seen in control (0.295 ±0.01 μmol/l) and camphor groups (0.308 ±0.01 μmol/l), respectively (Table 3). The highest and smallest values of testosterone were seen in olive oil (7.6250 ±3.693 ng/ml) and combined camphor and vitamin E groups (2.7500 ±1.108 ng/ml), respectively. No significance was observed in serum testosterone in groups (p= 0.30) (Table 3).

Discussion

In Asian and Islamic traditional medicine, it is believed that camphor can suppress sexual excitation, especially in males. Different and sometimes contradictory reports have been published on effects of camphor on genital system (Jamshidzadeh et al., 2006; Nikravesh and Jalali, 2004; Shahabi et al., 2013). Since little information has been published on the effects of camphor, the current study included quality of sperms, histological and histochemical studies, biochemistry tests and assessment of serum testosterone in mice exposed to camphor. Furthermore, protective role of vitamin E in camphor toxicity for testis was investigated. Hydroxylation of carbons nos. 5 and 8 (or 9) results in camphor hydroxy which consequently produces ketones and carbon dioxide. This 7-carbon dioxide can conjugate glucuronic acid (Koppel et al., 1982). Glucoronic acid plays three important roles in the body: 1) Detoxification through conjugation and elimination of toxicants, 2) Transportation of hormones and other important substances by combining with and releasing materials into target tissues, and 3) Synthesis of ascorbic acid (except in primates and guinea pigs). Camphor can prevent glucoronic acid activity by connecting to it (Rabl et al., 1997). Toxic effects of camphor reported in the current study can be associated to decreased glucoronic acid and consequently reduced detoxification capacity of the body (Rabl et al., 1997). For example, increased number of degenerated seminiferous tubules can be a consequence of released toxicants produced through camphor metabolism or due to the failure of body in detoxification of other toxicants (Rabl et al., 1997). Moreover, 4-Methyl-benzylidene camphor (4-MBC), an indicator of estrogenic activity, acts as a preferential ligand of estrogen receptor and includes a direct role in differentiation of sex organs and brain in both sexes (Durrer et al., 2007). The 4-MBC affects endocrine glands which are the locations for synthesis of various hormones including sex hormones (Saleha, 2009). Camphor is suggested as a disorganizer of endocrine glands and an agonist for estrogen hormone (Caserta et al., 2008).

Spermatogenesis is a complicated process and depends on function of endocrine and paracrine hormones and interaction between spermatogenic and Sertoli cells. Studies have shown that in addition to principal regulatory hormones of spermatogenesis such as testosterone, LH and FSH, 17-β-estradiol includes an important role in regulation of reproduction in males, as absence of estrogenic receptors in mice causes termination of spermatogenesis and induces infertility (Hess, 2003). Therefore, some changes following exposure to camphor such as decreased sperm number, increased im-

mature sperms, increased epithelial thickness of seminiferous tubules and failure to releasespermatids from germinal epithelium in treatment groups seem to occur due to disordered hormone balance in the body. Decreased inner diameter of seminiferous tubules has been observed in studies on animals receiving camphor; therefore, spermatogenesis cells are suggested to be poorly differentiated (Goel et al., 1985; Leuschner, 1997; Nikravesh and Jalali, 2004). This makes two reactions occur; first, wall thickness of seminiferous tubules increases and hence their inner diameter decreases and second, released cells into lumen decrease (Wing and Christensen, 1982). Results of the current study have revealed increased seminiferous epithelium thickness, in contrast to reports by other researchers. SI index showed an increased number of tubules containing spermatids in groups that received camphor. This might be due to the failure of seminiferous tubules to release spermatids from its germinal epithelium, as shown in previous reports (Jadhav et al., 2010; Nikravesh and Jalali, 2004). In a study by Jadhav et al. in 2010, effects of camphor on motility and viability of human sperms were investigated (Jadhav et al., 2010). Results showed that camphor could play a role in prevention of pregnancy through decreasing motility and viability of sperms. In the current study, sperms decreased in groups receiving camphor; similar to those in a previous study (Jadhav et al., 2010). Furthermore, vitamin E was found to prevent camphor negative effects on sperms, to some extent. The proportion of live sperms was also decreased. Decrease in sperms can be explained by increased degenerated tubules and decreased TDI. Release of immature germ cells into lumen was seen in the current study, as reported in another study (Pereira et al., 2012).

Effects of camphor on sexual parameters may be associated to mediators affecting sympathetic system. Camphor has been shown to inhibit secretion of catecholamines through blocking nicotin-acetylcholin receptors (Park et al., 2001). Role of sympathetic and parasympathetic systems on sexual parameters in males and inhibitory effect of camphor on secretion of catecholamines support the hypothesis that camphor can change sexual parameters including quality and quantity of sperms (Janjua et al., 2004). In a study by Shahabi et al. (2013) on the effects of camphor on sexual hormones, no changes in testosterone level were seen. However, an increase in LH and a decrease in FSH were observed in groups receiving camphor (Shahabi et al., 2013). In the current study, no significant differences were seen in serum testosterone within the groups. Furthermore, camphor has been shown to include no mutant effects (Gomes-Carneiro et al., 1998; Knezevic-Vukcevic et al., 2006). No significant differences were seen in number of sperms with defective DNA.

Olive oil is rich in phytoestrogens which contain phenol compounds (Owen et al., 2000; Carrion, 2010). Several studies have shown that these compounds can decrease serum testosterone, number and motility of sperms and structural changes in main and accessory genital glands (Weber et al., 2001; Roberts et al., 2000; Najafizadeh et al., 2013). In the current study, obvious changes were seen in morphometric, histologic and histochemical characteristics in groups that received olive oil. Major changes indicated unfavorable effects of olive oil on testis and sperm parameters. In histological studies, detached spermatogenic cells inside luminal space of seminiferous tubules, increased degenerated tubules, changes in diameter, decreased RI, increased reaction to alkaline phosphatase and Sudan black staining were observed in groups which used olive oil. In summary, although the precise mechanism of camphor is not well known, continuous administration of camphor has been shown to cause histological changes in testis and spermatogenesis. Furthermore, vitamin E as an antioxidant, can slightly moderate toxicity

of camphor in immature sperms, diameter of seminiferous tubule lumen and TDI indices. Further studies are needed to describe the effects of camphor on reproductive system.

Acknowledgments

This study was supported by grants from the university of Tehran.

References

1. Anczewski, W., Dodzuik, H., Ejchart, A. (2003) Manifestation of chiral recognition of camphor enantiomers by alphacyclodextrin in longitudinal and transverse relaxation rates of the corresponding 1:2 complexes anddetermination of the orientation of the guest inside the host capsule. Chirality. 15: 654-659.

2. Barzegari, F., Mirhosseini, M. (2012) Effect of persian hogweed (*Heracleum persicum*) on the morphological changes in mice testis and the level of hormone testostrone. Razi J Med Sci. 19: 18-24.

3. Budavari, S., O'Neil, M.J., Smith, A., Heckelman, P. E., Kinneary, J.F. (1996) The Merck index, an encyclopedia of chemicals, drugs, and biologicals. (12th ed.) Merck & Co. New Jersey, USA.

4. Carrion, Y., Ntinou, M., Badal, E., Olea europaea, L. (2010) In the north mediterranean basin during the pleniglacial and the early-middle Holocene. Quat Sci Rev. 29: 952-968.

5. Caserta, D., Maranghi, L., Mantovani, A., Marci, R., Maranghi, F., Moscarini, M. (2008) Impact of endocrine disruptor chemicals in gynaecology. Hum Reprod Update. 14: 59-72.

6. Chatterjie, N., Alexander, G.J. (1986) Anticonvulsant properties of spirohydantoins derived from optical isomers of camphor. Neurochem Res. 11: 1669-1676.

7. Durrer, S., Ehnes, C., Fuetsch, M., Maerkel, K., Schlumpf, M., Lichtensteiger, W. (2007) Estrogen sensitivity of target genes and expression of nuclear receptor co-regulators in rat prostate after pre-and postnatal exposure to the ultraviolet filter 4-methylbenzylidene camphor. Environ Health Perspect. 115: 42-50.

8. Ganesh, E., Chowdhury, A., Malarvani, T., Ashok-vardhan, N. (2012) Hepatoprotective effect of Vitamin- E & C in Albino rats. Int J Adv Lif Sci. 3: 21-26.

9. Gerald, G.B., Roger, K.F., Sumner, J.Y. (2002) Drugs in Pregnancy and Lactation. (6th ed.) Lippincott Williams and Wilkins. Philadelphia, USA.

10. Goel, H.C., Singh, S., Adhikari, J.S., Rao, A.R. (1985) Radiomodifying effect of camphor on the spermatogonia of mice. Jpn J Exp Med. 55: 219-223.

11. Gomes-Carneiro, M.R., Elzenszwalb, I.F., Paumgartten, F.J. (1998) Mutagenicity testing (+/-)-camphor, 1, 8-cineole, citral, citronellal, (-)-menthol and terpineol with the Salmonella/microsome assay. Mutat Res Genet Toxicol Environ Mutagen. 416: 129-136.

12. Heneweer, M., Muusse, M., van-den-Berg, M., Sanderson, J.T. (2005) Additive estrogenic effects of mixtures of frequently used UV filters on pS2-gene transcription in MCF-7 cells. Toxicol Appl Pharm. 208: 170-177.

13. Hess, RA. (2003) Estrogen in the adult male reproductive tract: a review. Reprod Biol Endocrinol. 1: 1-14.

14. Jadhav, M.V., Sharma, R.C., Rathore, M., Gangawane, A.K. (2010) Effect of *Cinnamomum camphora* on human sperm motility and sperm viability. J Clin Res lett. 1: 1-10.

15. Jamshidzadeh, A., Sajedianfardb, J., Nekooeianc A.K., avakolia, F., Omranid, G.H. (2006) Effects of Camphor on Sexual Behaviors in Male Rats. Iran Journal of Pharmaceutical Sciences. 2: 209-214.

16. Janjua, N.R., Mogensen, B., Andersson, A.M., Petersen, J.H., Henriksen, M., Skakkebaek, N.E., Wulf, H.C. (2004) Systemic absorption of the sunscreens benzophenone-3, octylmethoxycinnamate, and 3-(4-methyl-benzylidene) camphor after whole-body topical application and reproductive hormone levels in humans. J Invest Dermatol. 123: 57-61.

17. Kalantari Hesari, A., Shahrooz, R., Ahmadi, A., Malekinejad, H., Saboory, E. (2015) Crocin prevention of anemia-induced changes in structural and functional parameters of mice testes. J Appl Biomed. 53: 213-223.

18. Kheradmand, A., Alirezaei, M., Dezfoulian, O. (2013) Cadmium-Induced Oxidative Stress in the Rat Testes: Protective Effects of Betaine. Int J Pept Res Ther. 19: 337-344.

19. Koracevic, D., Koracevic, G., Djordjevic, V, Andrejevic, S., Cosic, V. (2001) Method for the measurement of anti oxidant activity in human fluids. J Clin Pathol. 54: 356-361.

20. Knezevic-Vukcevic, J., Vukovic-Gacic, B., Stevic, T., Stanojevic, J., Nikolic, B. Simic, D. (2006) Antimutagenic effect of essential oil of sage (*Salvia officinalis* L.) and its fractions against uv-induced mutations in bacterial and yeast cells. Arch Biol Sci. 57: 163-172.

21. Koppel, C., Tenczer, J., Schirop, T., Ibe, K. (1982) Camphor poisoning - abuse of camphor as a stimulant. Arch Toxicol. 51: 101-106.

22. Lattanzi, A., Iannece, P., Vicinanza, A., Scettri, A. (2003) Renewable camphor-derived hydroperoxide: synthesis and use in the asymmetric epoxidation of allylic alcohols. Chem Commun. 12: 1440-1441.

23. Leuschner, J. (1997) Reproduction toxicity studies of D-camphor in rats and rabbits. Arzneimittel- Forschung. 47: 124-128.

24. Libelt, E.L., Shannon, M.W. (1993) Small doses, big problems: a selected review of highly toxic common medications. Pediatr Emerg Care. 9: 292-297.

25. Liu, C.H., Mishra, A.K., Tan, R.X., Tang, C., Yang, H., Shen, Y.F. (2006) Repellent and insecticidal activities of essential oils from Artemisia princeps and *Cinnamomum camphora* and their effect on seed germination of wheat and broad bean. Bioresour Technol. 97: 1969-1973.

26. Maerkel, K., Durrer, S., Henseler, M., Schlumpf, M., Lichtensteiger, W. (2007) Sexually dimorphic gene regulation in brain as a target for endocrine disrupters: Developmental exposure of rats to 4-methylbenzylidene camphor. Toxicol Appl Pharm. 218: 152-165.

27. Mokhtari, M., Sharifi, E., Moghadamnia, D.

(2007) Effect of alcoholic extract of phoenix dactylifera spathe on histological change in testis and concentrations of LH, FSH and testosterone in male rat. IJBMS. 9: 265-271.

28. Najafizadeh, P., Dehghani, F., Panjeh-Shahin, M.R., Hamzei-Taj, S. (2013) The effect of a hydro-alcoholic extract of olive fruit on reproductive argons in male sprague-dawley rat. Iran J Reprod Med. 11: 293-300.

29. Nashev, L.G., Schuster, D., Laggner, C., Sodha, S., Langer, T., Wolber, G., Odermatt, A. (2010) The UV-filter benzophenone-1 inhibits 17beta-hydroxysteroid dehydrogenase type 3: Virtual screening as a strategy to identify potential endocrine disrupting chemicals. Biochem Pharmacol. 79: 1189-1199.

30. Nikravesh, M.R., Jalali, M. (2004) The effect of camphor on the male mice reproductive system. Urol J. 4: 268-272.

31. Owen, R., Mier, W., Giacosa, A., Hull, W., Spiegelhalder, B., Bartsch, H. (2000) Identification of lignans as major components in the phenolic fraction of olive oil. Clin Chem. 46: 976-988.

32. Park, T.J., Seo, H.K., Kang, B.J., Kim, K.T. (2001) Noncompetitive inhibition by camphor of nicotinic acetylcholine receptors. Biochem Pharmacol. 61: 787-793.

33. Rabl, W., Katzgraber, F., Steinlechner, M. (1997) Camphor ingestion for abortion (case report). Forensic Sci Int. 89: 137-140.

34. Pereira, M.D.L., Rodrigues, N.V., Costa, F.G. (2012) Histomorphological evaluation of mice testis after co-exposure to lead and cadmium. Asian Pacific J Reprod. 1: 34-37.

35. Reynolds, J.E.F. (1996) Martindale, the extra pharmacopeia. (31st ed.) Royal pharmaceutical society. London, Uk.

36. Rezvanfar, M., Sadrkhanlou, R., Ahmadi, A., Shojaei-Sadee, H., Rezvanfar, M., Mohammadirad, A., Salehnia, A., Abdollahi, M. (2008) Protection of cyclophosphamide-induced toxicity in reproductive tract histology, sperm characteristics, and DNA damage by an herbal source; evidence for role of free-radical

toxic stress. Hum Exp Toxicol. 27: 901-910.

37. Rezvanfar, M., Shahverdi, A.R., Ahmadi, A., Baeeri, M., Mohammadirad, A., Abdollahi, M. (2013) Protection of cisplatin-induced spermatotoxicity, DNA damage and chromatin abnormality by selenium nano-particles. Toxicol Appl Pharmacol. 266: 356-365.

38. Roberts, D., Veeramachaneni, D.R., Schlaff, W.D., Awoniyi, C.A. (2000) Effects of chronic dietary exposure to genistein, a phytoestrogen, during various stages of development on reproductive hormones and spermatogenesis in rats. Endocrine. 13: 281-286.

39. Saleha, Y.M.A. (2009) Evaluation of camphor mutagenicity in somatic cells of pregnant rats. Asian J Biotechnol. 1: 111-117.

40. Schlumpf. M., Schmid, P., Durrer, S., Conscience, M., Maerkel, K., Henseler, M., Gruetter, M., Herzog, I., Reolon, S., Ceccatelli, R., Faass, O., Stutz, E., Jarry, H., Wuttke, W., Lichtensteiger, W. (2004) Endocrine activity and developmental toxicity of cosmetic UV filters--an update. Toxicology. 205: 113-122.

41. Shahabi, S., Jorsaraei, S.G., Moghadamnia, A., Barghi, E., Zabihi, E., Golsorkhtabar-Amiri, M., Maliji, G., Sohan-Faraji, A., Abdi-Boora, M., Ghazinejad, N., Shamsai, H. (2013) The effect of camphor on sex hormones levels in rats. Cell J (Yakhteh). 16: 231-234.

42. Weber, K., Setchell, K., Stocco, D., Lephart, E. (2001) Dietary soy-phytoestrogens decrease testosterone levels and prostate weight without altering LH, prostate 5alpha-reductase or testicular steroidogenic acute regulatory peptide levels in adult male Sprague-Dawley rats. J Endocrinol. 170: 591-599.

43. Wing, T.Y., Christensen, A.K. (1982) Morphometric studies on rat seminiferous tubules. Am J Anat. 165: 13-25.

44. Yu, S.C., Bochot, A., Bas, G.L., Chéron, M., Mahuteau, J., Grossiord, J.L., Seiller, M., Duchêne, D. (2003) Effect of camphor/cyclodextrin complexation on the stability of O/W/O multiple emulsions. Int J Pharm. 261: 1-8.

16

Analysis of DNA isolated from different oil sources: problems and solution

Nemati, Gh.[1,4]**, Shayan, P.**[2,3*]**, Kamkar, A.**[1]**, Eckert, B.**[3]**, Akhondzadeh Basti, A.**[1]**, Noori, N.**[1]**, Ashrafi Tamai, I.**[5]

[1]*Department of Food Hygiene and Quality Control, Faculty of Veterinary Medicine University of Tehran, Tehran, Iran*

[2]*Department of Parasitology, Faculty of Veterinary Medicine University of Tehran, Tehran, Iran*

[3]*Research Institute of Molecular Biological System Transfer, Tehran, Iran*

[4]*Nestlé Iran, Agriculture Service Department, Tehran, Iran*

[5]*Department of Microbiology, Faculty of Veterinary Medicine University of Tehran, Tehran, Iran*

Key words:

adulteration, genomic DNA, PCR, Soya, vegetable oils

Correspondence

Shayan, P.
Department of Parasitology,
Faculty of Veterinary Medicine
University of Tehran, Tehran,
Iran

Email: pshayan@ut.ac.ir

Abstract:

BACKGROUND: One of the major aspects of traceability in food authenticity assessment is to explore practical methods to find the origin of food. **OBJECTIVES:** The aim of the present study was to find a DNA based method for authentication and traceability of food, which are of great importance in health management. **METHODS:** Four different DNA extraction methods were applied to obtain high pure DNA in some oil samples including olive oil, sunflower, canola and soybean oil to improve the traceability. The isolated DNA was analyzed by PCR using common primer pair, derived from the region harboring 18S rRNA/5.8S rRNA genes. Extraction methods were developed based on specific binding of DNA molecules to the silica membrane (column) or resin. **RESULTS:** Our results showed that amplifiable DNA could only be extracted from olive oil in method 1, whereas the isolated DNA from other samples needed to be purified. In method 2, by pre-treating oil with PBS and subsequent precipitation with Isopropanol, the amplification of isolated DNA was observed in sunflower, crude canola and olive oil. To remove the contaminants more effectively, method 2 was combined with chloroform and resin/Isoporopanol precipitation as method 3. Interestingly, the extracted DNA from all examined oil samples could be amplified with the mentioned primers. To eliminate the disadvantages of chloroform, method 4 was set up by direct usage of lysis and binding buffer. The extracted DNA from all refined oil samples could be amplified successfully. **CONCLUSIONS:** Based on our findings, the major problem in DNA extraction from oils is the PCR inhibitors in extracted DNA, which can be resolved by the presented methods 3 and 4.

Introduction

Vegetable oils play significant roles in human consumption, chemical, pharmaceutical and cosmetic industries. The presence of various vegetable oils with a wide variety of nutritional values and difference in prices provides a potential tendency for adulteration in oil composition. Therefore the authentication and traceability of food are of great importance in health management. European Commission defines traceability as the ability to trace and follow food, feed, and ingredients through all stages of production, processing and distribution (http://ec.europa.eu/food/food/foodlaw/traceability/index_en.htm). For this purpose valid methods and gold standards must be developed.

The conventional methods for identifying the traceability of the oils are proton transfer reaction mass spectrometry (PTR-MS) (Van Ruth et. al., 2010), nuclear magnetic resonance spectroscopy (NMR) (Vigli et al., 2003), high performance liquid chromatography (HPLC) (Fasciotti et al., 2010) and gas chromatography (GC) (Burian et al., 2011). Recently, (Mossoba et al., 2017) reported a new spectroscopic method (FT-NIR spectroscopic method) for identifying the adulteration in olive oil. Temiz et al. (2017) decribed the synchronous fluorescence spectroscopy for detection of adultration in tahini. Since the chemical composition of vegetable oils may differ among seasons and growing area, the use of chemical markers for authenticity assessment of the oils can be be associated with some problems (Gimenez et al., 2010). In recent years, there has been an increasing consideration towards the application of methods based on the analysis of DNA regarding food authentication (Mafra et al., 2008), to support or complement the methods based on the chemical markers (Gimenez et al., 2010, (Uncu et al., 2017, Vietina et al. 2013, Kumar et al. 2011).

For the DNA analysis different meth-ods were developed. The first method used for DNA extraction from oil samples was based on cetyltrimethylammonium bromide (CTAB). Although this method was used in many studies (Busconi et al., 2003, Consolandi et al., 2008, Gimenez et al., 2010, Martin-lopes et al., 2008, Muzzalipo et al., 2002, Testolin et al., 2005) the purity of the extracted DNA was not very high (Nikolic et al., 2014). Therefore, some investigators have modified the CTAB method with Hexane and chloroform in order to obtain high pure DNA (Consolandi et al., 2008, Gimenez et al., 2010). Although the modified CTAB method had a better effect on the purity of extracted DNA, recently many researchers have used the DNA extraction method based on the specific binding of DNA to the silica membrane such as Nucleospin food kit (Consolandi et al., 2008), Nucleospin plant kit (Martin-Lopes et al., 2008), QIAamp DNA Stool kit (Ayed et al., 2009, Costa et al., 2010, Testolin et al., 2005) and DNeasy Plant mini kit (Testolin et al., 2005) were also used. Some studies were performed with kits based on magnetic separation method such as Wizard Magnetic Purification System for food (Breton et al., 2004, Consolandi et al., 2008, Testolin et al., 2005).

Common problems in DNA extraction from oil which nearly all previous studies showed, were the low amount and purity of DNA in oil samples. It is a routine practice to refine crude oil prior to market for human consumption. Refinement process includes physical and chemical steps. Chemical steps including degumming, neutralization, washing, bleaching and deodorization, are applied on crude oil to remove unpleasant odor and color. The oil extraction and refinement processing cause defragmentation of genomic DNA (Gryson et al., 2004). On the other hand, food samples contain some components such as polysaccharides and phenolic components which can act as inhibitors for polymerase chain reaction(Pinto et al. 2007). Taken together, the extracted DNA for different oils can be accompanied with some PCR inhibitors. In the present study, the residual genomic DNA in different oil samples were extracted with 4 DNA extraction methods in order to obtain high pure DNA to improve traceability of the oil samples.

Materials and Methods

Samples and reagents: This study included a total of seven different refined and crude vegetable oils (crude/refined sunflower oil, crude/refined canola oil, crude/refined soybean oil and refined olive oil). Refined olive oils were supplied from Etka factory (Iran-Gilan). Crude and refined (canola, soybean and sunflower) oils were supplied from Margarine factory (Iran-Tehran). The origin of the oil samples was confirmed by GC analysis at the corresponding factory. Olive leaf and soybean seeds were used as positive control for PCR analysis. All used kits (lysis buffer, Binding buffer, Wash buffer, Resine and column) were provided by research group Molecular Biological System transfer (MBST, Iran/Germany). The abovementioned buffers could be used from other commercial kits such as Quiagen as well.

DNA extraction from olive leaf and seed of soybean

For extraction of DNA from plant materials (olive leaf and soybean seed) as positive control for primer analysis, Rapid DNA isolation kit from plant material was used.

Briefly, each sample (1cm2 olive leaves and 2 embryo of soybean seed that was grounded to fine powder), was added to 1.5 ml test tube and mixed thoroughly with 300 µl lysis buffer. Sample was supplemented with 20µl proteinase K and incubated at 56 °C for 2 hours. The mixture was centrifuged for 5 minutes at 8000 x g (Eppendorf, 5810R, Germany) and the supernatant transferred into a new sterile test tube. In the next step, 540µl binding buffer was added to the solution, mixed well and incubated for 10 min at 70 °C. The mixture was centrifuged for 5 min at 8000 x g and the supernatant transferred spin column A. The column was centrifuged for 1 min at 8,000 x g. The spin column A was removed. 410µl absolute ethanol (Merck, Germany) was added to the mixture and transferred into a spin column B. The column B was centrifuged for 1 min at 8,000 x g. Subsequently, the column was washed twice by using 500 µl wash buffer. Finally, the column was centrifuged for a further 2 min at 8000 x g to remove the ethanol completely. The genomic DNA was eluted with 40µl prewarmed sterile water (70 °C).

DNA extraction method 1: This method was based on the specific binding of DNA to the silica based membrane placed in the column. For extraction of DNA from oil, one milliliter of each sample (crude/refined sunflower oil, crude/refined canola oil, crude/refined soybean oil and refined olive oil) was added to 1.5 ml test tube and mixed thoroughly with 300 µl lysis buffer. The mixture was incubated at 70 °C for 1 hour, vortexed for 1 minute and centrifuged for 5 minutes at 8000 x g (Eppendorf, 5810R, Germany). The lower phase plus interphase was transferred into a new sterile test tube. The sample was supplemented with 20 µl proteinase K and incubated at 56 °C for 20 minutes. In the next step, 540 µl binding buffer was added to the solution, mixed well and incubated for 10 min at 70 °C. After addition of 410 µl absolute ethanol (Merck, Germany) to the mixture, the mixture was transferred into a spin column. The column was centrifuged for 1 minute at 8,000 x g. Subsequently, the column was washed twice using 500 µl wash buffer. Finally, the column was centrifuged for a further 2 min at 8000 x g to remove the ethanol completely. The genomic DNA was eluted with 40µl prewarmed sterile water (70 °C).

The extracted DNA was analyzed on 1% agarose gel, visualized using ethidium bromide or SYBR green dye using UV-transilluminator. The quantity of the extracted DNA was additionally analyzed by spectrophotometer under OD260.

DNA extraction method 2: Method 1 was improved by dilution of oil using PBS and subsequently DNA precipitation using Isopropanol. For extraction of DNA from oil, 5 mL of each oil sample (crude/refined sunflower oil, crude/refined canola oil, crude/refined soybean oil and refined olive oil) was used. Briefly, five ml oil sample was diluted with 5 ml PBS (8 g of NaCl, 0.2 g of KCl, 1.44 g of Na2HPO4, 0.24 g of KH2PO4, pH 8.0 in 1000 ml aqua bidest, Merk, Germany) and 1 ml tween 80 (Merck, Germany) and incubated at 70 °C for 3 h with occasional shaking. After that, the emulsified solution was centrifuged at 4000 x g (Eppendorf, 5810-Germany) for 20 minutes. After centrifugation, 3 separated phases were observed. The top supernatant layer, which consisted of oil, was discarded carefully. The remaining two layers (middle and bottom) were transferred into a sterile 15 ml tube. The precipitation of DNA was achieved by adding of 0.1 volume of Sodi-

um Acetate (3M, pH= 5.5) and 1 volume Isopropanol (Merck, Germany), incubation at -20 °C for 20 min and subsequently centrifugation. The precipitated DNA was washed twice with 70% ethanol (Merck, Germany), re-suspended in 180 µl lysis buffer and incubated at 70 °C for 10 min. After that, 20 µl proteinase K was added to the solution and the solution was incubated for 1 h at 56 °C. Subsequently, 360µl binding buffer was added to the solution, mixed well and incubated for 10 min at 70 °C. After adding 270 µl absolute ethanol (Merck, Germany) to the solution, the mixture was transferred into a spin column. The column was washed twice with wash buffer and the DNA was eluted in 40 µl sterile double distilled water.

The extracted DNA was analyzed on 1% agarose gel, visualized using ethidium bromide or SYBR green dye using UV-transilluminator. The quantity of the extracted DNA was additionally analyzed by spectrophotometer under OD260.

DNA extraction method 3: Method 2 was improved by washing the oil suspension with chloroform and replacingthe column through the silica base resin. For extraction of DNA from oil, 5 mL of each oil sample (crude/refined sunflower oil, crude/refined canola oil, crude/refined soybean oil and refined olive oil) was used. Briefly, five ml oil sample was diluted with 5 ml PBS and 1 ml tween 80 (Merck, Germany) and incubated at 70 °C for 3 h with occasional shaking. After that, the emulsified solution was centrifuged at 4000 x g (Eppendorf, 5810-Germany) for 20 minutes. After centrifugation, 3 separated phases were observed. The top supernatant layer, which consisted of oil, was discarded carefully. The remaining two layers (middle and bottom) were washed twice with 5 ml chloroform for 5 min at

4000 x g. The top supernatant layer, which consisted of PBS solution containing DNA, was transferred into a new tube. The precipitation of DNA was achieved by adding 0.1 volume of Sodium Acetate (3M, pH= 5.5), 1 volume Isopropanol (Merck, Germany) and 60 µl resin, incubation at -20 °C for 20 min and subsequent centrifugation. The DNA precipitant was then re-suspended in 300 µl lysis buffer and 540 µl binding buffer and transferred into a sterile 1.5 ml tube and incubated at 70 °C for 10 min. After the incubation time, 410 µl absolute ethanol (Merck, Germany) and 30 µl resins was added to the same mixture and incubated in room temperature for 1 h. The former solution was centrifuged for 5 min at 8,000 x g, and the supernatant was discarded. Resins were washed twice with wash buffer and the genomic DNA was eluted with 40 µl sterile water.

The extracted DNA was analyzed on 1% agarose gel, visualized using ethidium bromide or SYBR green dye using UV-transilluminator. The quantity of the extracted DNA was additionally analyzed by spectrophotometer under OD260.

DNA extraction method 4: To avoid chloroform, the fourth method was developed. For extraction of DNA from oil, 3 ml of each oil sample (crude/refined sunflower oil, crude/refined canola oil, crude/refined soybean oil and refined olive oil) was used. Briefly, three milliliters of oil sample was diluted with 1500 µl lysis buffer and 2700 µl binding buffer and incubated at 70 °C for 3 h with occasional shaking. The solution was centrifuged for 20 min at 4000 x g (Eppendorf, 5810R, Germany). After centrifugation, 3 separated phases could be observed. The top supernatant layer, which consisted of oil, was discarded carefully. The remaining two layers (middle and bottom) were transferred into a sterile 15 ml tube. 2050 µl absolute ethanol (Merck, Germany) and 60 µl resin were added to the same mixture and incubated at room temperature for 1 h. After centrifugation, the supernatant was discarded completely. Collected resins were washed twice with wash buffer. DNA was eluted with 40 µl sterile water.

The extracted DNA was analyzed on 1% agarose gel, visualized using ethidium bromide or SYBR green dye using UV-transilluminator. The quantity of the extracted DNA was additionally analyzed by spectrophotometer under OD260.

DNA purification: In some samples, the extracted DNA was further purified. For purification of extracted DNA, 100 µl of DNA was used. A hundred micro liters of DNA sample was diluted with 200 µl of binding buffer (purification Kit). After the addtion of 150 µl absolute ethanol (Merck, Germany) to the solution, the mixture was transferred into a purification spin column. The column was washed twice with wash buffer and the DNA was eluted in 40 µl double distilled sterile water.

Polymerase chain reaction: Amplifications by PCR were carried out by 1, 2 or 5 µl of DNA solution respectively. The PCR was performed on 100 µl total volume including 1 x PCR buffer, 2.5 U Taq Polymerase (Cinagene, Iran), 2 µl of each sense and antisense primer (20 mM, MWG, Germany), 200 µM of each dATP, dTTP, dCTP and dGTP (Fermenta) and 1.5 mM MgCl2 in automated thermocycler (MWG, Germany) with the following program: 5 min incubation at 95 °C to denature double strand DNA, 35-38 cycles of 45 s at 94 °C (denaturing step), 45 s at 56-60 °C (annealing step) and 45 s at 72 °C (extension step). Finally, PCR was completed with an additional extension step for 10 min. The common primers were derived from the corresponding region harboring 18S rRNA/5.8S rRNA genes registered under accession numbers of KF767534 (from nucleotide 3466 to 3803) for sunflower, KF704394 (from nucleotide 7 to 338) for canola, FJ609734 (from nucleotide 27 to 320) for soy bean and AJ585193 (from 26 to 341) for olive. The nucleotide sequence for forward primer was 5`TGCGGAAGGAT-CATTGTCG3`and for reverse primer was 5`ATTTCGCTACGTTCTTCATCGATGC 3. The nucleotide sequences of the used primers were identical to the corresponding sequence of the mentioned genes in the genomic DNA occurring in different used oil species. The PCR products were analyzed on 1.8% agarose gel in 0.5 x TBE buffer (5.4 g Tris base, 2.75 g boric acid and 2 ml of 0.5 M EDTA, pH 8.0 in 1000 ml aqua bidest) visualized using ethidium bromide or cyber green dye using UV-transilluminator.

PCR product purification and sequence analysis: PCR products were purified from the salts and proteins using PCR purification kit. Briefly, 200 µl binding buffer was added to 100 µl PCR product solution. After adding 150 µl absolute ethanol (Merck, Germany) to the sample, the mixture was applied into the column. The column was washed twice with 500 µl washing buffer and PCR product was eluted from the column using 100 µl elution buffer. The purified PCR product was then send to Taka-pousit Company (Iran-Tehran) for sequence determination.

Results

In the present study, we extracted DNA from different vegetable oil samples using four methods. To examine the quality of primer, DNA was extracted from olive leaf and soybean and subsequently amplified successfully by common primer pair derived from the region harboring 18S rRNA/5.8S rRNA gene. First, the DNA was extracted from different mentioned oil sources using DNA extraction kit, based on the specific binding of DNA to the silica based membrane placed in the column. In this method, DNA was extracted from 1ml of each oil sample. Our experiments showed that using this method, the amplifiable DNA can be extracted from refined olive oil. The amplification was performed using common primer pair derived from 18S rRNA and 5.8S rRNA genes resulting in PCR product of 316 bp in length (Fig. 1, A and A´). The amplifiable DNA could not be extracted from sunflower oil (crude, refined), canola oil (crude, refined) and soybean oil (crude, refined) (table 1). It seems that one of the main problem in DNA extraction from oil is the purity of the extracted DNA, therefore the purity of the extracted DNA was measured by spectrophotometer and found that the amplifiable DNA extracted from olive oils had no detectable DNA amount and the amount of unamplifiable DNA extracted from above-mentioned oils were between 11.5 ± 0.2 and 17.8 ± 0.4 ng µl-1 (Table 2). Interestingly, the analysis of measured DNA on agarose gel showed no detectable DNA bands. Therefore the extracted DNA with high OD260 was first purified using DNA purification kit and subsequently amplified by PCR. Fig. 1 (part B) showed that after purification of DNA, the Sunflower DNA could be amplified by PCR. Interestingly, in such cases, the purification process could not bring the OD260 to undetectable, the DNA could also not be amplified (data not

Table 1. DNA from different oils was extracted with 4 different methods and amplified with common primer pair. - was negative in PCR, + was positive in PCR. NT: not tested sample, C: crude oil, R: refined oil.

Oil / Extraction methods	Refined Olive oil	Sunflower oil		Canola oil		Soybean oil	
		C	R	C	R	C	R
Method 1 DNA	+	-	-	-	-	-	-
Method 2 DNA	+	+	+	+	-	-	-
Method 3 DNA	+	+	+	+	+	+	+
Method 4 DNA	+	+	+	+	+	+	+

Table 2. The DNA extracted from different oils was analyzed by spectrophotometry. ND: not detected.

	Refined Olive oil	crude Sunflower oil	Refined Sunflower oil	Crude Canola oil	Refined Canola oil	Crude Soybean oil	Refined Soybean oil
Method 1 DNA (ng/µL)	ND	11.5 ± 0.2	14.2 ± 0.4	13.4 ± 0.3	17.8 ± 0.4	17.1 ± 0.5	15.3 ± 0.3
Method 2 DNA (ng/µL)	ND	ND	ND	ND	17.2 ± 0.3	16.3 ± 0.2	14.8 ± 0.4
Method 3 DNA (ng/µL)	ND	ND	ND	ND	ND	ND	ND
Method 4 DNA (ng/µL)	ND	ND	ND	ND	ND	ND	ND

shown). To reduce the inhibitory factors for DNA polymerase, the oil was first emulsified with PBS and the DNA was subsequently precipitated using Isopropanol (method 2). After this procedure, the extracted DNA from refined olive, refined/crude sunflower and crude canola oil could be successfully amplified using the mentioned primer pair (Table 1). Figure 1 (part C) showed the PCR products of 337 bp, 316 bp and 332 bp in length for refined sunflower, refined olive and crude canola oils, respectively. The extracted DNA from refined or crude soybean oil and refined canola oil could not be amplified using the mentioned primer pair (Table1). To eliminate the PCR-inhibitors from DNA extracted from soybean oil and refined canola oil, the third DNA extraction method was developed. For this aim, the oil was first emulsified with PBS and the mixture was centrifuged and after separating the top supernatant layer (oil), the mixture was washed with chloroform (method 3). Subsequently, the DNA was precipitated with Isopropanol in presence of resin. The precipitated DNA was then purified using resin Kit. Interestingly, DNA extracted from all examined vegetable oils using third method, could be amplified by PCR (Table1). Figure 1(part D) showed the PCR products of 293 bp, 337 bp, 332 bp and 316 bp in length for refined/ crude soybean oil, refined/ crude sunflower oil, refined/ crude canola oil and refined olive oil respectively. To avoid the use of chloroform, in the next experiment, we extracted DNA from all used oil samples by method 4. The amplifiable DNA could be extracted from all examined oil samples (Table1, Fig. 1, E and E´). Our results showed that the most important

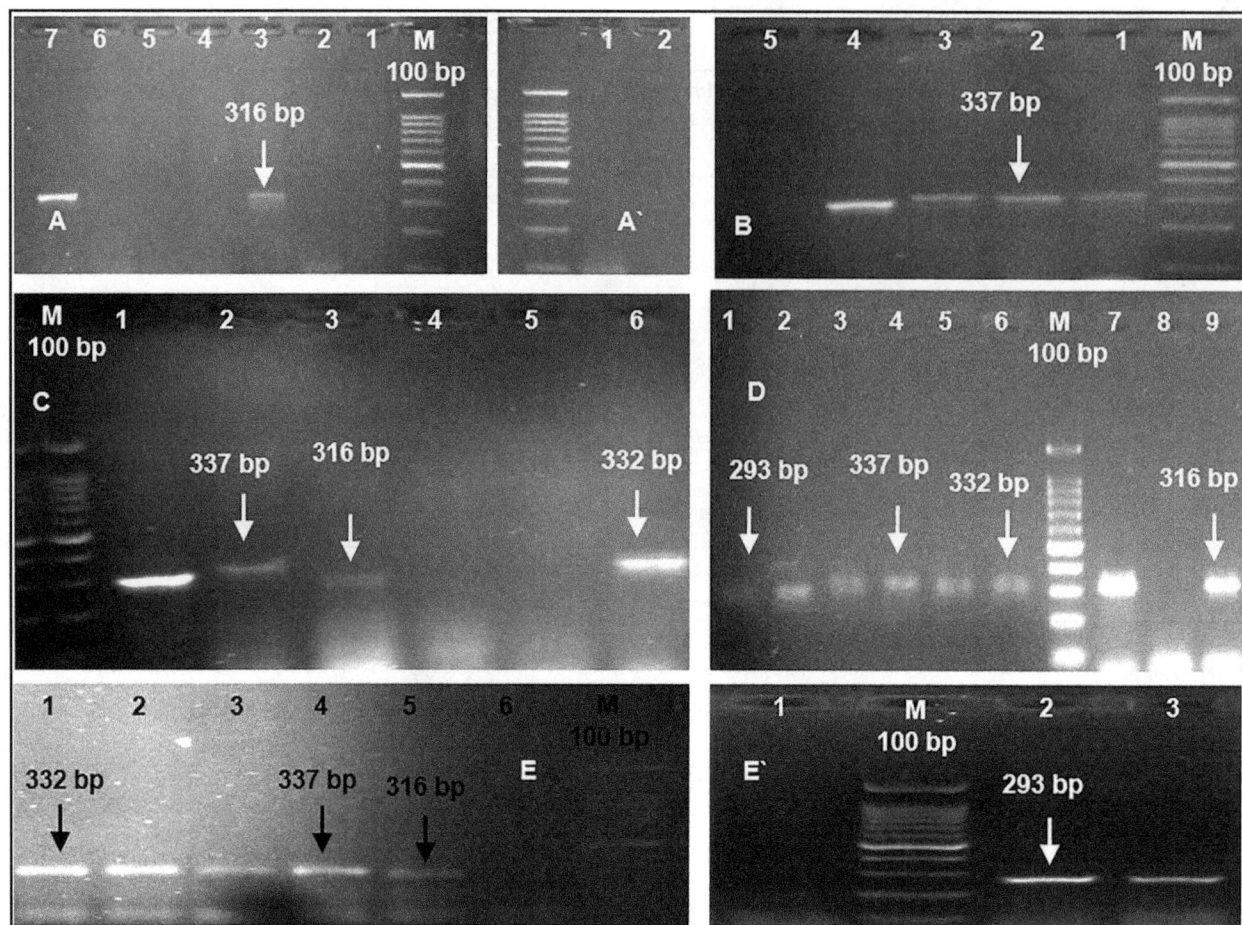

Figure 1. Agarose gel electrophoresis of PCR products achieved by amplification of DNA extracted from refined olive oil, refined/ crude canola oil, refined/ crude sunflower oil and refined/ crude soybean oil with 4 different methods. A: PCR of 0.5 μl DNA extracted with method 1 from refined (lane 2) and crude sunflower oil (lane 4), refined olive oil (lane 3), refined a (lane 5) and crude canola oil (lane 6), lane 7 was positive control (olive leaf) and lane 1 was negative control. A´ (continue method 1): from refined (lane 1) and crude soybean oil (lane 2). B: PCR of 0.5,2,5 μl DNA extracted with purification MBST kit from refined sunflower oil (lane 1, 2, 3 respectively),PCR of 0.5 μl of DNA extracted from refined olive oil(lane 4), negative control (lane 5). C: PCR of 0.5 μl DNA extracted with method 2 from crude sunflower oil (lane 2), refined olive oil (lane 3), refined (lane 4) and crude soybean oil (lane 5), crude canola oil (lane 6) and lane 1 was positive control (olive leaf). D: PCR of 0.5 μl DNA extracted with method 3 from refined (lane 1) and crude soybean oil (lane 2), refined (lane 3) and crude sunflower oil (lane4), refined (lane 5) and crude canola oil (lane 6), refined olive oil (lane 9), lane 7 was positive control (olive leaf) and lane 8 was negative control. E: PCR of 0.5 μl DNA extracted with method 4 from refined (lane 1) and crude canola oil (lane 2), refined (lane 3) and crude sunflower oil (lane 4), refined olive oil (lane 5) and lane 6 was negative control. E´ (continue method 4): from refined (lane 2) and crude soybean oil (lane 3) and lane 1 was negative control.

problem with DNA extraction from vegetable oils is the purity of extracted DNA. Sequence analysis showed 100% homology between the sequenced PCR products of canola oil and sunflower oil with corresponding sequences registered in GenBank under accession numbers KF704394 and KF767534 respectively. Additionally, we amplified successfully the extracted DNA from refined/ crude soybean oil with the primer pair derived from lectin gene (Nikolic et al. 2014) to confirm the specificity of the extracted DNA (data not shown).

Discussion

One of the major aspects of traceability in food authenticity assessment is to explore practical methods to find the origin of food through its whole production procedure. Therefore, some chemical methods such as proton transfer reaction mass spectrometry (PTR-MS) (Van Ruth et al. 2010), nuclear magnetic resonance spectroscopy (NMR) (Vigli et al. 2003), high performance liquid chromatography (HPLC) (Fasciotti et al., 2010) and gas chromatography (GC) (Burian et al., 2011) were developed. One of the most important problems of such methods is seasonal and growing area variations which can lead to the change in the chemical components of the vegetable oils. This change can affect the validity assessment of these methods. Such problems can be solved by genetic traceability analysis. It is important to emphasize that the genetic analysis alone can not be used as a gold standard method, because in some cases such as determination of the growing areas with cultivars it cannot be performed by genetic analysis. Therefore, the application of the chemical and genetic methods can complete each other and be used as gold standard methods for traceability.

Some oils such as olive oil have essentially been a topic of authenticity and traceability studies due to their high price value. Some investigators used PCR method based on microsatellite markers for identifying the single cultivar virgin olive oils (Busconi et al., 2003, Testolin et al., 2005). In recent years, many different methods have been applied to determine the suitable DNA extraction techniques (Costa et al., 2010., Gimenez et al., 2010, Nikolic et al., 2014, Pauli et al., 1998). Nicolic et al.(2014) reported that the isolated DNA from crude soybean oil by using CTAB method was not pure enough to be amplifiable by PCR (Nikolic et al., 2014). The most recommended method for the DNA extraction from oil was described as the method based on the specific binding of the DNA to silica membrane (Costa et al., 2012, Nikolic et al., 2014) which was also confirmed by the present study. The superiority of this extraction method is due to less loss of DNA in the DNA extraction compared with the CTAB method. Gimenez et al. (2010) showed the purity of DNA extraction was increased by use of CTAB method combined with hexane and chloroform extraction.

In the current study, we extracted successfully amplifiable DNA from various vegetable oil samples by methods 3 and 4. We believe that the purity of DNA extracted from vegetable oils is responsible for the successful PCR amplification. The spectrophotometric examination showed that the undetectable DNA by OD^{260} could be amplified by PCR, whereas the concentration of unamplifiable DNA was between 11.1 ± 0.2 and 17.8 ± 0.4 ng μl^{-1}. Therefore, we are of the opinion that the high measured absorbance by OD^{260} in DNA samples extracted from some oils was associated with the contaminants and not with the DNA, since the analysis of the extracted DNA with high amount of the DNA showed no detectable DNA bands by agarose gel electrophoresis.

To reduce the contaminant, the DNA was purified using PCR purification kit. Interestingly, the purification of some DNA samples lead to amplification of DNA by PCR. This means that the purity of DNA is the most critical aspect by DNA extraction methods. To obtain pure DNA from oil samples, we used method 2. With this method only the extracted DNA from olive oil, sunflower and crude canola oil could be amplified by PCR. It seems that more contaminant could be removed from the DNA samples by this method. In order to remove PCR inhibitors from different oil samples, method 3 was used. In this method chloroform as solvent of organic molecules (non DNA) was used. Interestingly, DNA extracted from all examined vegetable oils could be amplified by PCR. The absorbance of OD^{260} nm by all DNA samples extracted from different oils was not detectable. This means that the purity of DNA in the sample is decisive for amplification of DNA by PCR and not necessarily the low amount of DNA in samples. To avoid the use of chloroform in DNA extraction method, method 4 was developed. This method could also be performed successfully by all oil samples. Our results were in agreement with the results of Costa et al. (2012) regarding the low amount of DNA in vegetable oils, but we believe that the low amount of DNA is not responsible for the lack of PCR amplification. Our results support the reported results of Nicolic et al. (2014) and Costa et al.(2010) according to the importance of the purity of DNA by PCR amplification.

Our results showed that in all DNA samples extracted from different oils, DNA could be amplified with primer pairs resulting in PCR product of 293 to 337 bp. It is assumed that refining processes (chemical and mechanical steps, the deodorization phase (240 °C), acidified with phosphoric acid and neutralized with NaOH) cause DNA fragmentations (Costa et al., 2010). Therefore, some investigators used primer pairs for their study to amplify small PCR products about 150 bp in length (Costa et al., 2010, Nikolic et al., 2014). Costa et al. (2010) reported that they could amplify the DNA from oil with only primer pair giving PCR product of 103 bp in length but not those with 118 bp or 120 bp (Costa et al.

2010). Nikolic et al.(2014) recommended the use of DNA region with approximately 150 bp in length for processed food by PCR analysis (Nikolic et al., 2014). Even though in this study we were able to detect PCR product with 337 bp in length, we also follow the suggestion of Costa et al. (2010) and Nikolic et al. (2014) to amplify the small DNA region for processed food traceability because we used a multicopy DNA region (18S rRNA and 5.8S rRNA) and the others most probably used another gene with less copy number in genome.

Conclusion: Based on our findings, the major problem in DNA extraction from oils is the PCR inhibitors in extracted DNA. According to our study, the best methods for DNA extraction from oil was that method which was able to remove the PCR inhibitors. Methods 3 and 4 could be used as suitable DNA extraction methods for all oil samples.

Acknowledgements

We thank Mrs Narges Amininia and Mr. Abbas Gerami from the faculty of Veterinary Medicine for their assistance.

References

Ayed, R.B., Grati-Kamoun, N., Moreau, F., Rebaï, A. (2009) Comparative study of microsatellite profiles of DNA from oil and leave of two Tunisian olive cultivars. Eur Food Res Technol. 29: 757-762.

Breton, C., Claux, D., Metton, I., Skorski, G., Bervillé, A. (2004) Comparative study of methods for DNA preparation from olive oil samples to identify cultivar SSR alleles in commercial oil samples: possible forensic applications. J Agric Food Chem. 52: 531-537.

Busconi, M., Foroni, C., Corradi, M., Bongiorni, C., Cattapan, F., Fogher, C. (2003) DNA extraction from olive oil and its use in the identification of the production cultivar. Food Chem. 83: 127-134.

Consolandi, C., Palmieri, L., Severgnini, M., Maestri, E., Marmiroli, N., Agrimonti, C., Baldoni, L., Donini, P., De Bellis, G., Castiglioni, B. (2008) A procedure for olive oil traceability and authenticity: DNA extraction, multiplex PCR and LDR–universal array analysis. Eur Food Res Technol. 227: 1429-1438.

Costa, J., Mafra, I., Amaral, J. S., Oliveira, M. (2010) Monitoring genetically modified soybean along the industrial soybean oil extraction and refining processes by polymerase chain reaction techniques. Food Res Int. 43: 301-306.

Costa, J., Mafra, I., Amaral, J. S., Oliveira, M. B. P. (2010) Detection of genetically modified soybean DNA in refined vegetable oils. European Food Res Technol. 230: 915-923.

Costa, J., Mafra, I., Oliveira, M. (2012) Advances in vegetable oil authentication by DNA-based markers. Trends Food Sci Technol. 26: 43-55.

Fasciotti, M., Pereira Netto, A.D. (2010) Optimization and application of methods of triacylglycerol evaluation for characterization of olive oil adulteration by soybean oil with HPLC–APCI–MS–MS. Talanta. 81: 1116-1125.

Giménez, M. J., Pistón, F., Martín, A., Atienza, S. G. (2010) Application of real-time PCR on the development of molecular markers and to evaluate critical aspects for olive oil authentication. Food Chem. 118: 482-487.

Gryson, N., Messens, K., Dewettinck, K. (2004) Influence of different oil-refining parameters and sampling size on the detection of genetically modified DNA in soybean oil. J AOCS. 81: 231-234.

Kumar, S., Kahlon, T., Chaudhary, S. (2011) A rapid screening for adulterants in olive oil using DNA barcodes. Food Chem. 127: 1335-41.

Mafra, I., Ferreira, I. M., Oliveira, M. B. P. (2008) Food authentication by PCR-based methods. European Food Res Technol. 227: 649-665.

Martins-Lopes, P., Gomes, S., Santos, E., Guedes-Pinto, H. (2008) DNA markers for Portuguese olive oil fingerprinting. J Agric Food Chem. 56: 11786-11791.

Mossoba, M.M., Azizian, H., Fardin-Kia, A.R., Karunathilaka, S.R., Kramer, J.K. (2017) First application of newly developed FT-NIR spectroscopic methodology to predict authenticity of extra virgin olive oil retail products in the USA, Lipids. doi: 10.1007/s11745-017-4250-5.

Muzzalupo, I., Perri, E. (2002) Recovery and characterisation of DNA from virgin olive oil. Europ Food Res Technol. 214: 528-531.

Nikolic, Z., Vasiljevic, I., Zdjelar, G., Đordevic, V., Ignjatov, M., Jovicic, D., Miloševic, D. (2014) Detection of genetically modified soybean in crude soybean oil. Food Chem. 145: 1072-1075.

Pauli, U., Liniger, M., Zimmermann, A. (1998) Detection of DNA in soybean oil. Zeitschrift für Lebensmitteluntersuchung und-Forschung A. 207: 264-267.

Pinto, A.D., Forte, V., Guastadisegni, M.C., Martino, C., Schena, F.P., Tantillo, G. (2007) A comparison of DNA extraction methods for food analysis. Food Control. 18: 76-80.

Temiz, H.T., Tamer, U., Berkkan, A., Boyaci, I.H. (2017) Synchronous fluorescence spectroscopy for determination of tahini adulteration. Talanta. 167: 557-562.

Testolin, R., Lain, O. (2005) DNA extraction from olive oil and PCR amplification of microsatellite markers. J Food Sci. 70: C108-C112.

Uncu, A.T.,Uncu, A.O., Frary, A., Doganlar, S. (2017) Barcode DNA length polymorphisms vs fatty acid profiling for adulteration detection in olive oil. Food Chem. 221: 1026-1033.

Van Ruth, S., Villegas, B., Akkermans, W., Rozijn, M., Van der Kamp, H., Koot, A. (2010) Prediction of the identity of fats and oils by their fatty acid, triacylglycerol and volatile compositions using PLS-DA, Food Chem. 118: 948-955.

Vietina, M., Agrimonti, C., Marmiroli, N. (2013) Detection of plant oil DNA using high resolution melting (HRM) post PCR analysis: a tool for disclosure of olive oil adulteration. Food Chem. 141: 3820-6.

Vigli, G., Philippidis, A., Spyros, A., Dais, P. (2003) Classification of edible oils by employing 31P and 1H NMR spectroscopy in combination with multivariate statistical analysis. A proposal for the detection of seed oil adulteration in virgin olive oils. J Agric Food Chem. 51: 5715-5722.

17

Effects of *Aloe vera* crude extract on growth performance and some hemato-immunological indices of *Oncorhynchus mykiss* in farm scale

Alishahi, M.*, **Tulaby Dezfuly, Z., Mesbah, M., Mohammadian, T.**

Department of Clinical Sciences, Faculty of Veterinary Medicine, Shahid Chamran University of Ahvaz, Ahvaz, Iran

Key words:

Aloe vera, growth indices, hematological parameters, immune response, Rainbow trout

Correspondence

Alishahi, M.
Department of Clinical Sciences, Shahid Chamran University of Ahvaz, Ahvaz, Iran

Email: alishahim@scu.ac.ir

Abstract:

BACKGROUND: The immunostimulating effect of *Aloe vera* in mammals has been documented, but few works were done on effect of *A. vera* on fish health and immune responses. **OBJECTIVES:** In this study the effect of oral administration of *A. vera* on growth indices, hematological parameters and immune responses of rainbow trout were investigated. **METHODS:** One thousand five hundred rainbow trout fingerlings (20 ± 2 g, Mean ± SD) were divided into five groups, each in triplicate, in farm scale. Group 1 were adopted as control and fed with non-supplemented feed, groups 2 to 5 were fed with diet supplemented by 0.05%, 0.1%, 0.2% and 0.5% *A. vera* extract respectivly for 60 days. Growth indices (SGR, FCR, PWG, FER, PER and CF) were calculated in day 30 and 60. Blood samples were taken in day 60 and hematological parameters including: PCV, Hb, RBC, WBC, MCH, MCV, MCHC as well as immunological parameters including: Lysozyme and serum bactericidal activity, serum total protein and globulin were compared among the groups. **RESULTS:** Results showed that all calculated growth indices (except CF) and all mentioned immunological parameters were significantly increased in fish fed with 0.1% and 0.2% *A. vera* supplemented food (G3 and G4) compared to control group ($p<0.05$). Hematological parameters, HB, RBC, WBC and PCV showed a significant enhancement in G3 and G4 compared to control ($p<0.05$), but MCV, MCH and MCHC showed no significant changes ($p>0.05$). **CONCLUSIONS:** It can be concluded that oral administration of 0.1% and 0. 2% *A. vera* crud extract in food (G3 and G4) can improve growth indices, stimulate non-specific immune responses and affect some hematological parameters positively in rainbow trout.

Introduction

With the worldwide growth of fish production and popularity of intensive cultivation systems, fish are subjected to many diseases which lead to considerable losses and decrease in fish production (Phillip et al., 2006). The increasing pressure on the aquaculture to reduce or eliminate feed antibiotics as disease treatment or growth enhancers has initiated new research to find safe and efficient natural alternatives. This new generation of feed additives includes natural sources, particularly herbs and their essential oils and extracts (Brenes and Roura, 2010).

Immunotherapy is an approach that has been actively investigated in recent years as a method for decreasing the economical loss of diseases occurrence and increasing the overall profit of aquaculture (Chi et al., 2016; Guardiola et al., 2016). Interest in the use of immunostimulants as an alternative to the drugs, chemicals and antibiotics currently being used for fish diseases is growing because immunostimulants are inexpensive, environmentally friendly, more available in different parts of the world and enhance the innate (or non-specific) immune response which has a more important role in fish immunity (Galeotti, 1998; Sakai, 1999; Guardiola et al., 2016). So the use of immunostimulants for prevention of diseases in fish is considered an alternative and promising area (Sakai, 1999). There is a growing interest in the use of medicinal herbs as immune stimulants in aquaculture (Brenes and Roura, 2010) and the immunostimulating effects of herbal medicines in various fish species has been reported (Pugh et al., 2001). Abdy et al. (2017) showed that in comparison with traditional adjuvants such as Freund's adjuvant, *Aloe vera* gel could be used as a natural adjuvant with similar or even greater positive effects on vaccination of common carp. Herbal additives contain substances which also increase appetite and digestion (Barreto et al., 2008). Many studies have been published that confirm that the addition of plants or their extracts in the diets has a beneficial effect to improve growth parameters and protect from diseases in aquaculture (Sasmal et al., 2005; Johnson and Banerji, 2007, Sudagar

et al., 2010; Zanuzzo et al., 2017).

Aloe vera inner gel consists primarily of water and polysaccharides (pectin, cellulose, hemi cellulose, glucomannan, acemannan and mannose derivatives). Acemannan is considered as the main functional component of *Aloe vera* and is composed of a long chain of acetylated mannose (Lee et al., 2001).The physiological activity of *Aloe vera*'s polysaccharides has been widely reported. (Pugh, 2001; Tan and Vanitha, 2004). The refined polysaccharide has been shown to act as an immunostimulant, displaying adjuvant activity as well as stimulate hematopoiesis (Abdy et al., 2017).

Zanuzzo et al. (2017) found that dietary *A. vera* for 10 days prior to transport stress and infection with heat killed *Aeromonas hydrophila* either improved or prevented loss of innate immune activity in pacu (*Piaractus mesopotamicus*) after stressful handling and a bacterial infection. The results of research done by Mesbah & Mohammadian (2016) have demonstrated that the oral administration of *Aloe vera* (specifically 0.2%) in shirbot (*Barbus grypus*) compared with Echinacea can enhance some of the non-specific immune responses.

In another study the combination of methanolic extracts of herbal mix composed of *V. trifolia*, *S. crispus* and *A. vera* extracts in daily diet significantly improved growth of Oreochromis sp. juveniles and also reduced the mortalities post challenge with *S. agalactiae* (Manaf et al., 2016).

Although the immune modulatory potentials of *Aloe vera* in mammals, particularly in human and some other species have been well confirmed (Tan and Vanitha, 2004), few works were done on the effect of *Aloe vera* on fish (Kim et al., 1999; Alishahi et al., 2010). Iran has one of the highest rates of cold water fish culture in Asia and the world since 2005 and Rainbow trout is the main cultured species in Iran (FAO, 2012). So in this study the effects of Aleo vera crude extract on some growth indices, hematological and immunological parameters of *Oncorhynchus mykiss* were investigated.

Materials and Methods

Fish: One thousand five hundred rainbow trout fingerlings with average body weight of 20 ± 2 g were obtained from a rainbow trout hatchary in Chaharmahl bakhtiyari province, Iran. The experiment was done in in Cheshmeh Sarab Rainbow trout farm in the suburb of Koohrang, Chaharmahl bakhtiyari province. In order for acclimatization of fish, they were kept in farm condition prior to the beginning of the experiment for 30 days. Water quality factors were recorded during the experiment as: temperature 11±1 °C; Dissolved oxygen 8-9.5 ppm; pH 7.9-8.5, $NH_3 < 0.01$ mg/L, $NO_2 < 0.1$ mg/L.

Experimental Food preparation: The commercial Rainbow trout food (Faradaneh Co, Iran) (FFT1|:40% protein, 12% lipid, 3% fiber as, 6% moisture, 7% Ash) as a basal diet and *Aloe vera* extract (Baridj Essence Co, Iran) were mixed. For this purpose, initially granulated food was made into paste by adding distilled water to it, then 0.05, 0.1, 0.2 and 0.5% (w/w) *Aloe vera* extract was added to food and homogenized with electric mixture. Finally food was pelleted by means of a special meat grinder. This method was used for Control food without supplementation with *Aloe vera*. Prepared experimental foods were packed in nylon bags, labeled and stored at 4 °C until use.

Experimental design: Fishes were randomly divided into 5 groups (each in triplicate) and transferred into 15 pools (1.2×10m), the compositions of the feeds were as follows: Group 1: 0% *Aloe vera* as control group, Group 2: 0.05% *Aloe vera*, Group 3: 0.1% *Aloe vera*, Group 4: 0.2% *Aloe vera*, Group 5: 0.5% *Aloe vera*.

Assessment of growth performance: Percentage Weight Gain (PWG), Specific Growth Ratio (SGR), Food Conversation Ratio (FCR), Food Efficiency Rate (FER), Protein Efficiency Ratio (PER) and Condition Factor (CF) were calculated according to the following equations in day 30 and 60:

PWG (g/fish) = [Average final weight - Average initial weight] / initial weight

SGR (%/day) = [final body weight - initial body weight] × 100 / experimental period (day).

FCR = Food intake / weight gain.

FER = Body weight gain / Food intake.

PER = Body weight gain/ Total protein intake

CF = [Body weight / (Total length) 3] × 100

(All of the fish weights in top equations were calculated in gram unit).

Blood and serum sampling: At the end of experimental period, after 2 days off feeding, 20 fish from each group for biometric assay, 5 fish for hematological assay and 5 fish for immunological assay were collected from each group. Blood samples were taken from caudal vein after anesthetizing fish with MS-222 (FINQUEL, USA, Washington) by sterile syringe. Hematological parameters were measured after sampling on the same day. Remained blood samples were centrifuged (4000 rpm for 15 min), sera separated and stored at -20 °C until the desired tests were done.

Hematological assays: Hemoglobin (Hb) measurement was determined by the cianometa-haemoglobin method. Packed cell volume (PCV) was determined by centrifuging micro haematocrit in 10000g for 10 min, according to the method that was used for mammals and birds (Feldman et al., 2000). Total Red Blood Cell was calculated by Neubauer haemocytometer after diluting in Natt–Herrick solution (Thrall, 2004). Mean Corpuscular Volume (MCV), Mean Corpuscular Haematocrit (MCH) and Mean Corpuscular Haematocrit Concentration (MCHC) were calculated by using the standard formulas as follow (Thrall, 2004):

MCV (μm^3 cell^{-1}) = (Packed cell volume as percentage/RBC in millions cell mm^3)× 10

MCH (pg cell^{-1}) = (Hb in g 100 ml^{-1}/ RBC in millions cell mm^3)×10

MCHC (g 100 ml^{-1}Hct) = (Hb in g100 mL^{-1}/packed cell volume as percentage) ×100

The blood sample was diluted with Natt–Herrick solution to determine Total White Blood Cell (TWBC) by using Neubauer haemocytometer chamber, then the Total WBC was calculated by this formula (Thrall 2004):

TWBC = (total white cell counted in 9 big square + 10%) × 200

For Differential count of leukocytes, the blood smear on glass microscope slides was stained with Gimsa and one hundred WBC were calculated and the percentage of different types of leucocytes was determined following the method of Schaperclaus (Schaperclaus et al., 1991).

Immunological analysis (Serum lysozyme activity): The lysozyme activity was measured using photoelectric colorimeter equipped with attachment for turbidity measurement. A series of dilution was prepared by diluting the standard lysozyme from hen egg-white (Sigma) and mixed with Micrococcus lysodeikticus (Schroeter) (Sigma) suspension for establishing the calibration curve. Ten μl of standard solution or serum were added to 200 μl of micrococcus suspension (35 mg of Micrococcus dry powder/95 ml of 1/15 M phosphate buffer + 5.0 ml of 1M NaCl solution). The changes in the extinction were measured at 546 nm by measuring the extinction immediately after adding the solution which contained the lysozyme (start of the reaction) and after a 20 min incubation of the preparation under investigation at 40 °C (end of the reaction). The lysozyme content is determined on the basis of the calibration curve and the extinction measured (Thrall, 2004).

Serum bactericidal activity (SBA): Serum bactericidal activity was measured by the method described previously by Kajita et al. (1990) with slight modification. A. hydrophila AH04 (live, washed cells) was suspended in the 0.1% gelatin-veronal buffer (GVBC2) (pH 7.5, containing 0.5 mM ml-1 Mg2+ and 0.15 mM ml^{-1} Ca2+) to make a concentration of 1 ×10^5 cfu ml^{-1}. Serum was diluted at a ratio of 3 part buffer and 1 part serum v: v, then bacterial suspension was mixed with diluted serum and incubated for 90 min at 25 °C with shaking. 5 μl of this mixture on TSA plates in triplicate was incubated at 25 °C for 24 h. The number of viable bacteria was calculated by counting the colonies and results were reported in the form of calculated bacteria colonies.

Serum total protein and globulin measurements: Total protein and albumin concentrations were determined (Zist Shimi kit, Iran) according to Nayak et al. (2008). The albumin content was estimated spectrophotometrically using a standard kit (Glaxo, India). The globulin content was estimated by

Table 1. Results of growth indices in different groups at 30 and 60 days of experiment. (Group 1: control and groups 2 to 5 were fed with diet supplemented by 0.05%, 0.1%, 0.2% and 0.5% *A. vera* extract respectivly). Significant differences with control at level of 0.05 are marked by * sign.

	Group	PWG	SGR	FCR	FER	PER	CF
Day 30	1	71.36±8.56	0.93±0.08	1.55±0.14	64.22±9.63	1.76±0.21	1.52±0.16
	2	78.52±9	1±0.08	1.47±0.1	62.74±5	1.86±0.28	1.6±0.18
	3	93.78±13.32*	1.15±0.1*	1.22±0.13*	70.86±8.5*	2.24±0.33*	1.42±0.14
	4	100.16±14.22*	1.2±0.12*	1.14±0.12*	75.48±11.32*	2.41±0.29*	1.43±0.12
	5	83.77±11.9	1.06±0.1	1.35±0.15	61.87±9.28	2.02±0.24	1.48±0.13
Day 60	1	162.01±19.44	0.84±0.07	1.77±0.16	56.44±8.46	1.61±0.19	1.77±0.2
	2	187.07±22.44*	0.92±0.08	1.6±0.15	62.74±9.41	1.79±0.21	1.75±0.2
	3	210±25.2*	0.98±0.04*	1.41±0.09*	70.86±5*	2.02±0.11*	1.62±0.14
	4	222±31.52*	1.01±0.1*	1.32±0.13*	75.48±12.83*	2.16±0.34*	1.55±0.19
	5	181.28±20	0.9±0.03	1.61±0.08	61.87±9	1.76±0.13	1.55±0.16

Table 2. Effect of different concentration of *A. vera* on hematological parameters. (grouping is the same as Table 1). Significant differences with control at level of 0.05 are marked by * sign.

Group	PCV (%)	HB	WBC count (×10³ cell/mm3)	RBC count (×10⁶ cell/mm3)	MCV (fl)	MCH (%)	MCHC (%)
1	32.42±4.6	4.47±1.4	12.23±2.05	1.21±0.08	290.55±44.50	40.72±8.65	12.69±3.92
2	36.00±5.43	4.68±0.85	12.49±1.22	1.26±0.15	290.35±53.57	37.99±8.16	13.11±2.09
3	43.17±6.98*	5.50±1.26	13.68±1.88	1.26±0.12	322.74±46.32	43.95±9.93	12.94±2.85
4	47.33±4.48*	6.41±1.56*	15.15±1.65*	1.43±0.10*	306.18±54.48	44.75±11.13	13.48±2.77
5	39.50±7.67	5.08±1.53	13.32±2.27	1.29±0.17	293.78±67.73	37.66±12.45	12.75±2.93

subtracting the albumin content from total protein content.

Statistical analysis: Completely Randomized design was used in this study. For statistical analysis of data, SPSS version 16 software was used. Growth indices, haematological and immune parameters were analyzed using the one way ANOVA to determine the differences between the means and Duncan multiple range test was used to test the significance among the means, $p<0.05$ was accepted as significant.

Results

Growth indices: Results of growth indices are shown in Table 1. Percentage Weight Gain showed a significant difference between groups ($p<0.05$). Group fed with 0.1 and 0.2% *A. vera* showed a significant difference with other groups in the 30th day and

in the end of period, Group fed with 0.05, 0.1 and 0.2% *A. vera* had significant increase ($p<0.05$). Other growth indices except CF were significantly improved in Groups fed with 0.1 and 0.2% *A. vera* in both phases of experiment (day 30 and 60) ($p<0.05$). Condition Factor did not show any significant change among different groups over the experiment period ($p \geq 0.05$).

Hematological parameters: The results of hematological parameters are shown in Table 2. Packed cell Volume (PCV) increased significantly ($p<0.05$) in Group 3 and Group 4. In Hb measurement, white blood cell count and red blood cell count showed a significant difference in group fed with 0.2% *A. vera* supplemented feed. MCV, MCH and MCHC showed no significant differences in *A. vera* treated groups.

Immunological parameters (Lysozyme activity): The lysozyme activity in all

Table 3. Immunological parameters in experimental groups. (grouping is the same as Table 1). Significant differences with control at level of 0.05 are marked by * sign.

Group	Lysozyme activity (U/ml/min)	Bactericidal activity(cfu/plate)	Total protein (g/dl)	Total globulin (g/dl)
1	127.23±9.38	181.33±19.4	5.01±0.41	2.12±0.31
2	122.87±7.38	176.26±12.34	4.95±0.54	2.05±0.35
3	140.54±10.3*	171.5±14.41	5.85±0.62*	2.45±0.19
4	142.33±8.48*	156.63±15.6*	6.11±0.64*	3.13±0.37*
5	131.5±7.67	177.08±16.55	5.1±0.57	2.16±0.12

groups fed with *Aloe vera* is shown in Table 3. Group 3 and 4 showed a significant marked increase in lysozyme activity compared with control group.

Serum bactericidal activity: The result of serum bactericidal activity is presented in Table 3. Inactivated bacterial colony percentages enhanced significantly in group 4 (p<0.05). The other group showed increase during experiment but the differences were not statically significant (p>0.05).

Total protein and Total globulin: The levels of total protein and total globulin showed significant increase in 0.1% and 0.2% *A. vera* enriched diet compared to control group. No significant differences were seen in 0.05% and 0.5% *A. vera* enriched diet and control group (Table 3). Serum albomin level was not affected by different level of *Aloe vera* (p>0.05).

Discussion

Since rainbow trout is the only cold water species with high economic value cultured in the Iran aquaculture industry, attempts to enhance the immune response of the fish against various diseases, especially unknown diseases is increasing. Due to various reasons, specifically the hygienic, environmental and economic disadvantages of antibiotics, lack of efficient vaccine against different pathogens and more important role of non-specific immunity than specific immunity in fish, recently a strong tendency

for using the immune stimulants especially those with herbal origin has been established in the aquatic animals (Iwama, 1996; Sakai, 1999; Alishahi, 2010 and 2012).

In this study the effects of crude extract of *A. vera* on growth, immune and hematologic factors in Rainbow trout were investigated and the results showed that groups fed with food supplemented with 0.1 and 0.2% *A. vera* had positive effect on growth performance indices. The beneficial effects of *A. vera* extract seems to be dose dependent, as shown in our results, increasing the *A. vera* extract in diet up to a specific concentration (0.2%), causes the Food Conversion Ratio (FCR) to decrease, but increasing the extract in diet up to 0.5% causes declining SGR and PER and increasing FCR. Concentration of 0.5% did not induce any significant changes and it is probably because of the possible effects of *A. vera* on taste and appearance of diet.

No change in condition factor of fish in different groups indicates that no change in obesity has occurred. In other words, while total body weight has increased in groups 3 and 4 fishes were not obese. Effects of Immune-stimulants in the improvement of fish growth factors have been reported after administration of beta-glucan and bacterial LPS (Selvaraj et al., 2006), chitosan (Gopalakannan et al., 2006) Levamisole (Alvarez et al., 2006) and Ergosan (Gioacchini et al., 2008). Chi et al. (2014) reported the growth stimulation capacity of a medicinal plant, ryopteris crassirhizoma (a fern species in the genus Dryopteris), as a food additive in grass carp. Alishahi et al. (2012) reported the positive effect of Echinacea purpurea on the growth indices of rainbow trout. In fact, according to many reports, improvement in growth factors after oral administration of *A. vera* can be because of enhancement of immune response of fish (Chi et al., 2014).

Despite the increase in most of the blood factors in group fed on diet with 0.1% *A. vera*, only PCV increase was significant (p< 0.05). This result shows no effect of *A. vera* on the size and content of hemoglobin in red blood cells. Unlike warm-blooded animals, in cold-blooded animals, especially fish, blood factors are considerably affected by various environmental and external parameters such as stress, temperature, season, nutrition, etc. Thus there is not a completely fixed pattern for blood factors or immune status in fish (Iwama, 1996). But based on the results and by comparison of results of treatments with control group it can be claimed that *A. vera* extract can generally stimulate the hematopoiesis, or reduce the destruction of the blood cells by unknown mechanism. Different results about effects of immune stimulant on fish hematological parameters have been reported previously. Some researchers reported immune stimulant function on fish hematological parameters to be ineffective (Sakai, 1999); whereas conversely, the others reported changes in hematological parameters with the use of some immune stimulants such as vitamin C)Kajita, 1990; Marian, 2004). In a previous study, oral administration of *A. vera* gel in common carp led to increase in hematopoiesis (Alishahi and Abdy, 2013).

Increasing white blood cell counts can be caused by non-specific immune stimulation in fish. Since white blood cells, particularly Band T lymphocytes have a major role in the fish immune system, changing the number of these cells affected by immune stimulants seems reasonable. Many non-specific humoral immune components of fish are released by white blood cells. Increasing humoral factors were influenced by enhancing leukocytes. Increasing number of white blood cells in cases of vaccines administration and immunostimulants usage has been reported (Kajita et al., 1990, Marian, 2004; Sakai, 1999). Selvaraj et al. (2005) reported similar results after administration of ß-glucan in common carp. Increase in leukocyte numbers by using immunostimulants has been seen in other researches in various fishes (Khaksary Mahabady, 2006). Similar results were reported in tilapia, and many hematological indices including WBC count were increased under the effect of dietary *A. vera* (Gabriel et al., 2015). In contrast, although Dotta et al. (2014) reported an increase in hematocrit of Nile tilapia fed with *A. vera*, no significant increase was observed in WBC count.

Lysozyme is a valuable fish protein and one of the most important components of non-specific immunity. This enzyme destroys peptide glycan layer of gram positive bacteria and activates complement system and phagocytes (Sakai, 1999).

In this study, serum lysozyme activity levels in fish fed on concentrations of 0.1 and 0.2% *A. vera* showed a significant increase compared to control group. It seems that increasing concentration of lysozyme in blood serum in fish is related to white cell stimulation because the origin of lysozyme is leukocytes (Alvarez, 2006). Increasing lysozyme activity after administration of immune stimulants, vaccines and some probiotics in fish has been reported) Swain et al., 2006; Yuan et al., 2007). The lysozyme activity levels in Carassius auratus (Chen et al., 2003), yellow croaker (Jian and Wu, 2003) and common carp (Jian and Wu, 2004) have been enhanced after administration of herbal stimulant. Alishahi et al. (2010) reported that oral administration of *A. vera* extract in the level of 0.5% significantly increases serum Lysozyme activity in common carp.

Lower number of counted live bacteria in groups fed with 0.2% *A. vera* is than the control group means less survival of the bacteria in vitro and shows higher serum bactericidal activity. There are some similar studies that indicate the increasing serum bactericidal activity after administration of immune stimulant that matches the results of present study. In common carp enhanced serum bactericidal activity after oral administration of *A. vera* extract was reported in a study conducted by Alishahi et al. (2010), in addition Divyagnaneswari et al. (2007) in tilapia, Misra et al. (2006) in Indian major carp and Katija et al. (1990) in rainbow trout reported increase of serum bactericidal activity after administration of biological immunostimulants.

Serum total protein and globulin are a good indicator for determining the activation of immune system (Siwicki et al., 1994). The levels of total protein and Ig increased in 0.1% and 0.2% *A. vera* enriched diet compared to control group. Some herbal immunostimulants were reported to increase total protein as well as total globulin in fish (Sukumaran et al., 2016), in contrast, there are some reports which indicate lack of any influence of immunostimulant on serum proteins (Ispir and Mustafa 2005; Misra et al., 2006). The increase in serum protein content might be related to an increase of WBC and proteins like serum lysozyme, complement factors and bactericidal peptides (Misra et al., 2006).

As a general conclusion, based on these results it can be argued that the oral administration of 0.1- 0.2% concentration of the crude extract of *A. vera* improved investigated growth factors, stimulated non-specific immune and had a good effect on hematological factors.

Acknowledgments

This work was financially supported by the research council of Shahid Chamran University of Ahvaz, Ahvaz, Iran.

References

Abdy, E., Alishahi, M., Tollabi, M., Ghorbanpour, M., Mohammadian, T. (2017) Comparative effects of *Aloe vera* gel and Freund's adjuvant in vaccination of common carp (*Cyprinus carpio* L.) against *Aeromonas hydrophila*. Aquacult Int. 25: 727–742.

Alishahi, M., Abdy, E. (2013) Effects of different levels of *Aloe vera* L. extract on growth performance, hemato-immunological indices of *Cyprinus carpio* L. Iran J Vet Sci Technol 5: 33–44.

Alishahi, M., Ghorbanpour, M., Peyghan, R. (2012) Effects of *Viscum album* Linnaeus and *Nigella sativa* Linnaeus extracts on Some immune responses of Common carp *Cyprinus carpio* Linnaeus. Asian Fish Sci. 25: 15-28

Alishahi, M., Ranjbar, M.M., Ghorbanpour, M., Peyghan, R., Mesbah, M., Razijalali, M. (2010) Effects of dietary *Aloe vera* on specific and nonspecific immunity of Common carp (*Cyprinus carpio*). J Vet Res. 4: 85-91.

Alvarez-pellitero, P., Stija – Bobadilla, A., Bermuolez, R., Quiroga, M.I. (2006) Levamisole activates several innate immune factors in *Scophthalmus moximus* (Teleostei). Int J Immunopathol Pharmacol. 19: 727-738.

Barreto, M.S.R., Menten, J.F.M., Racanicci, A.M.C., Pereira, P.W.Z., Rizzo, P.V. (2008) Plant extracts used as growth promoters in broilers. Braz J Poultry Sci. 10: 109-115.

Brenes, A., Roura, E. (2010) Essential oils in poultry nutrition: Main effects and modes of action. Anim Feed Sci Tech. 158: 1-14.

Chen, X., Z. Wu, Z., Yin. J., Li, L. (2003) Effects of four species of herbs on immune function of *Carassius auratus gibelio*. J Fish Sci China. 10: 36-40.

Chi, C., Giri, S.S., Jun, J.W., Kim, H.J., Yun, S., Kim, S.G., Kim, G., Chang, S.P. (2016) Immunomodulatory effects of a bioactive compound isolated from *Dryopteris crassirhizoma* on the Grass Carp *Ctenopharyngodon idella*. J Immunol Res. 1: 1–10.

Divyagnaneswari, M.D., Christybapita, A., Dinakaran, R. (2007) Enhancement of nonspecific immunity and disease resistance in *Oreochromis mossambicus* by *Solanu mtrilobatum* leaf fractions. Fish Shellfish Immunol. 23: 249-259.

Dotta, G., de Andrade, J.I., Tavares Gonc¸ alves, E.L., Brum, A., Mattos, J.J., Maraschin, M., Martins, M.L. (2014) Leukocyte phagocytosis and lysozyme activity in Nile tilapia fed supplemented diet with natural extracts of propolis and Aloe barbadensis. Fish Shellfish Immunol. 39: 280-284.

Feldman, B.F., Zinkl, J.G., Jain, N.C. (2000) Schalm's Veterinary Hematology. (5th ed.) Lippincott Williams & Wilkins. London, UK.

Food and Agriculture Organization, FAO. (2012) FAO Statitical Yearbooks. FAO Pub.

Gabriel, N.N., Qiang, J., He, J., Ma, X.Y., Kpundeh, M.D., Xu, P. (2015) Dietary *Aloe vera* supplementation on growth performance, some haemato-biochemical parameters and

disease resistance against *Streptococcus iniae* in tilapia (GIFT). Fish Shellfish Immunol. 44: 504–514.

Galeotti, M. (1998) Some aspects of the application of immunostimulants and a critical review of methods for their evaluation. J Appl Ichthyol. 14: 189–199.

Gioacchini, G., Smith, P., Carnevali, O. (2008) Effects of Ergosan on the expression of cytokine genes in the liver of juvenile rainbow trout (*Oncorhynchus mykiss*) exposed to enteric red mouth vaccine. Vet Immunol Immunopathol. 123: 215–222

Gopalakannan, A., Arul, V. (2006) Immunomodulatory effects of dietary intake of chitin, chitosan and levamisole on the immune system of *Cyprinus carpio* and control of *Aeromonas hydrophila* infection in ponds. Aquaculture. 255: 179–187.

Guardiola, F.A., Porcino, C., Cerezuela, R., Cuesta, A., Faggio, C., Esteban, M.A. (2016) Impact of date palm fruits extracts and probiotic enriched diet on antioxidant status, innate immune response and immune-related gene expression of European seabass (*Dicentrarchus labra*), Fish Shellfish Immunol. 52: 298–308.

Ispir, U., Mustafa, D.M. (2005) A Study on the Effects of Levamisole on the Immune System of rainbow trout (*Oncorhynchus mykiss*, Walbaum). Turk J Vet Anim Sci. 29: 1169-1176.

Iwama, G., Nakanishi, T. (1996) The Fish Immune System. Chapter 3: Innate Immunity in Fish. Academic Press, London, UK.

Johnson, C., Banerji, A. (2007) Influence of extract isolated from the plant *Sesuviumportulacastrumon* Growth and Metabolism in Freshwater Teleost, *Labeo rohita* (Rohu). Fishery Tech. 44: 229-234.

Kajita, Y., Sakai, M., Atsuta, S., Kobayash, M. (1990) The immunonodulatory effects of levamisole on rainbow trout, *Oncorhynchus mykiss.* Fish Pathol. 25: 93-98.

Khaksary Mahabady, M., Ranjbar, R., Arzi, A., Papahn, A.A., Najafzadeh, H. (2006) A comparison study of effects of Echinacea extract and levamisole on phenytoin-induced cleft palate in mice. Regul Toxicol Pharmacol. 46: 163-166.

Kim, K.H., Hwang, Y.J., C. Bai, S. (1999) Resistance to *Vibrio alginolyticus* in juvenile rockfish (*Sebastes schlegeli*) fed diets containing different doses of aloe. Aquaculture. 180: 13–21.

Lee, J.K., Lee, M.K., Yun, Y.P., Kim, Y., Kim, J.S., Kim, Y.S., Kim, K., Han, S.S., Lee, C.K. (2001) Acemannan purified from *Aloe vera* induces phenotypic and functional maturation of immature dendritic cells. Int Immunopharmacol. 1: 1275–1284.

Manaf, S.R., Daud, H.M., Alimon, A.R., Mustapha, N.M., Hamdan, R.H. (2016) The Effects of *Vitex trifolia*, *Strobilanthes crispus* and *Aloe vera* herbal-mixed dietary supplementation on growth performance and disease resistance in red hybrid Tilapia (*Oreochromis* sp.), J Aquac Res Dev. 7(425), 2.

Marian, M.P. (2004) Growth and immune response of juvenile greasy groupers (Epinephelus tauvina) fed with herbal antibacterial active principle supplemented diets against Vibrio harveyi infections. Aquaculture. 237: 9-20.

Mesbah, M., Mohammadian, T. (2016) Effects of dietary *Aloe vera* and Echinacea on some nonspecific immunity in shirbot (*Barbus grypus*), Iran J Aquat Anim Health. 2: 24-36.

Misra, C.K., Das, B.K., Mukherjee, S.C., Meher, P.K. (2006) The immunomodulatory effects of tuftsin on the non-specific immune system of Indian Major carp, Labeo rohita. Fish Shellfish Immunol. 20: 728-738.

Nayak, S.K., Swain, P., Nanda, P.K., Dash, S., Shukla, S., Meher, P.K., Maiti, N.K. (2008) Effect of endotoxin on the immunity of Indian major carp, *Labeo rohita*. Fish Shellfish Immunol. 24: 394–399.

Phillip, H.K., Evans, J. J., Shoemaker, A.C., Pasnik, D.J. (2006) A vaccination and challenge model using calcein marked fish. Fish Shellfish Immunol. 20: 20-28.

Pugh, N., Ross, S.A., ElSohly, M.A., Pasco, D.S. (2001) Characterization of aloeride, a new highmolecular-weight polysaccharide from with potent immunostimulatory activity. J. Agric Food Chem. 49: 1030-1034.

Sakai, M. (1999) Current research status of fish immunostimulants. Aquaculture. 172: 63-92.

Sasmal, D., Babu, C.S., Abraham, T.J. (2005) Effect of garlic (*Allium sativum*) extract on the growth and disease resistance of Carassius auratus. Indian J Fish. 52: 207-214.

Schaperclaus, W., Kulow, H., Schreckenbach, K. (1991) Hematological and serological technique. In: Fish Disease, Oxonian Press. Kothekar, V.S. (ed.). New Delhi, India. p. 71-108.

Selvaraj, V., Sampath, K., Sekar, V. (2005) Administration of yeast glucan enhances survival and some non-specific and specific immune parameters in carp (*Cyprinus carpio*) infected with *Aeromonas hydrophila*. Fish Shellfish Immunol. 19: 293-306.

Selvaraj, V., Sampath, K., Sekar, V. (2006) Adjuvant and immunostimulatory effects of β-glucan administration in combination with lipopolysaccharide enhances survival and some immune parameters in carp challenged with *Aeromonas hydrophila*. Vet Immunol Immunopathol. 114: 15–24

Sudagar, M., Hosseinpoor, Z., Hosseini, A. (2010) The use of citric acid as attractant in diet of grand sturgeon (*Huso huso*) fry and its effects on growing factors and survival rate. AACL Bioflux. 3: 311-316.

Sukumaran, V., Park, S.C., Giri, S.S. (2016) Role

of dietary ginger Zingiber officinale in improving growth performances and immune functions of *Labeo rohita* fingerlings, Fish Shellfish Immunol. 57: 362–370.

Swain, P., Dash, S., Sahoo, P.K., Routray, P., Sahoo, S.K., Gupta, S.D., Meher, P.K., Sarangi, N. (2006) Non-specific immune parameters of brood Indian major carp *Labeo rohita* and their seasonal variations. Fish Shellfish Immunol. 22: 38-43.

Tan, B.K., Vanitha, J. (2004) Immunomodulatory and antimicrobial effects of some traditional Chinese medicinal herbs: a review. Curr Med Chem. 11: 1423–1430.

Thrall, M.A. (2004) Veterinary Hematology and Clinical Chemistry. Lippincott Williams & Wilkins, USA. p. 241, 277-288, 402.

Yuan, C., Li, D., Chen, W., Sun, F., Wu, G., Gon, Y., Tang, J., Shen, M., Han, X. (2007) Administration of a herbal immunoregulation mixture enhances some immune parameters in carp (*Cyprinus carpio*). Physiol Biochem. 33: 93- 101.

Zanuzzo, F.S., Sabioni, R.E., Montoya, L.N.F., Favero, G., Urbinati, E.C. (2017) *Aloe vera* enhances the innate immune response of pacu (*Piaractus mesopotamicus*) after transport stress and combined heat killed *Aeromonas hydrophila* infection, Fish Shellfish Immunol. 65: 198-205.

18

Radiological and histological assessment of the ossification centers of pectoral limb in quail

Alizadeh, S.[1*], Veshkini, A.[2], Rezaei, M.[1]

[1]*Department of Clinical Sciences, Faculty of Veterinary Medicine, Urmia Branch, Islamic Azad University, Urmia, Iran*

[2]*Department of Clinical Sciences, Faculty of Veterinary Medicine, Tehran Branch, Islamic Azad University, Tehran, Iran*

Key words:

histology, ossification centers, quail, radiography, wing

Correspondence

Alizadeh, S.
Department of Clinical Sciences, Faculty of Veterinary Medicine, Urmia Branch, Islamic Azad University, Urmia, Iran

Email: s_alizadeh01@yahoo.com

Abstract:

BACKGROUND: The growth and differentiation of skeletal pectoral limb girdle, wing and the ossification centers in these regions after hatching were investigated in some groups of quails. **OBJECTIVES:** The aim of this study was to determine the age of physical maturity and radiological and histological assessment of the ossification centers of pectoral limb in quail. **METHODS:** 14 quails after hatching were reared in similar and standard conditions and sampled once every 7 to 90 days. **RESULTS:** According to radiological and histological results, differentiation of the wing in quail commences with the appearance of centers of undeveloped cartilages in diaphyseal humerus, radius, and ulna at the end of 7 days, and also carpal regions at the beginning of the 14 days. The growth sequence in humerus, radius, ulna, carpus, metacarpus, and digits are observed in various stages that the high growth is related to the maximum cartilaginous activity and their ossification stages and humerus keeps its growth connection constant with the length of the whole wing skeletal, although its growth scale lessens after the 21st day. The histological results were evaluated based on prepared tissue sample from the proximal humeral portion. Lack of bone marrow was observed in the all 1st day`s tissue samples and bone marrow conformation was commenced after 7th day. The growth plate was not observed in all the samples and this issue is complementary to the information obtained from radiographic examination. **CONCLUSIONS:** According to this study, time, which could be as the completion of the ossification process and the formation of all parts of the pectoral limb girdle and wing is 70 days after hatching.

Introduction

Numerous studies have been done about the forming of the ossification centers in birds before and after hatching. There are studies about quail before hatching and embryonic period but there is no fundamental investigation on the time and place of the ossification centers after hatching while there is little information about the wing skeletal on quail (*Coturnix japonica*).

The anatomy of bird wings and the patterns related to it is widely studied (Alexander 1983, Rubin and Lanyon 1984). There have been many attempts for the analysis of the factors involved in controlling the differentiation of it (Hamilton 1961, Rayner 1979, Livezey and Zusi 2007). Most of these studies are about domestic poultry (*Gallus domesticus*) (Sullivan 1962, Koch 1973). As there is a great deal of information about the development of skeleton in *Gallus domesticus*, we can consider them to compare with the results of this study on quail. Such a comparison between the two species which have been classified under various branches of Galliformes is important (Blom and Lilja 2004).

The development of long bones in poultry from the histogenesis process of all the wing skeletal parts to the differentiation of mesenchymal cells to chondroblasts and osteoblasts are described in considerable detail (Guedes, de Abreu Manso et al. 2014).

Lansdowne's study has surveyed the differentiation of mesenchymal cells to chondroblasts and osteoblasts and the development method of cartilage and bone structure in humerus and wing skeleton considering the age of the quail embryo (Lansdown 1969).

Hogg's study that was done on *Gallus domesticus* showed the time of appearance of ossification centers after hatching in different parts of the wing skeleton (Hogg 1980).

In this study the formation process of the ossification centers in the skeletal of pectoral limb girdle and wing quail after hatching with using radiography and histology tests were investigated in all quails during different days.

Materials and Methods

This study was performed on quail (*Coturnix japonica*) after hatching. Fourteen quails (8 male and 6 female) with the age of 1 day to the end of investigation period were maintained in the same standard conditions such as diet, temperature, humidity (49%) and lighting (12:12). The assigned technique included processing the radiographic stereotype with normal radiography film. The radiography machine was Dean 44 X-Ray machine, KV 40-110 and mAs 0.1-200 and focal-film distance 100 cm.

For radiography of the specimens the lateral and VentroDorsal positions were used. Radiography was performed in the 1st and 7th days and then once at the end of the second, third, fourth, fifth, sixth, seventh, eighth, and ninth week and after the ninth week until the full maturity stage and completion of skeletogenesis, radiography of specimens was done every 14 days once. Subsequent radiography, curing periods of each cage a bird was selected randomly and was euthanized by sodium pentobarbital and for histological analysis of the ossification centers it was transmitted to laboratory of the Veterinary Faculty of Science and Research Branch of Tehran.

Along with radiology, histopathology examination was spotted for further and accurate study in this issue wherein tissue specimens were prepared and rapidly fixed in neutral buffered formalin 10%. Thereafter, conventional paraffin wax embedding technique was performed in fixed specimens. Then, the sections were cut into 5 microns thickness and were stained by Hematoxyline and Eosin (H&E) and Periodic Acid Schiff (PAS) staining methods. Study of the ossification centers on the specimens continued until 90 days after hatching.

Results

The observation of ossification time in

Table 1. The observation of ossification in the pectoral limb girdle in the radiology.

Area	Days after hatching												
	84	77	70	63	56	49	42	35	28	21	14	7	1
Scapula	+	+	+	+	+	+	+	+	+	+	+	+	-
Clavicle	+	+	+	+	+	+	+	+	+	+	+	+	-
Coracoid	+	+	+	+	+	+	+	+	+	+	+	+	-
Sternum	+	+	+	+	+	+	+	+	+	+	+	-	-

Table 2. The observation of ossification in the wing bones based on radiology.

Area	Days after hatching												
	1	7	14	21	28	35	42	49	56	63	70	77	84
Head of humerus	-	-	-	-	-	-	-+	+	+	+	+	+	+
Dorsal tubercle of humerus	-	-	-	-	-	-	-	-	-+	+	+	+	+
Venteral tubercle of humerus	-	-	-	-	-	-	-	-+	-+	+	+	+	+
Humerus	-	+	+	+	+	+	+	+	+	+	+	+	+
Venteral condyle of humerus	-	-	-	-	-	-	-	-+	-+	-+	+	+	+
Dorsal condyle of humerus	-	-	-	-	-	-	-	-+	-+	-+	+	+	+
Radius	-	+	+	+	+	+	+	+	+	+	+	+	+
Ulna	-	+	+	+	+	+	+	+	+	+	+	+	+
Radial carpal bone	-	-	-+	+	+	+	+	+	+	+	+	+	+
Ulnar carpal bone	-	-	-+	+	+	+	+	+	+	+	+	+	+
Metacarpus II	-	-	-	-	-+	-+	-+	+	+	+	+	+	+
Metacarpus III	-	+	+	+	+	+	+	+	+	+	+	+	+
Metacarpus IV	-	+	+	+	+	+	+	+	+	+	+	+	+
Proximal phalanx of digit II	-	+	+	+	+	+	+	+	+	+	+	+	+
Distal phalanx of digit II	-	+	+	+	+	+	+	+	+	+	+	+	+
Proximal phalanx of digit III	-	+	+	+	+	+	+	+	+	+	+	+	+
Distal phalanx of digit III	-	+	+	+	+	+	+	+	+	+	+	+	+
Phalanx of digit IV	-	+	+	+	+	+	+	+	+	+	+	+	+

pectoral limb girdle and sternum (Scapula, Clavicle, Coracoids, Humerus): In the first day after hatching these bones were not seen in any of the samples because they were cartilaginous and 7 days later were observed in all cases.

Sternum: It was not observed until the seventh day in all of the samples. After the 14th day, it was observed in all specimens. The beginning of ossification in the pectoral girdle is shown in Table 1.

The observation of Ossification time in the wing bones (Head of humerus): It was not observed in all of the specimens until the 35th day. It was observed at day 42 in more than 90% and after day 49 in all spec-imens.

Dorsal tubercle of humerus: In the all of specimens, ossification time was not observed until the 49th day. Instead, it was observed at day 56 in more than 90% of specimens and after the 56th day in all specimens.

Ventral tubercle of humerus: The ossification time was not seen in all of the specimens until the 42nd day wherein it was observed at day 49 in 80%, day 56 in 95% and after day 63 in all specimens.

Humerus: In the first day after hatching this bone was not observed in all of the samples because it was cartilaginous and was observed in all specimens after the 7th day.

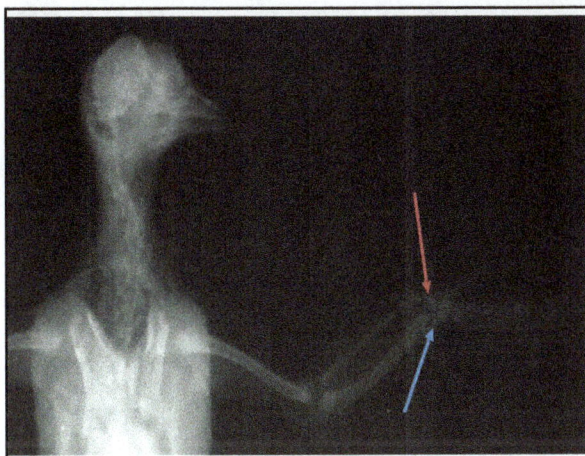

Figure 1. Radial carpal bone (Red arrow) and Ulnar carpal bone (Blue arrow) in 21st day.

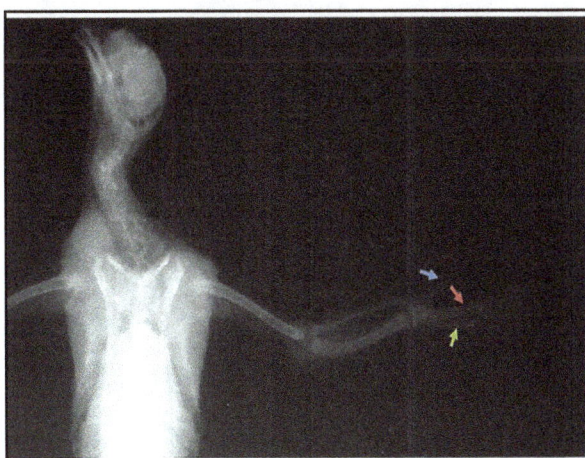

Figure 2. Metacarpal Bone: Metacarpus II (Blue arrow), Metacarpus III (Red arrow), Metacarpus IV (Green arrow) in 21st day.

Ventral condyle of humerus: In all of the samples, the ventral condyle was not observed until the 42nd day in the humerus. The ossification time at day 49 was 60% and at day 56 was 85%.

Dorsal condyle of humerus: Until the 42nd day, the dorsal condyle of humerus was not clarified in all of the specimens. It was observed at day 49 in 60%, day 56 in 85%, the 63rd day in 95%, and after the 70th day in all of the samples.

Radius: The radius was not observed after hatching in the first day in the all of samples owing to it being cartilaginous wherein it was observed in all specimens after the

7th day.

Ulna: Until the 7th day of hatching, the ulna was not seen and afterward it was detected through radiology in all of the samples.

Ulnar carpal bone: The ulnar carpal bone was not observed until the 7th day in all of the samples. Thereafter, the forenamed bone was observed in more than 95% of samples and after the 21st day in 100% of the specimens (Fig. 1).

Metacarpus II: The metacapus II was not observed in the all of samples until the 21st day. It was observed at day 28 in 50%, at day 35 in 80%, at day 42 in 95%, and after the 49th day in all of the samples.

Metacarpus III: In the first day after hatching, the metacarpus III was not determined based on radiology in all of the specimens due to cartilaginous structure and it was observed in all specimens after the 7th day.

Metacarpus IV: In all specimens, metacarpus IV was not seen in the first day after hatching because it was cartilaginous and it was observed in all specimens after day 7 (Fig. 2).

Proximal and distal phalanx of digit II: In the first day after hatching these bones were not observed in any of the samples because they were cartilaginous and after the 7th day they were observed as joined together, but after the 21st day they were separable.

Proximal and distal phalanx of digit III: The forenamed bones were not observed during the first day after hatching in all of the specimens owing to their structure which was cartilaginous, but after the 7th day they appeared as joined together. Finally, after day 21 they were recognizable.

Phalanx of digit IV: In the first day af-

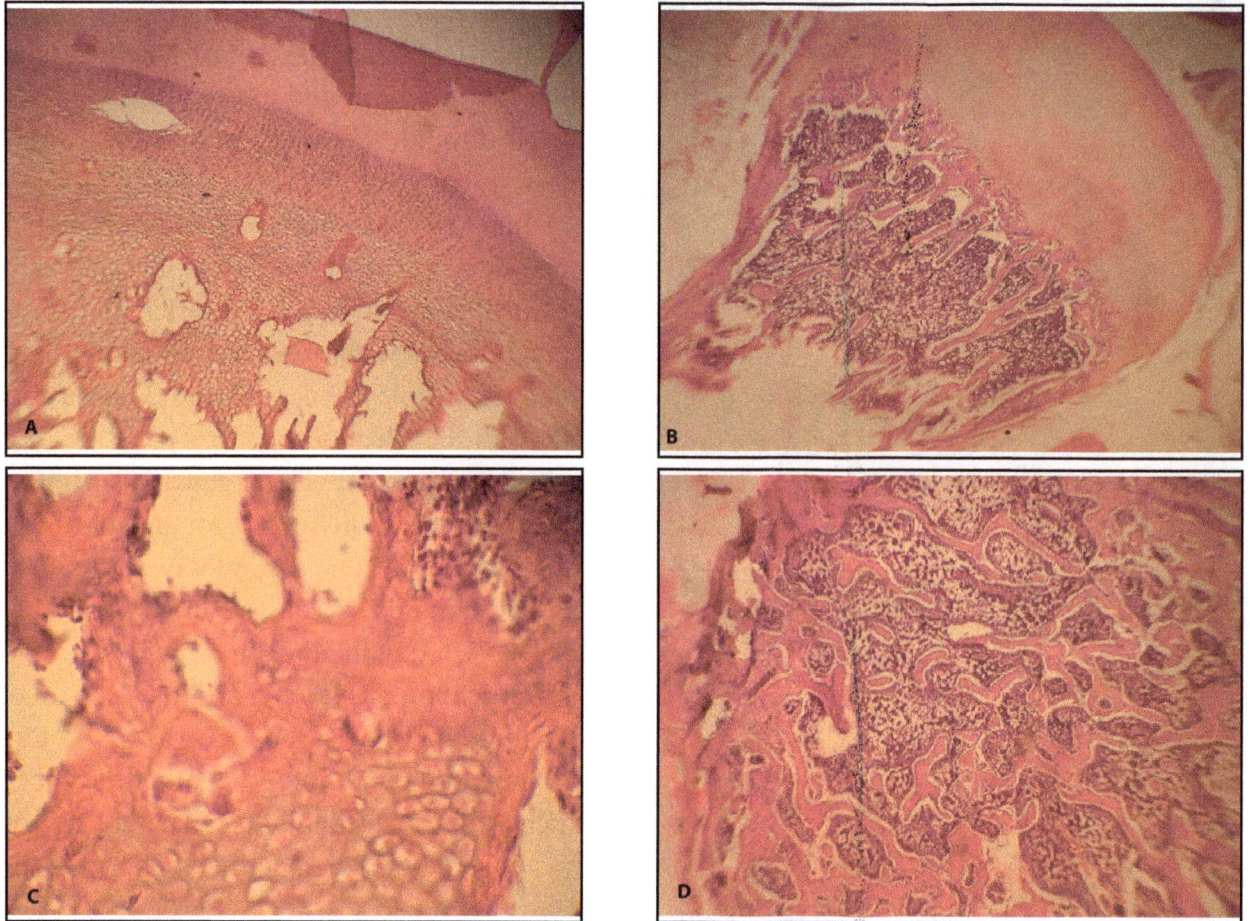

Figure 2. aFigure 3. The histological section of the proximal humerus. A. Conversion of cartilage into bone area. 21 d. B. Epiphyseal plate has been shown in this micrograph. 28 d. C. Conversion of cartilage into bone area. 42 d. D. Cancellous bone area. 56 d. (40×H&E).

ter hatching this bone was not observed in any specimen because it was cartilaginous and after day 7 it was observed as joined to proximal of digit III. After the 21st day, these two were separable. The ossification starting time of wing bones is shown in Table 2.

In the histopathology examination, the formation of bone marrow was not observed until the 7th day in all of the samples, but it was formed after day 7. Furthermore, the growth plate was not seen in all of the histopathologic samples and this issue is in accordance with radiographic examination. In addition, the bones lengthening seems to commence from epiphysis cartilage (Figs. 3, 4).

Discussion

Several studies have been performed with respect to skeletal development in the birds such as *Gallus domesticus*, (Blom and Lilja 2004, Maxwell 2008) but there is not any published evidence regarding skeletal development in quail; hence, we try to compare the development of wing skeleton in this bird with *Gallus domesticus* in this study. The general formula in digit ossification in birds is 1:2:1.(Maxwell and Larsson 2009) But the formula observed in this study was usually 2:2:1 that was observed in further studies of past researchers about chicken (Seki, Kamiyama et al. 2012). It seems that only Bellairs et al (1960) uses

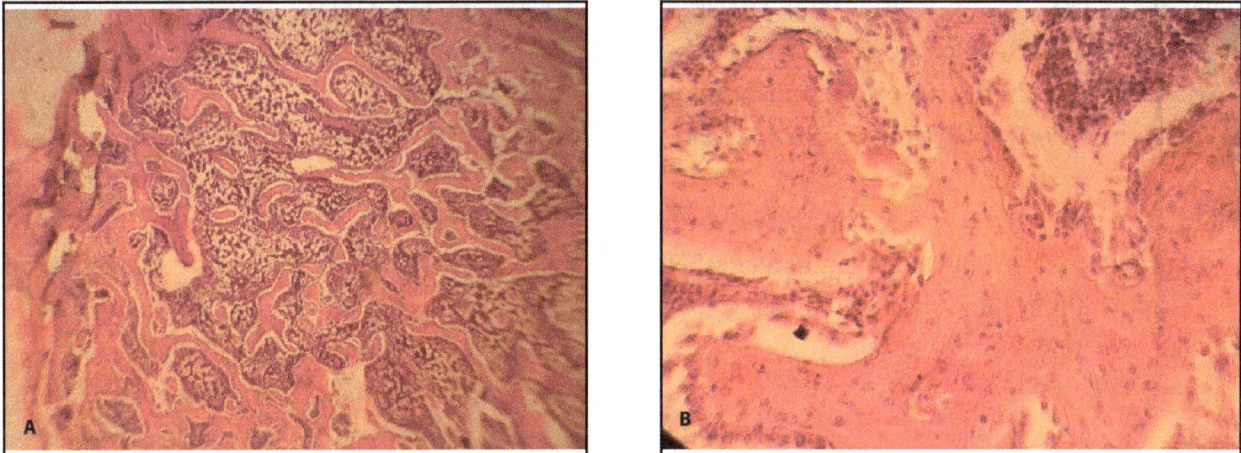

Figure 4. The histological sections of the proximal humerus. A. The cancellous bone area. B. There are a lot of active osteoblasts in this micrograph. 70 d. (40×H&E).

this formula specifically for *Gallus domesticus* and it was confirmed in few birds studied in this investigation (Bellairs and Jenkin 1960). On the other hand, the formula 2:3:2 is also discussed for *Gallus domesticus* that was not seen in the specimens of this study, although it may be mentioned for the inferior row of phalanges that exists as an extra and in the embryo but it is synthesized with the proximal row later.

For adult birds the formula 2:3:2 is also mentioned. Maybe the fuse time of the carpus and manus is after hatching which is in contrast with the findings of past researchers (Yasuda 2004). According to Schinz et al (1973) about 1 or 2 months after hatching the chicken metacarpus ossifies which is at the end of the 7th day for metacarpus III and IV and the end of the seventh week for metacarpus II in quail in all specimens (Mitgutsch, Wimmer et al. 2011).

It seems that less attention is paid to the development of the digits in birds, however, it can be said that the first center of ossification in digits area of wing skeleton in quail is about the end of the first week.

It is probable that the development of skeletal in distal portions of quail wing happens around the end of the first week with special mention of development in metacarpus, and digit area. Such a speed can have little result in the development of the carpus area.

The formation process of pectoral limb girdle and wing bones in quail (*Coturnix japonica*) and chicken have few differences but the growth pattern is similar in both. In this study, the ossification of the long bones of the wing was begun after the 7th day and the ossification was finished at the end of the 63rd day. The growth plate was not observed in the pectoral limb girdle and wing bones. According to this study it seems time, which could be as the completion of the ossification process and the formation of all parts of the pectoral limb girdle and wing is 70 days after hatching.

Acknowledgments

This study was supported by Faculty of Veterinary Medicine, Urmia Branch, Islamic Azad University, Urmia, Iran.

References

Alexander, R. (1983) Allometry of the leg bones of moas (Dinornithes) and other birds. J Zool. 200: 215-231.

Bellaairs, A.D'A., Jenkin, C.R. (1990) The skeleton of birds. In: Biology and Comparative Physiology of Birds. New York and London Academic Press. New York, USA. 52: 241-255.

Blom, J., Lilja C. (2004) A comparative study of growth, skeletal development and eggshell composition in some species of birds. J Zool. 262: 361-369.

Guedes, P.T., De Abreu Manso, P.P., Caputo, L.F.G., Cotta-Pereira, G., Pelajo-Machado, M. (2014) Histological analyses demonstrate the temporary contribution of yolk sac, liver, and bone marrow to hematopoiesis during chicken development. Plos one. 9: e90975.

Hamilton, T. (1961) The adaptive significances of intraspecific trends of variation in wing length and body size among bird species. Evolution. 15: 180-195.

Hogg, D.a. (1980) A re-investigation of the centres of ossification in the avian skeleton at and after hatching. J Anat. 130: 725-743.

Lansdown, A.B.G. (1969) An investigation of the development of the wing skeleton in the quail (Coturnix c. japonica). J Anat. 105: 103-114.

Livezey, B.C., Zusi, R.L. (2007) Higher-order phylogeny of modern birds (Theropoda, Aves: Neornithes) based on comparative anatomy. II. Analysis and discussion. Zool J Linn Soc. 149: 1-95.

Maxwell, E.E. (2008) Comparative embryonic development of the skeleton of the domestic turkey (*Meleagris gallopavo*) and other galliform birds. Zoology. 111: 242-257.

Maxwell, E.E., Larsson, H.C. (2009) Comparative ossification sequence and skeletal development of the postcranium of palaeognathous birds. Zool J Linn Soc. 157: 169-196.

Mitgutsch, C., Wimmer, C., Sánchez-Villagra, M.R., Hahnloser, R., Schneider, R.A. (2011) Timing of ossification in duck, quail, and zebra finch: intraspecific variation, heterochronies, and life history evolution. Zool Sci. 28: 491-500.

Rayner, J.M.V. (1979) A vortex theory of animal flight. Part 2. The forward flight of birds. J Fluid Mech. 91: 731-763.

Rubin, C.T., Lanyon, L. (1984) Regulation of bone formation by applied dynamic loads. J Bone Joint Surg Am. 66: 397-402.

Seki, R., Kamiyama, N., Tadokoro, A., Nomura, N., Tsuihiji, T., Manabe, M., Tamura, K. (2012) Evolutionary and developmental aspects of avian-specific traits in limb skeletal pattern. Zoolog Sci. 29: 631-644.

Koch, T. (1973) Anatomy of the chicken and domestic birds. Zoolog Sci. 22: 201-215.

Sullivan, G. (1962) Anatomy and embryology of the wing musculature of the domestic fowl (Gallus). Aust J Zool. 10: 458-518.

Yasuda, M. (2004) The anatomical atlas of Gallus, University of Tokyo Press. Tokyo, Japan. 2: 556-580.

19

Cecal cannulation in horse; an experimental study

Safaee Firouzabadi, M.S.[1], Haji Hajikolaei, M.R.[1*], Baniadam, A.[1], Ghadrdan Mashhadi, A.R.[1], Ghorbanpoor, M.[2]

[1]*Department of Clinical Sciences, Faculty of Veterinary Medicine, Shahid Chamran University of Ahvaz, Ahvaz, Iran*

[2]*Department of Pathobiology, Faculty of Veterinary Medicine, Shahid Chamran University of Ahvaz, Ahvaz, Iran*

Key words:

cannulation, cecum, emergency, horse, surgery

Correspondence

Haji Hajikolaei, M.R.
Department of Clinical Sciences, Faculty of Veterinary Medicine, Shahid Chamran University of Ahvaz, Ahvaz, Iran

Email: mhajih@scu.ac.ir

Abstract:

BACKGROUND: In order to analyze the cecum-colon ecosystem and the treatment of the cecal impaction and hindgut acidosis, cecal cannulation is needed. It is essential to select a simple, fast and inexpensive cecal cannulation method. Because of different complications in general anesthesia, the standing surgery is known as a better option for the horse emergency surgery. **OBJECTIVES:** The objective of the present study was to design a simple, fast and inexpensive cecal cannulation method in standing horses. **METHODS:** For this purpose, at first a cannula with approximately 7cm, 2cm and 2.6cm in length, internal and external diameters, respectively was designed. Immediately before the standing surgery, the horses were sedated with xylazine (1mg/kg) and morphine (0.3 mg/kg). After incising the subcutaneous tissue, the external abdominal oblique, internal abdominal oblique and transverse abdominis muscles were opened by grid incision. The peritoneum was bluntly perforated and the abdomen was exposed. The muscles were separated only enough to permit one hand to enter the abdomen. The cecum was readily identified by palpation of the cecal base and the dorsoventrally oriented tenia. At this stage, a purse string was secured on the serosal surface of the cecum by nylon and a stab incision was made. Then the cannula was inserted into the cecum and the suture was tightened. **RESULTS:** The surgery was successfully performed for all horses, however, some complications such as increasing body temperature, transient signs of colic, ileus, pneumoperitoneum, subcutaneous emphysema and necrosis of the borders of the skin in the sutural places were detected. All complications were alleviated by proper nursing management. **CONCLUSIONS:** The surgical method was successfully terminated. Therefore, the method is recommended as a simple and inexpensive emergency surgical method for cecum in order to conduct different investigation, diagnosis and treatment techniques.

Introduction

It is essential to understand and describe the feed degradation mechanisms in the equine digestive system in general, and in the hindgut ecosystem in particular. The cecum-colon ecosystem is very important for analysis or investigation of the nutritional status of the horse. Besides, the importance of this ecosystem has not been fully investigated yet, and few studies have focused on deeply on the effect of the hindgut microbial population on the nitrogen and energy requirements of the horse (Santos et al., 2010). However, there are some studies about the performance of the cecal cannulation in horses related to different nutritional, physiologic or pharmacologic aspects which require sampling of cecal contents. Cecal disorders and ingesta movements within the equine cecum have been monitored by endoscopy through a cecal fistula (Boyd, 1988).

The pathogenesis of the cecal dysfunction is not determined and it is multifactorial. As a result, a singular treatment of the cecal dysfunction is often treated by bypass procedures after the initial disease identification. However, because of the decreased prognosis and increased cost caused by the bypass procedure of the caecum, this procedure should be retained and used only for the chronic cecal impactions, reiterated laparotomies and evidence of chronic leakage. The first time dysfunction cases with no prior history of chronic colic, seem to have a good prognosis with typhlotomy alone as many horses appear to get back normal function (Roberts and Sloned, 2000).

General anesthesia has some drawbacks and it is more costly. In the anesthetized horses, the shifts of the muscle planes and difficult anesthetic recovery may lead to the dehiscence of the stoma which is created by the surgery. Today, the available drugs for standing chemical restraint have made standing surgery a better option than it was before. Most of the standing surgery procedures are originally described (Beard et al., 2014). The purpose of this report is to present a simple, fast and inexpensive cecal cannulation method, as a new emergency surgery method, in standing horses to study the effects of dietary change from hay to concentrate on biochemical parameters of blood, cecum and cecal bacterial population.

Materials and Methods

Designed cannula: The cannula with retaining flanges and caps (Fig. 1) is a modification of the Simmons design and is manufactured from sticks of an acetyl homopolymer plastic (Simmons and Ford, 1988). The research was performed in winter 2016 at the hospital of veterinary medicine, Shahid Chamran University of Ahvaz, Ahvaz, Iran.

The length of the designed cannula was approximately 7cm and its internal and external diameters were 2cm and 2.6cm respectively. In order to prevent the necrosis and crush of the cecal base, while it was placed between the convex part and the screw holder, the part of the cannula which was entered into the cecum was built in a convex shape. For the maintenance and the tuning of the screw holders in all of the external surface of the cannula, small threads having 1mm diameter, where lathed on it. In order to consolidate the internal screw holder on the cecum and the external screw holder on the skin by some retentive stitches, small holes were created in the screw holders. In order to prevent the leakage of the cecal discharges from its external part, a screw cap was used. This cap was made from the plastic with an external diameter, internal diameter and length 2.5cm, 2cm

Table 1. Surgical complications in each horse.

	Post surgery fever	Colic and ileus	Pneumoperito-neum	Subcutaneous Emphysema	Necrosis of the skin borders	Accumulation of granulation tissues
Horse1	_	_	+	+	_	+
Horse2	+	_	_	+	_	+
Horse3	+	_	_	+	_	+
Horse4	-	+	_	+	+	_

Table 2. Temperature in each horse.

Day / N. Horse	0	1	2	3	4	5	6
1	37.4	38.1	38.2	38.1	38	38	38.1
2	38	40	40.5	40.2	40	39	38.3
3	38	39.9	40.5	40.3	40	39.1	38.2
4	37.7	38.1	38.2	38	38	37.9	38

Table 3. Heart rate/min in each horse.

Day / N. Horse	0	1	2	3	4	5	6
1	36	39	45	42	40	39	37
2	40	45	49	45	43	41	39
3	43	46	50	48	46	44	42
4	38	40	44	43	40	38	38

Table 4. Respiratory rate /min in each horse.

Day / N. Horse	0	1	2	3	4	5	6
1	13	16	18	17	15	14	14
2	16	17	22	20	20	18	17
3	14	16	19	18	16	16	15
4	15	16	18	17	17	15	15

and 2.5cm respectively. In order to prevent the inflammatory reactions, the whole surface of the cannula which was directly connected to the body tissues was smoothed.

Animals: Four healthy Iranian horses (Stallion) with the average age of 10 years (range 7 to 13 years) and with a mean BW of 290 kg (range 270 to 320 kg) were used in this study. Horses were housed individually in box stalls. Alfalfa and water were available at all times and 1.5 kg of barley was offered to them twice daily. Feeding was withheld for 18 h prior to the surgery.

Surgical procedure: After shaving, a povidone iodine surgical scrub was used to aseptically prepare the right paralumbar fossa. Before draping, skin and flank muscles at the surgical site were desensitized by an inverted L block using 40 to 50 mL of 1% lidocaine per horse. Immediately before the standing surgery, horses were sedated with 1mg/kg of xylazine and 0.3 mg/kg of morphine intravenously (Smith, B.P., 2015). After draping, a skin incision was made from the middle of the last rib to the tuber coxa, beginning 5 cm ventral to the transverse process of the lumbar vertebrae extending for 10 to 15 cm. After incising the subcutaneous tissue, the external abdominal oblique, internal abdominal oblique and transverse abdominis muscles were opened by grid incision. The peritoneum was bluntly perforated and the abdomen was exposed. The muscles were separated only enough to permit one hand to enter the abdomen. The cecum was readily identified by palpation of the cecal base and the dorsoventrally oriented tenia (Fig. 2). At this stage, a purse string was secured on the serosal surface of the cecum by nylon suture 1 and a stab incision was made. Then the cannula was inserted into the cecum and the suture was tightened (Fig. 3). The first screw keeper was placed on the cannula and a few simple interrupted sutures were used for fixation of cecum to the holes of screw keeper. Then, the second screw keeper was placed on the cannula and a few simple sutures were used for fixation of skin to the holes of second screw keeper. The remaining incised skin was sutured by the simple pattern using nylon suture 1 (Fig. 4). The total duration of the surgery was 30 minutes for each horse. The vital signs of the horses were examined and recorded every day for the first few days after each surgical procedure. The existence of the clinical signs such as colic and fever was monitored and dictated with a specific monitoring interval. The intervals between the examinations were gradually extended as the horses were stabilized after the surgery until they were being monitored at 24-h intervals at the end of the first month after the surgery.

Medications: Immediately after the surgery, horses were intramuscularly injected procaine penicillin and dihydro-streptomycin b.i.d. at a dosage of 20000 IU/kg B.W for 7 days. Flunixin meglumine was injected at a dosage of 1.1 mg/kg intravenously, immediately after the surgery and continued for 5 days (Constable, 2017). Horses that required tranquilization for the surgical preparation were injected 0.05mg/kg of acepromazine intravenously (Smith, B. P. (2015). Antiseptic solutions (povidone-iodine 2%) were used to clean and wipe around the cannula and nitrofurazone ointment was applied around the wound for the skin protection.

Results

Surgical complications, temperature, respiratory and heart rate of 4 horses are shown in Table I to IV, respectively. The average temperature of the body of the horses before the surgery was 37.7 °C. Two horses became febrile (temperature >38.2°C), within 5 days after the surgery, which was attributed to inflammation at the surgical site (Table II).

One of the horses became recumbent with signs of colic and ileus (in physical examination) in the second day after the surgery. Oral fluids and electrolytes, three liters of mineral oil (paraffin) with a nasogastric tube, flunixin meglumine (1.1mg/kg, intravenously) for analgesia, solution of metoclopramide 0.3mg/kg in one liter of normal saline (infused over 30 min), were administrated. Eventually, the peristaltic and cecal movements were returned to normal.

After the surgery, pneumoperitoneum occurred in one of the horses. After sealing the skin, it recovered after 24 h.

Twelve hours after the surgery, subcutaneous emphysema was observed in all

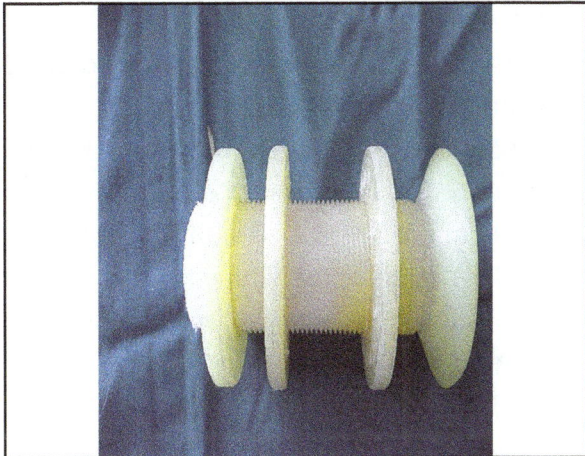

Figure 1. The cannula with retaining flanges and caps.

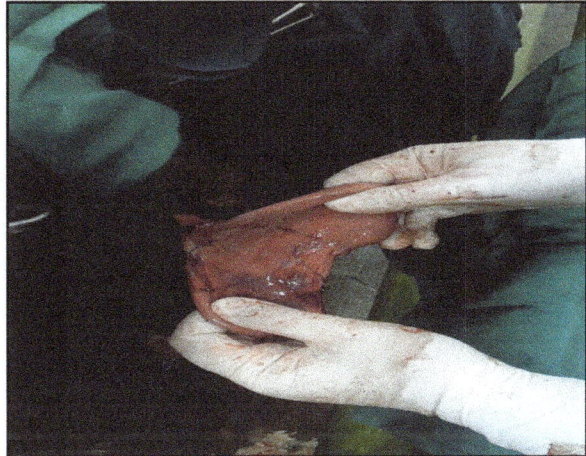

Figure 2. Identification of the cecum by palpation of the cecal base and the dorsoventrally oriented tenia.

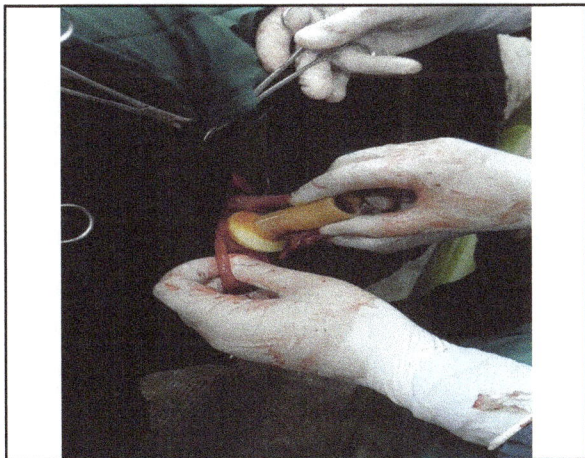

Figure 3. Insertion of the cannula into the cecum.

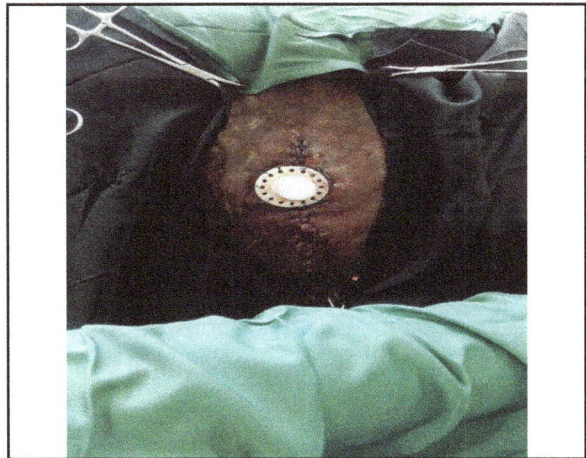

Figure 4. The cannula in place after fixation suture to the skin.

horses and continued up to 8 days after the surgery. It was soft and painless but was relieved spontaneously.

Excessive granulation tissue around the cannula caused opening of the skin sutures in two horses. To solve this problem, the edges of the wounds were refreshed and sutured again after granulation tissue excision. Fourteen days after the surgery, accumulation of the granulation tissue near the cannula caused error in sampling cecum secretion. To avoid this complication, the granulation tissue was removed by scalpel and normal saline solution substituted for povidone-iodine 2%.

Two months later, the cannula was re-moved by releasing the peripheral adhesions by similar anesthesia protocol in standing horses. The fistula was formed around the cannula. In this fistula, drains were placed to discharge secretions. Three weeks later, the healing of this fistula occurred by daily washing with normal saline. The health of the horses was followed after 8 months (at the time of writing the present article) of the second surgery. As a result, all of them are healthy and do not have any problem.

Discussion

In this experience, a fast method for cecal cannulation in standing horses was demonstrated. This method is similar to one of the reports (Beard et al., 2014) and differs from the other previous methods (Jasper and Cupps, 1950; Simmons and Ford, 1988). General anesthesia is more costly. Besides, the requirement for equipment and recovery facilities for the general anesthesia limits the location in which the procedure can be safely performed (Beard et al., 2014). Therefore, for sedation and analgesia of the standing horses, xylazine and morphine were utilized for the emergency surgery. One study revealed that the majority of after-hours equine admissions to a university hospital referral require medical intervention and are mostly due to the gastrointestinal disorders. Information resulted from this study can be used in emergency referral planning (Viljoen et al., 2009).

Post-operative ileus occurred in horses. Ileus can directly develop from diseases involving the digestive system, or it can be the result of diseases in other body systems, such as trauma to retroperitoneal structures or irritation of the peritoneum. Shock, electrolyte imbalances, hypoalbuminemia, peritonitis, endotoxemia, distension, ischemia or inflammation of the intestinal tract have all been implicated as contributing to the pathophysiology of ileus in the horse (Adams, 1988).

Because of having an antagonistic effect on dopaminergic DA2 receptors, metoclopramide prevents the inhibitory effect of dopamine on gastrointestinal smooth muscle. The prokinetic capacity of metoclopramide appears substantial, but its potential side effects, for clinical use, have to be considered. Unfortunately, horses showed transient excitement after the administration of metoclopramide. There are similar side effects such as sweating, excitement, and restlessness in humans (Koenig and Cote,

2006).

In diseases in which there is a leakage of air from the lungs or airways into the subcutaneous space, the subcutaneous emphysema can occur. The etiology of subcutaneous emphysema is varied . It could be resulted from the air entering through a cutaneous wound made surgically or accidentally. Treatment of subcutaneous emphysema is clinically important. Because, the disease can lead to a life-threatening pneumothorax if the pressure is great enough to migrate through the mediastinum into the pleural cavity. Similar to this experience, this complication successfully responded to the treatment with penicillin and antitetanic serum. This way, the subcutaneous emphysema was completely recovered within a week of treatment (Ghanem and Abdel-Galil, 2011).

Accumulation of granulation tissue near the cannula was removed by scalpel. One study showed that, wound healing of surgical resection of hyper granulation tissue was faster than the non-surgical resection. For example, the mean time of wound healing was 25 days in non-surgical removal of hypergranulation tissue subgroup while it was 20 days in surgical one (Bader and Eesa, 2011).

Closure of this fistula is resulted from the daily washing with normal saline. Cleaning is a vital part of the wound management. However, there are few studies that inform the development of protocols. Research has revealed that the use of antiseptic solutions may compromise the healing process and, as a result, the use of normal saline as a cleaning solution is widely recommended (Fernandez et al., 2001).

It seems that the technique described in this report is easy, fast and affordable. The application of this procedure is recommended to cannulate the cecum for emergency goals and any other diagnostic, therapeutic and researchable plans. Eventually, the success of the surgery and post-operative survival horses as noted in the results, is directly associated with wound management and nursing services. Although this study was conducted in healthy horses, because of the difference in sensitivity and even anatomical differences between horses with digestive disorders, especially colic and healthy horses, it is recommended that this method should be used in horses suffering from colic to be better measured.

Acknowledgments

The authors would like to acknowledge the research vice chancellors of Shahid Chamran University of Ahvaz for financial support.

References

Adams, S.B. (1988) Recognition and management of ileus. Vet Clin North Am Equine Pract. 4: 91–104.

Bader, O. A., Eesa, M. J. (2011) Treatment of hyper-granulated limb wounds in horses, Iraq. J Vet Sci. 25: 71-80.

Beard, W. L., Slough, T. L., Gonkel, C. D (2014) Technical note: A two-stage cecal cannulation technique in standing horses. J Anim Sci. 89: 2425–2429.

Boyd, J.S. (1988) Endoscopic observations of the effect of number of spasmolytic and analgesic drugs on equine caecal motility. Vet Anaesth Analg. 15: 17–38.

Constable, P.D., Hinchcliff, K.W., Done, H.S., Grunberg, W. (2017) Veterinary Medicine. (11th ed). Elsevier. China. p. 233.

Fernandez, R., Griffiths, R., Ussia, C. (2001) Wound cleansing: which solution, what technique? Primary Intention. 9: 51-58.

Ghanem, M., Abdel-Galil, S.A. (2011) Subcutaneous emphysema in equine due to different etiology with successful treatment protocols, Benha Vet Med J. 22: 185-192.

Jasper, D. E., Cupps, P. T. (1950) Cecostomy in the horse; a practical experimental procedure. J Am Vet Med Assoc. 117: 456–458.

Koenig, J., Cote, N. (2006) Equine gastrointestinal motility — ileus and pharmacological modification. Can Vet J. 47: 551–559.

Roberts, C. T., Sloned, E. (2000) Cecal impactions managed surgically by typhlotomy in 10cases (1988-1 998). Equine Vet J Suppl.32: 74-76.

Santos, A. S., Rodrigues, M. A. M., Bessa, R. J. B., Ferreira, L. M., Martin-Rosset, W. (2010) Understanding the equine cecum-colon ecosystem: current knowledge and future perspectives, Anim. 5: 48–56.

Simmons, H. A., Ford, E. J. (1988) Multiple cannulation of the large intestine of the horse. Br Vet J. 144: 449–454.

Smith, B.P. (2015) Large Animal Internal Medicine. In: Diseases of the Alimentary Tract. L. Hall, T. (5th ed.). Elsevier. USA. p. 723- 727.

Viljoen, A., Saulez, M. N., Donnellan, C. M., Bester, L., Gummow, B. (2009) After-hours equine emergency admissions at a university referral hospital (1998–2007): Causes and interventions. J S Afr Vet Assoc. 80: 169-173.

20

The effects of prolonged azathioprine administration on blood cells, lymphocytes and immunoglobulins of Iranian mixed-breed dogs

Hassankhani, M.[1], Aldavood, S.J.[1*], Khosravi, A.[2], Sasani, F.[3], Masoudifard, M.[4], Ansari, F.[5], Taheri, M.[6]

[1]Department of Small Animal Internal Medicine, Faculty of Veterinary Medicine, University of Tehran, Tehran, Iran

[2]Department of Microbiology, Faculty of Veterinary Medicine, University of Tehran, Tehran, Iran

[3]Department of Pathology, Faculty of Veterinary Medicine, University of Tehran, Tehran, Iran

[4]Department of Surgery and Radiology, Faculty of Veterinary Medicine, University of Tehran, Tehran, Iran

[5]Iranian Evidence-based Center of Excellence, Tabriz University of Medical Sciences, Tabriz, Iran

[6]Dr. Rastegar Research Laboratory, Faculty of Veterinary Medicine, University of Tehran, Tehran, Iran

Key words:

azathioprine, complete blood count, dogs, gamma globulin, lymphocyte

Correspondence

Ale-Davoud, S.J.
Department of Small Animal Internal Medicine, Faculty of Veterinary Medicine, University of Tehran, Tehran, Iran

Email: sja@ut.ac.ir

Abstract:

BACKGROUND: Azathioprine is an immunosuppressive agent that is used in a variety of dermatologic, digestive and hematologic disorders in both humans and small animals. **OBJECTIVES:** The effects of long term Azathioprine administration on complete blood count, rate of CD4+ and CD8+ lymphocytes, serum immunoglobulins and protein concentrations of mixed-breed dogs were evaluated in this study. **METHODS:** 24 healthy mixed-breed dogs were divided randomly into two equal control and treatment groups. Dogs in the treatment group received the therapeutic dose of Azathioprine for four months, while the dogs in the control group did not receive this drug. Peripheral blood samples were taken from both groups before and after the trial to check CBC, CD4+ and CD8+ lymphocytes and the concentrations of total protein, albumin, serum IgM and IgG. **RESULTS:** There was significant decrease in the levels of WBC, RBC, hematocrit and CD4 lymphocyte and double positive CD4/CD8 rates (all p values< 0.001), concentrations of total protein, albumin, serum IgG and IgM (P values: 0.014, 0.001, 0.007 and 0.041 respectively) in treatment group after the trial. **CONCLUSIONS:** Myelotoxicity induced by Azathioprine could be the probable cause of decrements in the rate of WBC and RBC. Decrease in the rate of dpCD4/CD8 might be due to decrement in dpCD4/CD8 progenitor cells and/or decrease in the activation rate of single positive T cells as the result of pharmacological effect of Azathioprine. Disrupted synthesis processes, from genes to proteins through Azathioprine might be the cause of decreases in the level of serum gamma globulins and protein.

Introduction

Azathioprine is an i mmunosuppressive drug used to treat immune-mediated dermatologic, digestive and hematologic disorders, to prevent rejections of transplants and to treat some types of leukemia in humans and dogs (Lennard et al 1987; Rinkardt and Kruth 1996; Sebbag et al 2000; Snow and Gibson 1995; Viviano 2013 and White et al 2000). Azathioprine is a purine analogue and 6-mercaptopurine (6-MP) prodrug (Aarbakke et al 1997 and Elion 1993). Azathioprine is rapidly absorbed following oral administration and then metabolized to 6-MP by a variety of enzymes (Lennard 1998) and only about 2 percent of Azathioprine is excreted unchanged in the urine (Stern et al 2005). It undergoes non enzymatic degradation due to reactions with sufahydryl compounds in the liver, erythrocytes and body tissues and is converted into 6-MP. Then 6-MP is metabolized by the variety of enzymes. Enzyme Hypoxanthine- Guanine Phosphoribosyl Transferase (HGPRT) converts 6-MP into 6-Thioinosine-5'-Monophosphate (TIMP). Other enzymes that are responsible for inactivating Azathioprine are Thiopurine Methyl Transferase (TPMT), Aldehyde Oxidase (AO) and Xanthine Oxidase (XO). Thiopurine Methyl Transferase (TPMT) results in TIMP methylation and MeTIMP, an inactive metabolite formation. Xanthine Oxidase (XO) oxidizes Azathioprine forming inactive 6-thiouric acid metabolite and Aldehyde Oxidase (AO) causes Azathioprine dehydroxylation forming inactive Hydroxylated 6-Thioguanine Nucleotide (Hydroxylated 6-TGN) metabolite.

Following the conversion of 6-MP to TIMP, TIMP is converted into 6-Thioguanosine-5'-monophosphate (TGMP) and then TGMP is converted to a 6-TGN metabolite, Deoxy-6-thioguanosine-5'-phosphate (dGS), due to effects of some kinases and reductases. dGS disrupts DNA/ RNA replication, transcription and translation processes as a false base resulting in cell cycle arrest and apoptosis (Stern et al 2005).

Xanthine oxidase (XO) and aldehyde oxidase (AO) enzymatic competition causes only 16% of Azathioprine dose converted into 6-MP. However, TPMT enzyme plays important roles in systemic distribution of 6-MP levels by metabolizing them into 6-Methylmercaptopurine (6-MMP) and MeTIMP. The most important cells affected by Azathioprine are the lymphocytes since these cells do not have Salvage Purine pathways in their metabolisms (Viviano 2013) and these abnormal purine metabolites are constantly used in DNA and RNA synthesis in lymphocytes (Maltzman and Koretzy 2003).

Researchers are still studying the effects of Azathioprine on dog's immune system changes. To the best of our knowledge, there is no published document regarding long term in vivo effects of Azathioprine administration on dogs, based on searching along databases up to now. The aim of this study was to evaluate the effects of long term administration of Azathioprine in therapeutic dose, which is recommended for treatment of Canine Inflammatory Bowel Disease (Papich 2016 and Plumb 2007), on mixed-breed dogs and assessment of hematologic, CD4+ and CD8+ lymphocyte percentages and the level of serum gamma globulins changes after this treatment period.

Materials and Methods

In this study, all institutional and national

guidelines for the care and use of animals were followed. Twenty-four mixed breed dogs, 12 males and 12 females, with age range of 1-2 years (mean ± SD: 17.16 ± 3.80 month), and average weight of 15.26 ± 2.93 kg (mean ± SD), were randomly divided into 2 equal groups as control and treatment. Before the trial, for health evaluation of dogs, all of them were clinically and paraclinically assessed by clinical examination, radiographic assessment of thoracic cavity and laboratory evaluation of CBC and blood biochemistry profile including: BUN, Creatinine, Alkaline Phosphatase, Alanine Aminotransferase, Aspartate Aminotransferase, serum total protein and albumin. After attaining assurance of the physical health of all dogs, each one received anti-parasitic drugs for external and internal parasitism as prophylaxis (Ivermectin, 0.4 mg/kg, SC and Praziquantel forte, 1 tablet for each 10 kg body weight, PO).

In the beginning of trial, 15 ml jugular venous blood samples were taken from all dogs. The sample was divided into three equal parts as one for complete blood count (CBC) in EDTA tube, one for CD4 and CD8 lymphocyte flow cytometry in heparinized tubes and one part to measure total protein, albumin and serum immunoglobulins in clotting tubes.

Then dogs of the treatment group received the therapeutic dose of Azathioprine that is indicated for treatment of Canine Inflammatory Bowel Disease (as a model for long term consumption of this drug) as 2 mg/kg, PO, once a day for 4 weeks, then 2 mg/kg, PO, every 48 h for 4 weeks and finally 1 mg/kg, PO, every 48 h for 8 weeks; while the dogs of the control group have not received this drug for a four month trial period. To prevent probable opportunistic infections, all dogs in both groups received Ivermectin (0.4 mg/kg, SC, monthly), and Cefixime (10 mg/kg, PO, q12h) and Coamoxyclave (15 mg/kg, PO, q12h) from the second month to the end of the trial.

Doses of all drugs including: Azathioprine, Ivermectin, Cefixime and Coamoxyclave were determined based on that documented in Saunder's Handbook of Veterinary Drugs (Papich 2016) and Plumb's Veterinary Drug Handbook (Plumb 2007).

In the whole of the trial, each dog was housed in separated individual cage with approximate dimensions of 2×2×1.5 m (length, width and height respectively) with ambient temperature of 20 to 25 degrees centigrade in the ward of Small Animal Hospital of School of Veterinary Medicine of Tehran University.

The diet of all dogs was the same during the whole period of the study and they were fed with Nutripet® dry food (Behindasht Co, Iran) as ad libitum water and food status. The amount of daily required feed for each dog was calculated based on amount of energy of dry food (kcal/100g) and total daily energy requirement as the following formula (Bermingham et al 2014):

Resting Energy Requirement (RER) = $70 \times \text{Body Weight}^{0.75}$

Total Energy Requirement (TER) = $1.5 \times \text{RER}$

At the end of trial, blood samples were taken from all dogs (15 ml from jugular vein) and equally divided into three tubes as the method in the initiation of the trial, to evaluate CBC, Flow cytometry of CD4 and CD8 lymphocytes and serum total protein, albumin and serum immunoglobulins (IgG and IgM) concentrations.

CBC: To count and differentiate blood cells, 5 ml of each dog's jugular vein blood sample in EDTA tube was sent to the Laboratory of the Small Animal Hospital of School of Veterinary Medicine of Tehran University. The RBC and WBC count were measured with Automated Hematology Analyzer (Celltacα, MEK-6450, NIHON KOHDEN®, Japan) and air dried blood smear stained with Giemsa's solution (Merck KGaA, Germany), evaluated microscopically (1000x magnification) for determination of different blood WBC percentages.

CD4+ and CD8+ lymphocytes flow cytometry: For flow cytometric assessment of CD4+ and CD8+ peripheral blood lymphocytes, 5 ml heparinized jugular vein blood sample from each dog was sent to Dr. Rastegar Laboratory of School of Veterinary Medicine of Tehran University.

To do so, Rat anti-dog CD4: FITC/CD8: RPE kit (AbD Serotec, Bio-Rad Co, USA) was used together with its isotype control, Rat IgG2a: FITC/ Rat IgG1: RPE (AbD Serotec, Bio-Rad Co, USA).

To perform the flow cytometry assay, 100 μl heparinized jugular vein whole blood was prepared. Then 10 μl of reconstituted (1 ml distilled water in each lyophilized cocktail) Rat anti-dog CD4: FITC/CD8: RPE and for isotype control, 10 μl of reconstituted (0.5 ml distilled water in each lyophilized cocktail) was added to each 100 μl heparinized whole blood sample. Then the antibody- whole blood mixture was properly mixed together and incubated for 30 min in room temperature. After that, 2-3 ml of 0.1x ammonium chloride based RBC lysis buffer for flow cytometry (Erythrolyse BUF04, AbD Serotec, Bio- Rad Co, USA) was added to each tube and incubated for 10 min at room temperature. Then each tube was centrifuged for 5 min in 400×g at 18-20 °C and its supernatant was discarded. There-

after each sample was washed with 2 ml of PBS/BSA and was centrifuged for 5 min in 400×g at 18-20 °C and its supernatant was discarded. Then the pellet cells were re-suspended in 0.2 ml PBS/BSA and finally each sample was analyzed with ParTEC-pas Flow Cytometry Machine (PARTEC, GmbH, Munster, Germany) and Flowmax® software. 10000 cells were counted in each run and primary gating of lymphocyte population was performed based on forward and side scattering light properties in linear scaling dot-plot (Fig. 1-A). Quadrant frame positioning was determined by means of isotype control analysis and ascertainment of negative cells population (Fig. 1-B). Finally, on lymphocyte gated population, the percentages of CD4+ and CD8+ lymphocytes were determined by means of analysis of traced events on FL1 (CD4: FITC) versus FL2 (CD8: RPE) channels in logarithmic scaling on dot-plot.

Total protein, albumin and globulin measurement: Serum total protein and albumin concentrations were measured by spectrophotometry kit (using Teb Gostaran Hayyan Iranian Co. Iran) with Automated Biochemistry Analyzer (Selectra ProM, ELITech Group) in Laboratory of Small Animal Hospital of School of Veterinary Medicine of Tehran University. The levels of serum globulins were calculated according to the difference between the concentrations of albumin and total protein.

Serum IgG and IgM measurement in dogs: Dog's serum total IgG and IgM were measured by Quantitative Sandwich ELISA assay using Abcam® Eliza Kits (canine IgG ELISA kit ab193768, canine IgM ELISA kit ab157702, Abcam, UK), in Dr. Rastegar Laboratory of School of Veterinary Medicine of Tehran University.

Table 1. Changes of the numbers of blood cells in the control and treatment groups, before and after the trial in Mean ± SD. A P value less than 0.05 is considered statistically significant. In the treatment group, the levels of WBC, RBC and Plt were significantly decreased after 4 months receiving Azathioprine. WBC: white blood cells, RBC: Red Blood Cells, Plt: Platelets.

		WBC (cell/µl)	RBC (cell/µl)	Plt (cell/µl)	
Control Group	Before	7666.67±3727.19	6241666.67±479504.16	423333.33±85634.88	
	After	9244.67±1920.29	6091666.67±519542.34	420833.33±80165.55	
	P Value	0.194	0.154	0.950	
Treatment Group	Before	9912.50±1911.11	6375000.00±771215.10	380000.00±93127.48	
	After	2679.17±2989.10	2708333.33±1098311.38	135250.00±61224.07	
	P Value	0.001	0.001	0.001	

Table 2. Changes of different WBC types numbers in the control and treatment groups, before and after the trial in Mean ± SD. A P value less than 0.05 is considered statistically significant. In the treatment group, after 4 months receiving Azathioprine, the levels of neutrophil, lymphocytes and monocytes were significantly decreased. Neut: Neutrophil, Lymph: lymphocyte, Band Neut: Band Neutrophil, Mon: Monocyte, Eos: Eosinophil.

		Neut. (cell/µl)	Lymph. (cell/µl)	Band Neut. (cell/µl)	Mon. (cell/µl)	Eos. (cell/µl)
Control Group	Before	5593.25±2173.35	2878.83±1191.94	20.25±47.50	50.92±78.24	38.83±78.76
	After	6256.50±1907.13	2780.58±823.01	16.75±40.72	103.83±93.08	86.50±94.26
	P Value	0.437	0.821	0.593	0.156	0.093
Treatment Group	Before	6360.92±1586.13	3368.17±978.47	26.58±6468	79.83±86.42	77.00±109.34
	After	1689.50±1802.60	948.80±1208.01	2.86±6.83	15.80±25.71	22.25±46.28
	P Value	<0.001	<0.001	0.258	0.019	0.161

Table 3. Changes of RBC's factors in the control and treatment groups, before and after the trial in Mean ± SD. A P value less than 0.05 is considered statistically significant. In the treatment group, after 4 months receiving Azathioprine, the levels of Hct and Hb were significantly decreased. Hct: Hematocrit, Hb: Hemoglobin.

		Hct (%)	Hb (g/dl)	MCV (fl)	MCH (pg)	MCHC (g/dl)
Control Group	Before	44.00±3.52	14.17±1.15	70.50±3.90	23.37±1.52	33.50±1.09
	After	42.83±3.86	14.28±1.10	70.42±4.44	23.37±1.52	33.50±0.90
	P Value	0.095	0.143	0.777	1	1
Treatment Group	Before	44.17±4.59	14.76±1.30	69.42±2.43	22.84±1.56	33.58±1.08
	After	18.91±8.12	6.29±2.67	69.42±2.27	22.47±1.41	33.50±2.54
	P Value	0.001	0.001	1	0.118	0.811

To do so, 5 ml of jugular vein blood sample from each dog, was collected into clotting tube. After clot formation, samples were centrifuged at 2000×g for 10 min at room temperature and their serums were separated. Then all reagents, working standard and samples were prepared as were directed in assay procedure of each kit.

For IgG measurement, 50 µl of pre-diluted serum samples (1/1×10^6) and different concentrations of serially diluted standard solutions (with concentrations of: 20, 10, 5. 2.5, 1.25, 0.63, 0.31 and 0 ng/ml) were added into the appropriate ELISA kit's wells. Then 50 µl of antibody cocktail was added to each well and the wells were incubated for 1 h at room temperature on plate shaker (400 rpm). After that, the wells were washed with wash buffer (3 times). Then 100 µl TMB - Substrate was added to each well and the wells were incubated 30 min in the dark in plate shaker (400 rpm).

Table 4. Percentages and intensities of blood cells changes in comparison to their reference intervals in the treatment group, after the trial. The total numbers of treatment group's members were 12 dogs. Sev: severe, Mod: Moderate.

Abnormality	Thrombocytopenia (PLT<15×10³ cell/µl)			Anemia (Hct<37)				Leukopenia (WBC<5000 cell/µl)		
Total Percentage (%)	58.3			100				75		
Severity	Severe (<50×10³ cell/µl)	Mod. (50-100×10³ cell/µl)	Mild (100-150×10³ cell/µl)	Very Sev. (<13)	Severe (13-19)	Mod. (19-29)	Mild (30-37)	Severe (<1700 cell/µl)	Mod. (1700-3500 cell/µl)	Mild (3500-5000 cell/µl)
Relative Percentage (%)	14	43	43	17	33	42	8	77	23	-
Total Percentage (%)	8.3	25	25	17	33	42	8	58	17	-

Table 5. Flow cytometric results of percentages of CD4+ and CD8+ blood lymphocytes and their changes before and after the trial in Mean ± SD. A P value less than 0.05 is considered statistically significant. In the treatment group, after 4 months receiving Azathioprine, the percentages of CD4+, dp-CD4/CD8, dn-CD4/CD8 and CD4+/CD8+ lymphocytes were significantly decreased. dp-CD4/CD8: double positive CD4/CD8 lymphocytes, dn-CD4/CD8: double negative CD4/CD8 lymphocytes, CD4+/CD8+: ratio of CD4+ lymphocytes to CD8+ lymphocytes.

		CD4+ (%)	CD8+ (%)	dp-CD4/CD8	dn-CD4/CD8	CD4+/CD8+
Control Group	Before	43.56±3.31	19.50±2.20	2.16±0.29	34.80±5.29	2.25±0.17
	After	43.17±3.14	20.19±2.08	2.13±0.31	34.51±4.85	2.16±0.17
	P Value	0.583	0.247	0.780	0.820	0.111
Treatment Group	Before	44.27±3.70	19.43±1.70	2.19±0.35	34.11±5.05	2.27±0.16
	After	34.71±2.56	20.29±2.61	0.52±0.23	44.47±3.56	1.74±0.27
	P Value	0.001	0.321	0.001	0.001	0.001

Table 6. Results of changes of serum proteins and immunoglobulins concentrations in the control and treatment groups, before and after the trial in Mean ± SD. A P value less than 0.05 is considered statistically significant. In the treatment group, after 4 months receiving Azathioprine, the levels of concentration of serum total protein, serum albumin, IgG and IgM were significantly decreased.

		Total Protein (g/dl)	Albumin (g/dl)	Globulin (g/dl)	IgG (g/dl)	IgM (g/dl)
Control Group	Before	6.57±0.53	3.31±0.46	3.27±0.25	1.29±0.28	0.16±0.06
	After	6.77±0.46	3.62±0.39	3.14±0.28	1.25±0.25	0.14±0.07
	P Value	0.228	0.081	0.297	0.954	0.271
Treatment Group	Before	6.52±0.53	3.47±0.45	3.06±0.24	1.16±0.29	0.18±0.06
	After	5.97±0.72	2.76±0.21	3.22±0.77	0.81±0.18	0.14±0.18
	P Value	0.014	0.001	0.520	0.007	0.041

Thereafter, 100 µl of stop solution was added to each well and then the optical density (OD) of samples and serially diluted solutions of standard were measured in 450 nm wavelength using ELISA Reader (BioTek®, ELx800 Absorbance Reader).

For IgM measurement, 100 µl of diluted serum samples (1/1×10⁴) and serially diluted solutions of standard (with concentrations of: 800, 400, 200, 100, 50, 25 and 0 ng/ml) were added to each well. After 30 min incubation at room temperature, each well was washed with wash buffer (3 times). Then 100 µl of Enzyme- Antibody conjugate was added to each well and the wells were incubated 30 min in dark at room temperature. After that, wells were washed again (3 times with wash buffer). Thereafter, 100 µl TMB

– Substrate was added into each well and was incubated for 10 min at room temperature. After 10 min, 100 µl of stop solution was added to each well and then the OD of each well was measured in 450 nm wavelength with ELISA Reader.

After OD recording, the standard curve of serially diluted standard solutions was prepared (for both IgG and IgM in separated curves). Then the recorded OD values of each pre- diluted canine serum sample were put into standard curve and immunoglobulin concentrations of them were submitted. Finally, the achieved values of immunoglobulins of each diluted sample were multiplied by their dilution factors to find out the immunoglobulins concentrations in each serum sample in g/dl unit.

Statistical analysis: The results were analyzed using SPSS Software V.16 (SPSS-Chicago, IL, USA). At the beginning, the normality of data was examined using Kolmogorov- Smirnov test. Then, Paired Sample- T Test was used to analyze the normal distributed possibilities and Wilcoxon Signed- Ranks test was used for those with non- normal distributed possibilities (numbers of Band neutrophils, Eosinophils, MCHC and values of IgM concentrations). The results were recorded as Mean ± Standard Deviation (Mean ± SD) and a P values less than 0.05 were considered as statistically significant.

Results

The results of blood cell count: The results of the statistical test show that the number of white blood cells (WBC), red blood cells (RBC) and the levels of hematocrit and hemoglobin are significantly decreased after the trial in the treatment group (Tables 1, 2 and 3). Also, comparison of hematologic results with their reference intervals (reference intervals submitted in Schalm's veterinary hematology, sixth edition (Weiss and Wardrop 2010)) shows that, in control group (before and after trial and in treatment group (before trial) all of the hematologic values were within their reference intervals range. But in the treatment group after the trial, 58.3, 100 and 75% of the dogs suffered from thrombocytopenia, anemia and leukopenia, respectively (Table 4). The results show concurrent thrombocytopenia in 66.6% of leukopenic individuals and concurrent lymphopenia in 88.9% of neutropenic ones in treatment group after the trial.

The results of peripheral blood CD4+ and CD8+ lymphocytes flow cytometry: Peripheral blood lymphocytes in the treatment and control groups before and after the trial are shown in Table 5. The results of statistical analysis show that the percentages of all blood lymphocyte subgroups except CD8+ lymphocytes were significantly different after the trial in a way that the percentages of CD4+ and double positive CD4/CD8 cells are decreased and the percentage of double negative cells are increased after Azathioprine administration (Fig. 2).

Measuring serum protein and immunoglobulins concentrations: The average and standard deviation of serum immunoglobulins and protein concentrations of the treatment and the control groups before and after the trial are shown in Table 6. The results of statistical analysis show significant decreases in total protein concentration, albumin, albumin to globulin ratio, and IgG and IgM concentrations of the treatment group after the trial compared with the results of this group before the trial. Com-

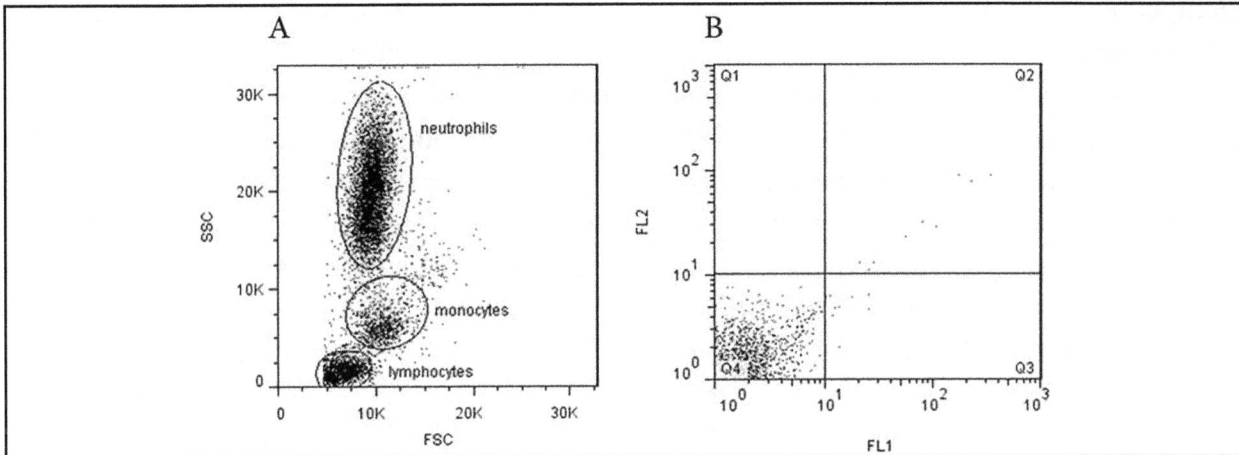

Figure 1- A: Forward versus side scattering properties of canine erythrolyzed whole blood in linear scaling dot- plot. Neutrophils, Monocytes and lymphocytes populations are gated based on forward (their size) and side (their granularity) scattering properties. Events for lysed RBC, debries and platelets are electronically excluded (with proper flow cytometer's threshold setting) during flow cytometer analysis. FSC: Forward Scattering, SSC: Side Scattering. B: Flow cytometric isotype control analysis (Rat IgG2a: FITC/ Rat IgG1: RPE) on Canine erythrolyzed whole blood and proper quadrant positioning for determination of negative population in dot- plot logarithmic scaling. FL1: Rat IgG2a: FITC, FL2: Rat IgG1: RPE. Q1: Area of CD8+ lymphocyte population, Q2: Area of Double Positive CD4/CD8, Q3: Area of CD4+ lymphocyte population and Q4: Area of Double Negative CD4/CD8 lymphocyte population.

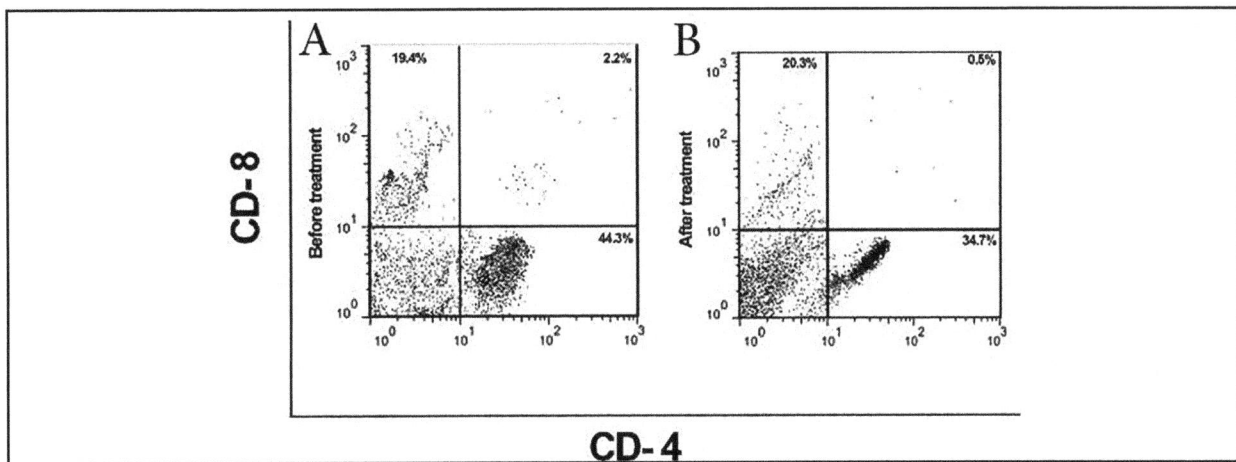

Figure 2. Representation of flow cytometric dot-plot percentages of CD4+, CD8+, double positive CD4/CD8 and double negative CD4/CD8 lymphocytes in lymphocyte gated population of canine erythrolyzed whole blood sample, A: before the trial and B: after the trial in one of the members of treatment group, using Rat Antidog CD4: FITC/CD8: RPE antibody cocktail.

parison of serum concentrations of IgG and IgM in members of treatment and controls groups, before and after the trial, with their reference intervals (Day 2010) shows that serum concentrations of IgG and IgM in control groups before and after the trial and in treatment group before the trial were between reference range, but in spite of significant decrease in their values in treatment group after the trial, only in 8.8% and 30% of individuals, concentrations of serum IgG and IgM were below reference intervals respectively.

Discussion

To the best of our knowledge, there is no published document regarding long term in vivo effects of Azathioprine administration on dogs up to now. In this study effects of long term administration of Azathioprine in therapeutic dose, which is recommended for treatment of Canine Inflammatory Bowel Disease on mixed-breed dogs were evaluated and hematologic, CD4 and CD8 lymphocyte percentages and the level of serum gamma globulins changes after four months of Azathioprine treatment were assessed.

Blood cells counting and differentiating results of this study demonstrate occurrence of myelosuppression with different severity in dogs of treatment group after the trial.

Rinkardt et al studied the effects of Azathioprine on dogs in a 14-day period in 1999 and stated that there were no changes in complete blood counts of the dogs that received Azathioprine (Rinkardt et al 1999). This was probably due to the short treatment period. The studies indicated that the therapeutic effects of Azathioprine began about 2 to 5 weeks after the start of IMHA treatment in humans and dogs (Al-Ghazlat 2009 and Fox 2013).

Campbell et al observed in a study on Azathioprine effects on the human patients with inflammatory bowel disease (IBD) that administering 2-5 mg/kg/day dose of Azathioprine for a year caused significant lymphopenia in the treatment group. Although the neutrophil counts were decreased in this group, the difference was not significant compared to the group who suffered from IBD but did not receive Azathioprine. There was also no significant difference between the platelet counts of the group that received Azathioprine and the group which did not (Campbell et al 1976).

Several clinical reports about bone marrow suppression, though in a few percentages of dogs and humans administered standard dose of Azathioprine, were published (Andersen et al 1998; Lennard and Lilleyman 1996; Lennard et al 1987; Snow and Gibson 1995; Stolk et al 1998). A wide range of disorders in counting blood cells such as leukopenia, neutropenia, thrombocytopenia, anemia and pancytopenia, with the most occurrence of lymphopenia were observed in these reports. In this study anemia and in the second place leukopenia were the most hematologic changes in dogs which received Azathioprine.

One of the enzymes involved in Azathioprine metabolism is TPMT enzyme. The average TPMT enzyme activities are 37.1, 2.8 and 35.7 nmol/bHb/h in dogs, cats and humans, respectively (Foster et al 2000; Tavadia et al 2000). The studies indicated that the activity of this enzyme is high in 88.6 %, moderate in 11.1% and low in 0.3 % of human population. In people with low activity level of this enzyme, Azathioprine metabolism caused the production of 6-MMP inactive metabolites to decrease and the production of 6-TGN active metabolites to increase. These people would suffer from toxicity and acute bone marrow suppression (Rinkardt and Kruth 1996; Rodriguez et al 2004). Human studies indicated that measuring TPMT enzyme activity in RBCs could be considered as a predictive factor for thioporine toxicity occurrence in those administering Azathioprine (Andersen et al 1998; Klemetsdal et al 1993; Lennard et al 1987; Snow and Gibson 1995; Stolk et al 1998). Nowadays, for minimizing Azathioprine induced toxicity, many physicians believe that TPMT enzyme activity should be evaluated phenotypically (measuring this enzyme in tissues like RBC) and/or genotypically (analyzing TPMT encoding genes) before treating with Azathioprine (Sebbag et al 2000; Stolk et al 1998; Tavadia et al 2000). On the other hand, Azathioprine dosage could be calculated based on TPMT enzyme activity level (Lennard and Lilleyman 1996; Lennard 1998).

Recent studies indicated that the variety and distribution of TPMT enzyme in dogs are similar to humans (Foster et al 2000; White et al 2000). Rodriguez et al in a study on 300 dogs in 2004 found out that TPMT enzyme activity is moderate in 58% and high in 42% of the studied dogs and none of them showed low enzyme activity (Rodriguez et al 2004). All studies on dogs have not indicated any low levels of TPMT activity (Rodriguez et al 2004; Stolk et al 1988; White et al 1984; White et al 2000). However, in another study dogs with moderate TPMT activity had significantly lower neutrophil counts after 4-week Azathioprine treatment and indicated that mild to moderate bone marrow suppression (severe neutropenia, leukopenia and thrombocytopenia) could occur in dogs with moderate TPMT activity (Rodriguez et al 2004). One possible explanation for these findings is that the threshold of TPMT activity at which dogs will experience myelotoxicity when receiving Azathioprine differs from the threshold in humans. Other possible causes include the existence of some mechanisms, other than TPMT enzyme, involved in Azathioprine mylotoxicity in dogs such as low activity levels of inosine triphosphate pyrophosphohydrolase (ITPP) (Fraser et al 1975; Lennard 2002) and xanthine oxidase (XO) or increasing concentration of methylated ribonucleotides (Dubinsky et al 2001) and/or idiosyncratic reactions (Giger et al 1985; Trepanier et al 2003).

In our study anemia and in the second place leukopenia were the most established hematologic changes. Studies on myelotoxicity effect of Azathioprine in humans showed that the most prevalent hematologic changes were Leukopenia, Anemia and thrombocytopenia respectively. Considering lack of salvage pathway for purine biosynthesis in lymphocytes and greater risk for leukopenia due to Azathioprine, from the aspect of the author of this article, this deference remains unexplained. Perhaps, the study of cumulative concentrations of Azathioprine and its metabolites in different canine bone marrow cell lineage and/or assessment of Azathioprine- related changes in hematopoietic and growth factors could explain these differences.

Studies on black and white races of humans in different geographical regions indicated high variety in TPMT enzyme activity in the populations (Gisbert et al 2007; Jang et al 1996; Lennard et al 1996; McLeod et al 1994). Kidd et al indicated that dog breeds including Giant Schnauzer and Alaskan Malamute had the most and least TPMT enzyme activity among the studied breeds of dogs, respectively (Kidd et al 2004).

In the current study, specific activities of TPMT, XO and ITPP enzymes were not measured. According to the high occurrence rate of blood cell changes in dogs treated with Azathioprine in this study, it was suggested to perform a more distributed study with various breeds of dogs including the mixed-breeds in Iran to measure and determine the activities of these enzymes. Also, it is necessary to evaluate and study the correlation between TPMT enzyme activities in main Azathioprine metabolizing tissues such as the liver with the activities of this enzyme in RBCs.

In the current study, significant decrements of CD4+ and Double Positive CD4+/CD8+ (dp-CD4/CD8) lymphocytes were observed in the treatment group after a 4-month Azathioprine administration period. In a study on the effects of administering Azathioprine for a short period, 14 days, in dogs, no changes in CD4+ and CD8+ lymphocytes were recorded (Rinkardt et al 1999). This was probably due to short administration period of Azathioprine since studies indicated that the shortest period needed to induce therapeutic effects of Azathioprine is two to five weeks (Al-Ghazlat 2009 and Fox 2013).

It could be concluded based on the results of the current study and revision of the previous studies that the reason of significant CD4+ lymphocyte decrement might be leukopenia occurrence followed by CD4+ and CD8+ lymphocyte decrements compared with the control group and/or decreasing the division and proliferation of T lymphocytes caused by Azathioprine administration in the treatment group.

In this study, there is significant decrease in percentages of dp-CD4/CD8 lymphocytes in treatment group after the trial.

Immature T cells were dp-CD4/CD8 lymphocyte. During the maturity process, these cells changed into single positive cells. Hence, it has been long thought that circulating mature T lymphocytes were CD4+ and/ or CD8+ (Bukowska-Straková et al 2006). Zuckermann et al was indicated in 1992 that there are mature T lymphocytes in peripheral blood of human, primate, swine, rats, mouse and chickens that are simultaneously dp-CD4/CD8 (Zuckermann et al 1992). This cell population was also found in the dogs (Alexander- Pires et al 2010; Otani et al 2008). The rate of this cell population was 2.5% in dogs (Blue et al 1985; Nascimbeni et al 2004), 2-9% in humans (Bismarck et al 2012) and about 60% in swine (Zuckermann 1999). It seems the rates of these cells are positively correlated with age (Bismarck

et al 2012; Zuckermann 1999; Zuckermann and Husmann 1996) while the gender might not effect on dp-CD4/CD8 rate (Bismarck et al 2012). Since dp-CD4/CD8 cells lack CD1 (surface marker of immature T cells) in humans, the population is considered mature (Zuckermann 1999). In dogs, these cells are in fact mature TCRαβ T cells and are divided into three groups as CD4bright CD8αbright, CD4dim CD8αbright and CD-4bright CD8αdim (Bismarck et al 2014).

The progenitor cells of dp-CD4/CD8 population are CD4 single positive T cells, single positive CD4 and single positive CD8 (with higher potency of CD8 Single Positive) and single positive CD4 and single positive CD8 (with higher potency of CD4 SPs) in swine, human and dogs, respectively (Bismarck et al 2014; Bismarck et al 2012; Saalmüller et al 2002).

In human and swine, the activation of T cells is directly correlated with becoming double positive (Saalmüller et al 2002; Sullivan et al 2001). In vitro developed canine dp-CD4/CD8 express high rate of CD25 in dog (Bismarck et al 2014). It is necessary to mention that CD25 is the alpha chain of interleukin 2 receptors that is expressed on activated T cells. In some clinical cases such as thymoma, allergy, transplantation (Bukowska-Straková et al 2006) and autoimmune diseases in humans, the rate of dp-CD4/CD8 has been increased (Alexander-Pires et al 2010; Bismarck et al 2014; Parel and Chizzolini 2004). Also, PBMC stimulation in dogs with parapox ovis, distemper virus, *Staphylococcus aureus* enterotoxin B, Concavalin A, IL-2 and Anti CD3 antibody resulted in increasing the population of this type of cells (Bismarck et al 2014; Fraser et al 1975 and Schütze et al 2009). The studies indicated that canine dp CD4+/CD8+ T cells probably belonged to memory/effector T cells (Bismarck et al 2014).

In this study, the decrement of dp-CD4+/CD8+ cell population might be due to decreasing population of CD4+ and CD8+ cells as the progenitors of dp-CD4+/CD8+ and/or decreasing the level of single positive T cell antigenic activation as a result of administering Azathioprine.

In our study, the concentrations of albumin and IgG and IgM globulins were significantly decreased after administering Azathioprine for four months in the treatment group.

Rinkardt et al performed a short 2-week study on dogs and concluded that Azathioprine could not affect the concentrations of plasma immunoglobulins (Rinkardt et al 1999). This is probably due to the limited time of study.

Also, in another study on the effects of Azathioprine on immunoglobulin synthesis in humans for a long period, it was indicated that the synthesis rates of IgG and IgM were decreased 33.4 and 40%, respectively but the decreasing level of immunoglobulin concentration was not significant compared to the prior of the study (Levy et al 1972).

Wolf et al indicated that administering 6-thioguanine could suppress the immunoglobulins in rabbits (Wolff and Goodman 1963). Also, Mott et al studied the turnover of the immunoglobulins and showed that administering 6-MP in young rabbits could result in hypoglobulinemia (Mott et al 1968). The results of these studies are in agreement with the current study. The reason of gamma globulin decrement in these studies might be due to reduction of their synthesis. However, it seems the decrement is dose-dependent so that it only occurred in higher doses of Azathioprine (Levy et al

1972; Mott et al 1968; Wolff and Goodman 1963).

In this study in spite of significant decrease in concentration of IgG and IgM in treatment group, after the trial (Table 6), only in 8.8% and 30% of individual levels were below reference range respectively. This may be due to longer serum half-life of IgG comparing to IgM (Abbas et al 2015 and Bergeron et al 2014).

The decrement of serum proteins such as albumin and gamma globulins could be due to Azathioprine and its metabolites-related disruption in mechanisms such as DNA replication, transcription, translation and finally protein synthesis that are involved in synthesis of these proteins. Since occurrence of leukopenia is not required to suppress the synthesis of gamma globulins (Levy et al 1972), leukopenia might not be the definite cause of gamma globulin concentration's decrement in the current study.

Conclusion: It is concluded that Azathioprine can induce high rate occurrence of myelosuppression, decrease in CD4+, CD8+ and dp-CD4/CD8 peripheral blood lymphocytes percentages and decrement of serum IgG and IgM concentrations in Iranian mixed large breed dogs. Whereas some factors including: enzymes such as TPMT, ITPP, XO and breed differences, can possibly contribute in Azathioprine associated myelosuppression, it is suggested there is a correlation between these factors and Azathioprine associated myelotoxicity evaluated in more distributed and specified studies. Decrease in the rate of dpCD4/CD8 might be due to induced apoptosis in peripheral blood lymphocytes or decrement in dp-CD4/CD8 progenitor cells and/or decrease in the activation rate of single positive T cells as the result of pharmacological effect of Azathioprine. Disrupted synthesis processes, from genes to proteins through Azathioprine might be the cause of decreases in the level of serum gamma globulins and protein.

Acknowledgments

We would like to acknowledge Dr. Amir Tavakoli, Dr. Mohammadreza Esmaeili Nejad, and Dr. Atefeh Sabagh for their support as veterinarians. We also appreciate Mr. Alireza Ghovati, Mr. Bijari and Mr. Vazifeh for their efforts and help at University of Tehran's Small Animal Hospital to perform this study.

References

Aarbakke, J., Janka-Schaub, G., Elion, GB. (1997) Thiopurine biology and pharmacology. Trends Pharmacol Sci. 18: 3-7.

Abbas, A.K., Litchman, A.H., Pillai, S. (2015) Antibodies and antigens. In: Cellular and Molecular Immunology. Abbas, A.K., Litchman, A.H., Pillai, S. (eds.). Elsevier Inc. Philadelphia, USA. p. 87-106.

Alexandre-Pires, G., de Brito, MT., Algueró, C., Martins, C., Rodrigues, O.R., da Fonseca, I.P., Santos-Gomes, G. (2010) Canine leishmaniosis. Immunophenotypic profile of leukocytes in different compartments of symptomatic, asymptomatic and treated dogs. Vet Immunol Immunopathol. 15; 137: 275-83.

Al-Ghazlat S. (2009) Immunosuppressive therapy for canine immune-mediated hemolytic anemia. Compendium (Yardley, PA). 31: 33-41.

Andersen, J.B., Szumlanski, C., Weinshilboum, R.M., Schmiegelow, K. (1998) Pharmacokinetics, dose adjustments, and 6-mercaptopurine/methotrexate drug interactions in two patients with thiopurine methyltransferase deficiency. Acta Paediatr. 1;87: 108-11.

Bergeron, M.L., McCandless, E.E., Dunham, S., Dunkle, B., Zhu, Y., Shelly, J., Lightle, S., Gonzales, A., Bainbridge, G. (2014) Comparative functional characterization of canine IgG subclasses. Vet Immunol Immunopathol. 157: 31-41.

Bermingham, E.N., Thomas, D.G., Cave, N.J., Morris P.J., Butterwick, R.F, German, A.J. (2014) Energy requirement of adult dogs: a meta- analysis. PLoS One. 9: e109681.

Bismarck, D., Moore, P.F., Alber, G., von Buttlar, H. (2014) Canine CD4(+)CD8(+) double-positive T cells can develop from CD4(+) and CD8(+) T cells. Vet Immunol Immunopathol. 15;162: 72-82.

Bismarck, D., Schütze, N., Moore, P., Büttner, M., Alber, G., Buttlar, H.V. (2012) Canine CD4+CD8+ double positive T cells in peripheral blood have features of activated T cells. Vet Immunol Immunopathol. 15;149:157-66.

Blue, M.L., Daley, J.F., Levine, H., Schlossman, S.F. (1985) Co-expression of T4 and T8 on peripheral blood T cells demonstrated by two-color fluorescence flow cytometry. J Immunol. 1;134: 2281-6.

Bukowska-Straková, K., Baran, J., Gawlicka, M., Kowalczyk, D. (2006) A false expression of CD8 antigens on CD4^+ T cells in a routine flow cytometry analysis. Folia Histochem Cytobiol. 1;44: 179-83.

Campbell, A.C., Skinner, J.M., Maclennan, I.C., Hersey, P., Waller, C.A., Wood, J., Jewell, D.P., Truelove, S.C. (1976) Immunosuppression in the treatment of inflammatory bowel disease. II. The effects of Azathioprine on lymphoid cell populations in a double blind trial in ulcerative colitis. Clin Exp Immunol. 24: 249-58.

Day, M.J. (2008) Immunodeficiency diseases. In: Clinical Immunology of the Dog and Cat. Day, M.J. (eds.). (2nd ed.) Manson Publishing Ltd. London, UK. p. 302.

Dubinsky, M.C., Hassard, P.V., Seidman, E.G., Kam, L.Y., Abreu, M.T., Targan, S.R., Vasiliauskas, E.A. (2001) An open-label pilot study using thioguanine as a therapeutic alternative in Crohn's disease patients resistant to 6-mercaptopurine therapy. Inflamm Bowel Dis. 7: 181-9.

Elion, G.B. (1993) The George Hitchings and Gertrude Elion Lecture. The pharmacology of Azathioprine. Ann N Y Acad Sci. 23;685: 400-7.

Foster, A.P., Shaw, S.E., Duley, J.A., Shobowale-Bakre, E.M., Harbour, D.A. (2000) Demonstration of thiopurine methyltransferase activity in the erythrocytes of cats. J Vet Intern Med. 1;14: 552-4.

Fox, L.E. (2013) Antineoplastic drugs. In: Handbook of Veterinary Pharmacology. Hsu, W.H.(ed.). Shinilbooks Company. Seoul, Republic of Korea. p. 569.

Fraser, J.H., Meyers, H., Henderson, J.F., Brox, L.W., McCoy, E.E. (1975) Individual variation in inosine triphosphate accumulation in human erythrocytes. Clin Biochem. 28;8: 353-64.

Giger, U., Werner, L.L., Millichamp, N.J., Gorman, N.T. (1985) Sulfadiazine-induced allergy in six Doberman pinschers. J Am Vet Med Assoc. 186: 479-84.

Gisbert, J.P., Gomollón, F., Cara, C., Luna, M., González-Lama, Y., Pajares, J.M., Maté, J., Guijarro, L.G. (2007) Thiopurine methyltransferase activity in Spain: a study of 14,545 patients. Dig Dis Sci. 1;52(5): 1262-9.

Hoshino, Y., Takagi, S., Osaki, T., Okumura, M., Fujinaga, T. (2008) Phenotypic analysis and effects of sequential administration of activated canine lymphocytes on healthy beagles. J Vet Med Sci. 70: 581-8.

Jang, I.J., Shin, S.G., Lee, K.H., Yim, D.S., Lee, M.S., Koo, H.H., Kim, H.K., Sohn, D.R. (1996) Erythrocyte thiopurine methyltransferase activity in a Korean population. Br J Clin Pharmacol. 1;42: 638-41.

Kidd, L.B., Salavaggione, O.E., Szumlanski, C.L., Miller, J.L., Weinshilboum, R.M., Trepanier, L. (2004) Thiopurine methyltransferase activity in red blood cells of dogs. J Vet Intern Med. 1;18: 214-8.

Klemetsdal, B., Straume, B., Wist, E., Aarbakke, J. (1993) Identification of factors regulating thiopurine methyltransferase activity in a Norwegian population. Eur J Clin Pharmacol. 1;44: 147-52.

Lennard, L., Lilleyman, J.S. (1996) Individualizing therapy with 6-mercaptopurine and 6-thioguanine related to the thiopurine methyltransferase genetic polymorphism. Therapeutic Drug Monitoring 1;18: 328-34.

Lennard, L., Van Loon, J.A., Lilleyman, J.S., Weinshilboum, R.M. (1987) Thiopurine pharmacogenetics in leukemia: Correlation of erythrocyte thiopurine methyltransferase activity and 6-thioguanine nucleotide concentrations. Clin Pharmacol Ther. 1;41: 18-25.

Lennard, L. (1998) Clinical implications of thiopurine methyltransferase-optimization of drug dosage and potential drug interactions. Ther Drug Monit. 1;20: 527-31.

Lennard, L. (2002) TPMT in the treatment of Crohn's disease with Azathioprine. Gut. 1;51(2): 143-6.

Levy, J., Barnett, E.V., MacDonald, N.S., Klinenberg, J.R., Pearson, C.M. (1972) The effect of Azathioprine on gammaglobulin synthesis in man. J Clin Invest. 51: 2233-38.

Maltzman, J.S., Koretzky, G.A. (2003) Azathioprine: old drug, new actions. J Clin Invest. 15;111: 1122-4.

McLeod, H.L., Lin, J.S., Scott, E.P., Pui, C.H., Evans, W.E. (1994) Thiopurine methyltransferase activity in American white subjects and black subjects. Clin Pharmacol Ther. 1;55: 15-20.

Mott, P.D., Wochner, R.D., Wolff, S.M. (1986) The Effect of 6-mercaptopurine on the turnover of I131-gamma globulin and I125-albumin in rabbits. J Pharmacol Exp Ther. 1;159: 211-5.

Nascimbeni, M., Shin, E.C., Chiriboga, L., Kleiner, D.E., Rehermann, B. (2004) Peripheral CD4+ CD8+ T cells are differentiated effector memory cells with antiviral functions. Blood 15;104: 478-86.

Otani, I., Ohta, K., Ishikawa, A., Yamada, T., Ishinazaka, T., Ohtaki, T., Tsumagari, S., Kanayama, K. (2008) Flow cytometric analysis of canine umbilical cord blood lymphocytes. J Vet Med Sci. 70: 285-7.

Papich, M.G. (2016) Saunder's Handbook of Veterinary Drugs, Small and Large Animals. (4th ed.) Elsevier Inc. USA.

Parel, Y., Chizzolini, C. (2004) CD4+ CD8+ double positive (DP) T cells in health and disease. Autoimmun Rev. 31;3: 215-20.

Rinkardt, N.E., Kruth, S.A., Kaushik, A. (1999) The effects of prednisone and Azathioprine on circulating immunoglobulin levels and lymphocyte subpopulations in normal dogs. Can J Vet Res. 63: 18-24.

Rinkardt, N.E., Kruth, S.A. (1996) Azathioprine-induced bone marrow toxicity in four dogs. Can Vet J. 37: 612-3.

Rodriguez, D.B., Mackin, A., Easley, R., Boyle, C.R., Hou, W., Langston, C., Walsh, A.M., Province, M.A., McLeod, H.L. (2004) Relationship between red blood cell thiopurine methyltransferase activity and myelotoxicity in dogs receiving Azathioprine. J Vet Intern Med. 1;18: 339-45.

Saalmüller, A., Werner, T., Fachinger, V. (2002) T-helper cells from naive to committed. Vet Immunol Immunopathol. 10; 87: 137-45.

Salavaggione, O.E., Kidd, L., Prondzinski, J.L.,

Szumlanski, C.L., Pankratz, V.S., Wang, L., Trepanier, L., Weinshilboum, R.M. (2002) Canine red blood cell thiopurine S-methyltransferase: companion animal pharmacogenetics. Pharmacogenetics 1;12: 713-24.

Schultze, A.E. (2010) Interpretation of canine leukocyte responses. In: Schalm's Veterinary Hematology. Weiss, D.J., Wardrop, K.J. (eds.). (6th ed.) Blackwell Publishing Ltd. Iowa, USA. p. 321-334.

Schütze, N., Raue, R., Büttner, M., Alber, G. (2009) Inactivated parapoxvirus ovis activates canine blood phagocytes and T lymphocytes. Vet Microbiol. 12;137: 260-7.

Sebbag, L., Boucher, P., Davelu, P., Boissonnat, P., Champsaur, G., Ninet, J., Dureau, G., Obadia, J.F., Vallon, J.J., Delaye, J. (2000) Thiopurine S-methyltransferase gene polymorphism is predictive of Azathioprine-induced myelosuppression in heart transplant recipients. Transplantation 15;69: 1524-7.

Snow, J.L., Gibson, L.E. (1995) The role of genetic variation in thiopurine methyltransferase activity and the efficacy and/or side effects of Azathioprine therapy in dermatologic patients. Arch Dermatol. 1;131: 193-7.

Stern, D.K., Tripp, J.M., Ho, V.C., Lebwohl, M. (2005) The Use of systemic immune moderators in dermatology: an update. Dermatol Clin. 23.2: 259-300

Stolk, J.N., Boerbooms, A.M., de Abreu, R.A., de Koning, D.G., van Beusekom, H.J., Muller, W.H., van de Putte, L. (1998) Reduced thiopurine methyltransferase activity and development of side effects of Azathioprine treatment in patients with rheumatoid arthritis. Arthritis Rheum.1;41: 1858-66.

Sullivan, Y.B., Landay, A.L., Zack, J.A., Kitchen, S.G., Al-Harthi, L. (2001) Upregulation of CD4 on CD8+ T cells: CD4dimCD8bright T cells constitute an activated phenotype of CD8+ T cells. Immunology 1;103: 270-80.

Tavadia, S.M., Mydlarski, P.R., Reis, M.D., Mittmann, N., Pinkerton, P.H., Shear, N., Sauder, D.N. (2000) Screening for Azathioprine toxicity: a pharmacoeconomic analysis based on a target case. J Am Acad Dermatol. 30;42: 628-32.

Trepanier, L., Cribb, A., Danhof, R., Toll, J. (2003) Clinical findings in 40 dogs with hypersensitivity associated with administration of potentiated sulfonamide. J Vet Intern Med. 17: 647-52.

Vedten, H. (2010) Laboratory and clinical diagnosis of anemia. In: Schalm's Veterinary Hematology. Weiss, D.J., Wardrop, K.J. (eds.). (6th ed.) Blackwell Publishing Ltd. Iowa, USA. p. 152-161.

Viviano, K.R. (2013) Update on immununosuppressive therapies for dogs and cats. Vet Clin North Am Small Anim Pract. 30;43: 1149-70.

Weinshilboum, R.M., Raymond, F.A., Pazmino, P.A. (1978) Human erythrocyte thiopurine methyltransferase: radiochemical microassay and biochemical properties. Clin Chim Acta. 2;85: 323-33.

White, S.D., Rosser, E.J. Jr., Ihrke, P.J., Stannard, A.A. (1984) Bullous pemphigoid in a dog: treatment with six-mercaptopurine. J Am Vet Med Assoc. 15;185: 683-6.

White, S.D., Rosychuk, R.A., Outerbridge, C.A., Fieseler, K.V., Spier, S., Ihrke, P.J., Chapman, P.L. (2000) Thiopurine methyltransferase in red blood cells of dogs, cats, and horses. J Vet Intern Med. 1;14: 499-502.

Wolff, S.M., Goodman, H.C. (1963) Effect of purine antimetabolites on serum globulins in the rabbit. Proc Soc Exp Biol Med. 1;112: 416-9.

Wu, Y., Cai, B., Feng, W., Yang, B., Huang, Z., Zuo, C., Wang, L. (2014) Double positive CD4+ CD8+ T cells: key suppressive role in the production of autoantibodies in systemic lupus erythematosus. Indian J Med Res. 140: 513-9.

Zuckermann, FA. (1999) Extrathymic CD4/CD8 double positive T cells. Vet Immunol Immunopathol. 15;72: 55-66.

Zuckermann, FA, Husmann, R.J. (1996) Functional and phenotypic analysis of porcine peripheral blood CD4/CD8 double-positive T cells. Immunology. 87: 500-12.

21

Effects of methylphenidate on the mice adrenal glands and lymphoid organs: Results of histochemical, histometrical and histopathological investigations

Fazelipour, S.[1*], Kiaei, M.[2], Adhami Moghadam, F.[3], Tootian, Z.[4], Sheibani, M.T.[4], Gharahjeh, M.R.[5]

[1]*Department of Anatomy, Islamic Azad University, Tehran Medical Sciences Branch, Tehran, Iran*

[2]*Pharmacist, Islamic Azad University, Tehran, Iran*

[3]*Department of Ophthalmology, Islamic Azad University, Tehran Medical Sciences Branch, Tehran, Iran*

[4]*Department of Basic Sciences, Faculty of Veterinary Medicine, University of Tehran, Tehran, Iran*

[5]*Medical Student, Islamic Azad University, Tehran Medical Sciences Branch, Tehran, Iran*

Key words:

adrenal gland, histopathology, lymphoid organs, methylphenidate, morphometry

Correspondence

Fazelipour, S.
Department of Anatomy, Islamic Azad University, Tehran Medical Sciences Branch, Tehran, Iran

Email: simin_Fazelipour@ yahoo.com

Abstract:

BACKGROUND: Considering the wide administration of methylphenidate and also its immunosuppressive effects on different organs, the importance of related microscopic studies is obvious. **OBJECTIVES:** Determining histological effects of methylphenidate on adrenal glands and lymphatic organs in mice. **METHODS:** A total number of 30 adult male Balb/C mice were provided, weighed and divided into one control and two experimental groups. The control group received water by gavages once a day, for 40 days. The experimental groups were orally administered MPH hydrochloride (2mg/kg and 10mg/kg body weight,) respectively. Animals were anesthetized and blood samples were collected through cardiac puncture for analysis of blood cells. Spleen, thymus, lymph nodes and adrenal glands were removed and processed for microscopic studies through hematoxylin and eosin staining. Spleen samples were processed for plasma cell count and staining (label antibody CD138*). The data were analyzed using analysis of variance (ANOVA) and $p < 0.05$ was considered significant. **RESULTS:** The changes in lymphoid organs provided morphological evidence for MPH induced immune suppression. Our findings showed increase in the number of megakaryocytes in spleen, neutrophils of peripheral blood and thickness in capsule of thymus and lymph node. Also, thickening of the adrenal cortex and medulla, decrease in the reticularis layer of adrenal cortex and medulla of thymus and decreasing lymphocytes in peripheral blood were significantly observed in experimental groups. Moreover, there were significant changes in serum cortisol. **CONCLUSIONS:** Regarding the resulted data indicating some pathologic, inhibitory and suppressive roles of methylphenidate on immune system and the studied organs, it is suggested that caution should be considered in prescription of this medication.

Introduction

Methylphenidate hydrochloride is one of the most frequently prescribed pediatric drugs for the treatment of attention deficit hyperactivity disorder. Besides its well-known addictive properties, amphetamine (AMPH) was found to influence the immune functions as a potent immunosuppressor. AMPH and its derivatives (eg. 3, 4- metylendodioxymethamphetamine and fenfluramine) cause a decrease in leukocyte and lymphocyte numbers in the peripheral blood (Freire-Garabal et al., 1991; Connor, 2004; Pacific et al 2001).

Amphetamines are found to suppress cytokine and antibody production, lymph proliferative responses, as well as to decrease in natural killer cells cytotoxicity and induction of cytotoxic T lymphocytes (Freire-Garabal et al., 1991; Connor, 2004; Nunez –Iglesias et al 1996; Richards et al., 2014).

It has been suggested that AMPH can act either directly on peripheral cells or indirectly by affecting neuroendocrine pathway. Acute and chronic AMPH administration also could cause a marked stimulation of the hypothalamic– pituitary – adrenal axis and sympathetic nervous system resulting in the elevation of glucocorticoids (cortisol) and catecholamines (epinephrine and norepinephrine) levels (Wrona et al., 2005; Seiden et al., 1993; Ruginsk et al., 2011; Zuloaga et al., 2015). Glucocorticoids and catecholamine are known to have strong immunomodulating properties (McEwen et al., 1997; Friedman and Irwin 1997).

It has been shown that in vitro effects of glucocorticoids are immunosuppressive, however, it is becoming increasingly evident that the in vivo effects of glucocorticoids are frequently different from in vitro treatment or treatment with synthetic glucocorticoids such as dexamethasone (Fleshner et al., 2001).

Cytogenetic effects have been observed in peripheral lymphocytes in children treated with MPH for 3 months raising questions about the genetic toxicity of this compound. MPH has been found negative in most genetox studies performed; however, no in vitro chromosome aberration data in human lymphocytes has been reported. A chromosomal aberration study in cultured human peripheral lymphocytes has shown that d, 1-methylphenidate (MPH, Ritalin) in concentrations up to 10 Mm neither induced structural nor numerical chromosome abnormalities (Suter et al., 2006).

Bryant et al. implanted 75 mg morphine pellets into mice and observed marked atrophy and reduced cellularity of the spleen and thymus, and an attenuated lymphocyte proliferative response to T-and B-cell mitogens, concavalin-A and bacterial lipopolysaccharide (LPS), respectively (Bryant et al., 1987).

AMPH injection has produced differential effects on leukocyte populations in the peripheral blood. It has also induced a marked lymphopenia together with an increase in LGL- NK cell number, (lymphocyte subset) as well as an increase in granulocyte and monocyte numbers. The total number of WBC remained unaffected. In the spleen, AMPH- induced changes were more uniform – all the leukocyte populations were decreased. Parallel to LGL number increase, NKCC was enhanced in the peripheral blood after injection of AMPH (Schedlowski et al., 1993; Gagnon et al., 1992; Witt et al., 2008).

Proliferation of human peripheral blood

mononuclear leukocytes (PBML) is measured in the presence or absence of amphetamines, and has revealed that the abuse of amphetamines, especially the designer drugs, may adversely affect the activity of immunoregulatory cells and might lead to a compromised immune system in amphetamine abuser (Gagnon et al., 1992).

Opioids and opioid agents are known to have profound immune suppressive effects. Results of the functional assays have shown that acute morphine administration inhibits peripheral blood lymphocyte activity and causes a definite decline in the peripheral blood lymphocyte counts in the rat (Flores et al., 1995; Liang et al., 2016).

The aim of the present study was to determine overall effect of methylphenidate on immune system. The assessments were based on histological and histochemical evaluation in the mice lymphoid organs. In order to investigate the indirect pathway related to the effects of methylphenidate on the adrenal cortex, its histological structure was investigated histometrically.

Materials and Methods

Animals and experimental design: Thirty male adult Balb/C mice, at three months of age and weighing 25-30 g, were randomly divided into 3 groups of 10 animals each. The animals were housed individually in the cages located in a pathogen free, temperature and humidity-controlled colony room which was maintained under a 12 hours day–night illuminating cycle with free access to food and water. Prior to the experiment, the animals were prepared for manipulations during a 1 week acclimatization in the Experimental Medical Research and Application Center of the Faculty of Medicine, Islamic Azad University.

The animals in the first group served as controls and received water without drug. Experimental groups received 2mg/kg and 10mg/kg body weight MPH respectively, as gavages for 40 days (Fazelipour et al., 2014).

WBC and leukocyte subsets: At the end of the administration period, blood samples from the hearts of the animals were taken into heparinized (100 IU heparin/ml blood) tubes. From each sample, four blood films were prepared, air dried and stained with Gimsa. Total WBC counts were determined using the hematology analyzer. The percentages of lymphocytes, granulocytes, and monocytes were determined by counting 200 WBC with a microscope Gimsa staining. The number of each leukocyte subset was calculated as WBC number × percentage of individual leukocyte subset.

Histological and Histochemical studies: The animals were sacrificed by cervical dislocation and spleens, thymuses, adrenal glands and lymph nodes were removed. Each sample was placed in 10% buffered formalin. Following the fixation, the tissue samples were processed using routine histological techniques. The spleen samples were fixed in alcoholic formalin and processed for plasma cell staining (label antibody CD 138*) (Dako-Denmark) and then splenic plasma cell counting.

For immunohistochemistry procedure, paraffin blocks were sectioned at 3 microns and after several hydration steps by H2O2 and alcohol, usage of antibody including secondary antibody as administered was implemented. In this method the dilution rate of 1:50 has been used.

Splenic plasma cells in unit area $(1.44 \times 10^4 \mu m^2$ tissue area) were determined by counting in 10 randomly selected subcapsular white pulp regions using an ocular square micrometer and the results were expressed as cell count/ unit area (pc/UA). Histometrical measurements on the spleens, adrenal glands and thymuses were done with the aid of an ocular linear micrometer. For this purpose, 10 tissue semi- thin sections, 5μm, were taken from each animal and the values were expressed as Mean ± SD.

Hormone analysis: Blood samples were collected from the hearts of all animals on day 40 after treatment and then serum specimens collected from these samples were frozen at -20 °C. After collection of all specimens, serum levels of cortisol were measured using ELFA (Enzyme Linked Fluorescent Assay) technique (Fardavard Company-France).

Statistical analysis: The results are presented as mean±SD. One way analysis of variance (ANOVA) followed by the post-hoc Tukey test were used for the statistical analysis and a value of $p < 0.05$ was considered significant.

Results

Spleen: Mean splenic plasma cell count of the MPH treated animals was lower than those of the controls ($p < 0.05$) (Table 1) (Fig. 1). Splenic megakaryocyte counts were relatively increased in the treatment group (Table 1) (Fig. 2).

Thymus: Lymphoid tissue of the thymus is organized as a dense cellular cortex with lesser cellular medulla. The thickness of the capsules was increased significantly ($p < 0.05$), though for the medulla it was decreased significantly ($p < 0.05$). Hassal corpuscles were rarely seen in the thymic medulla (Table 1) (Fig. 3).

Mesenteric lymphatic nodes: Mesenteric lymphatic nodes of the control group had larger cortical areas which were occupied by lymphoid follicles, paracortical zones formed by lymphatic cords and medullary areas containing large lymphatic sinuses. Some of the sinuses were with lymphocytes (Fig. 4). The thickness of the capsules of lymph nodes was significantly increased in treated groups ($p < 0.05$) (Table1).

Peripheral Blood: Percentage of the peripheral blood lymphocytes was declined significantly ($p < 0.05$). Significant ($p < 0.05$)) increases were also observed in neutrophil cell ratio of the methylphenidate treatment group (Table 2).

Adrenal glands: Adrenal glands of the control animals showed typical morphology with a larger cortical area and a centrally located medulla region. Overall thickness of adrenal cortex was increased in the experimental group compared to those of the controls. Statistical analysis showed that methylphenidate with different doses could increase thickness of the glomerulosa and fasciculate layers of the adrenal cortex, and decrease the reticularis layer. On the other hand, the thickness of capsule and also the medullary layer were increased significantly in the experimental groups (10 mg/kg) compared to those of the control group ($p < 0.05$). Significant changes in serum cortisol were observed in the MPH treated animals, however, no significant histopathological changes were seen in control specimens ($p < 0.05$) (Table 3).

Discussion

Methylphenidate hydrochloride is one of the most frequently prescribed pediatric drugs for the treatment of attention deficit

Table 1. The histometric characteristics of lymphoid organs in different groups. Group 1 mice received 2 mg/kg water. Groups 2 and 3 were treated with 2 mg/kg and 10 mg/kg MPH. respectively. The values from seven animals are expressed as mean ± SD. Different superscript letters in the same rows indicate a significant difference, p<0.05. PC/UA: plasma cell count/unit (1.44.104μm2) tissue area; MC/UA: Megakaryocyte count/unit (1.44.104 μm2) tissue area; TCT, Thymic capsule thickness; TM: Thymic Medulla; CD: capsule diameter.

Organs/parameters	Group 1	Group 2	Group 3
Spleen			
PC/UA	23.08±9.90[a]	9.67±4.43[b]	1.23±0.38[c]
MC/UA	0.42±0.27[a]	0.63±0.22[a]	2.46±1.30[b]
Thymus			
TCT(μm)	115.49±47.19[a]	281.39 ±77.70[b]	317.98±105.019[c]
TM (μm)	21969.83±86[a]	16342.41[b]	18479.58[c]
Lymph node			
CD (C/UA)	129,6±23.56[a]	363.41±86.18[b]	267.18±59.621[c]

Table 2. The Peripheral blood cells. Group 1: mice received water without drug. Group 2 and 3 were treated with 2 and 10 mg/kg MPH, respectively. The values from seven animals are expressed as mean ±SD. Different superscript letters in the same rows indicate a significant difference, p<0.05.

Organs/parameters	Group 1	Group 2	Group 3
Neutrophil			
(count/unit)	9.33± 4.13[a]	25.33± 10.25[b]	13.33 ± 3.20[a]
Lymphocyte			
(count/unit)	88.33± 4.80[a]	74.33 ± 9.99[b]	83.33 ± 3.88[a]
Monocyte			
(count/unit)	1± 0.89[a]	0[a]	0.67± 1.63[a]
Eosinophil			
(count/unit)	1.5± 1.22[a]	0.33± 0.81[a]	1.67± 1.96[a]

Table 3. The histometric characteristics of adrenal gland and cortisol in different groups. Group 1: mice received water without drug. Group 2 and 3 were treated with 2 and 10 mg/kg MPH, respectively. The values from seven animals are expressed as mean ±SD values. Different superscript letters in the same rows indicate a significant difference, p<0.05. ZGL: zona glomerulosa layer, ZFL: zona fasciculata layer, ZRL: zona reticularis layer, ML: Medullary layer.

Organs/parameters	Group 1	Group 2	Group 3
Capsule (μm)	15.42±2.43[a]	9.06±2.70[b]	14.64±5.50[a]
ZGL (μm)	28.28±7.70[a]	31.70±6.36[a]	47.76±10.23[b]
ZFL (μm)	109.84±26.99[a]	194.26±82.26[b]	210.08±40.99[b]
ZRL (μm)	172.97±52.43[a]	83.44±17.20[b]	114.78±32.12[b]
ML (μm)	918.45±123.99[a]	924.22±286.56[a]	996.60±243.47[b]
Cortisol (μg/dl)	2.95 ±1.12[a]	5.23 ±2.14[b]	7.1 ±2.94[c]

hyperactivity disorders.

From the results of the study it could be deduced that amphetamines as methylphenidate, can influence the peripheral blood and make significant changes in the number of leukocytes compared to the control group. Our study indicated that the number of lymphocytes, involved in immune functions, showed a significant decrease and the number of neutrophils was increased significantly compared to the control group, whereas the total percentage of leukocytes remained unaffected.

In a study by Gagnon et al. the effect of amphetamines on proliferation of leuko-

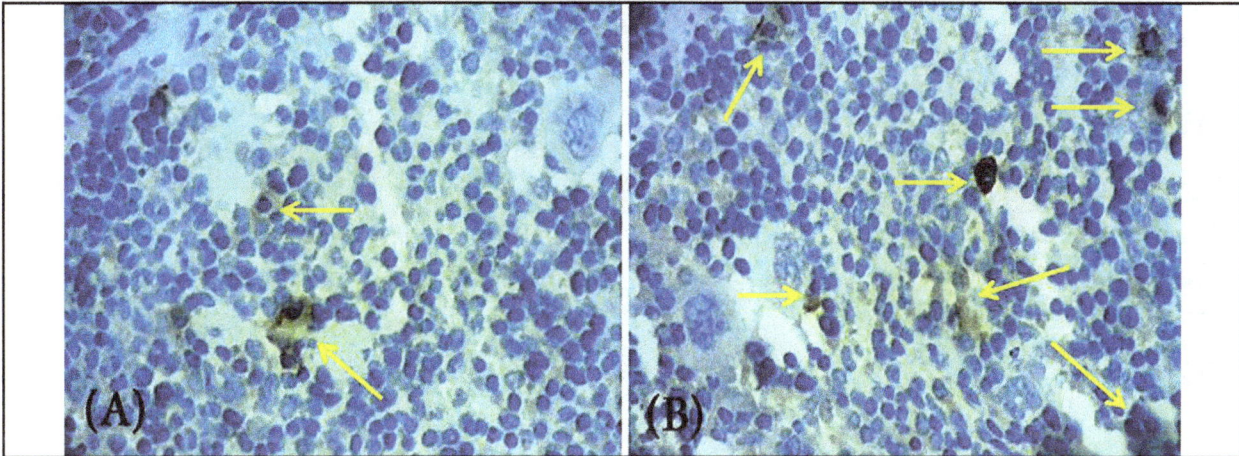

Figure 1. Photomicrograph of spleen (H&E, ×400); (A): Plasma cells, shown and stained with CD 138 antibody (arrows), in control group (B): Increased plasma cells, stained with CD 138 antibody (arrows), in experimental groups.

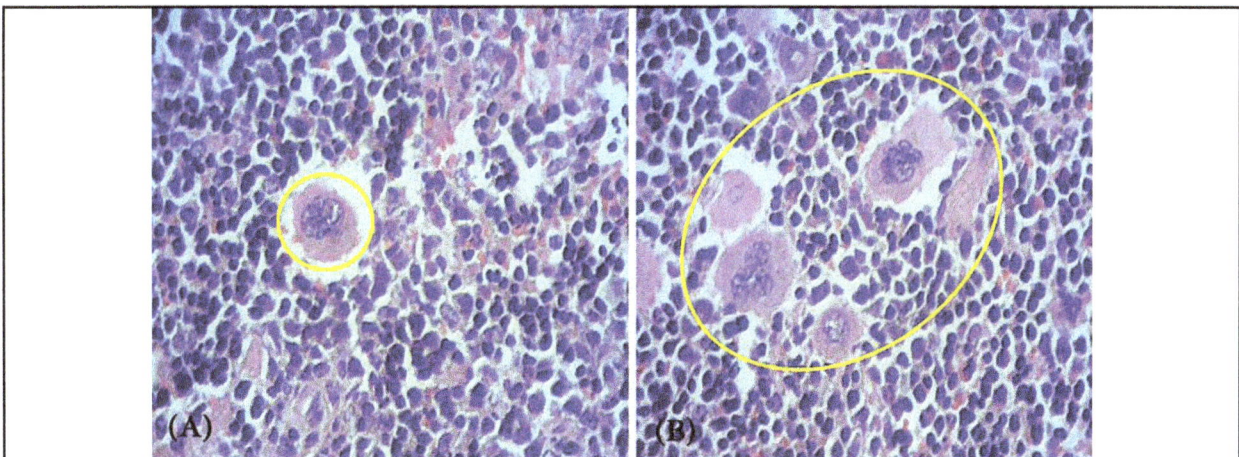

Figure 2. (A): Photomicrograph of a megakaryocyte (circle), in control group (H&E, ×400). (B): Photomicrograph of more megakaryocytes (ellipsoid), in experimental groups (H&E, ×400).

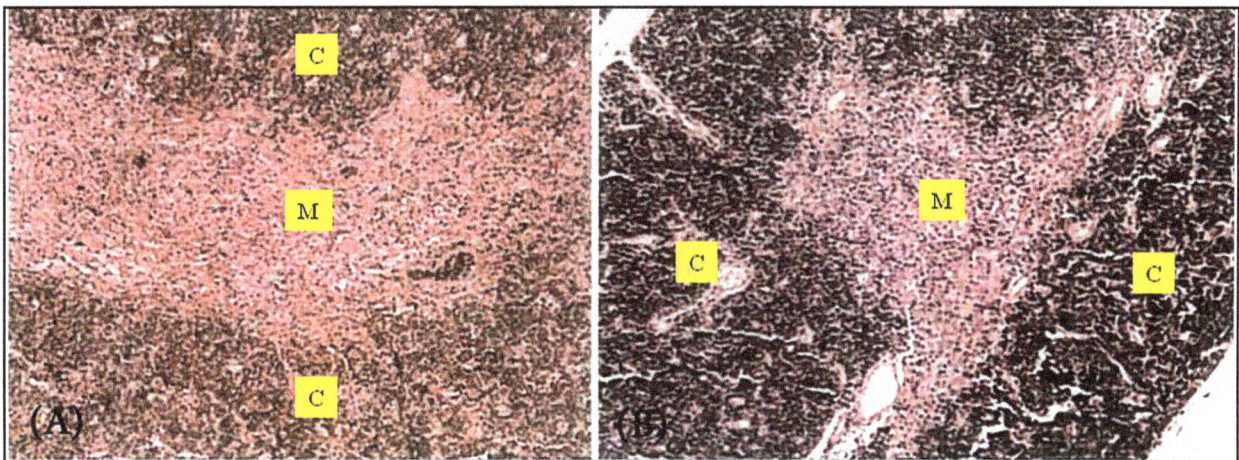

Figure 3. Photomicrograph of a thymic lobule (H&E, ×100); (A): Medullary thymus in control group with large medullary region (M); cortex (C); (B): More limited medullary region (M) in experimental groups; cortex (C).

cytes has been shown. Also different studies show a variety of effects on leukocytes of the peripheral blood and similar results have been reported by other investigators. Many studies have revealed that amphetamines can affect proliferation of immune

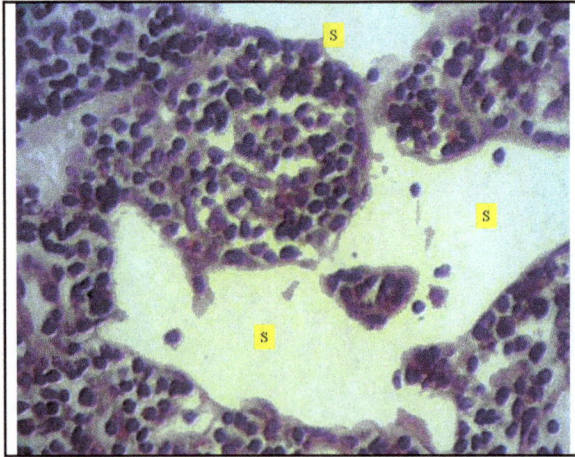

Figure 4. Photomicrograph of lymph node (H&E, ×400); Dilatation in medullary sinuses of lymph node (S) in experimental groups.

cells in other organs (Gagnon et al.,1992; Bredholt et al., 2013).

It has been stated that methylphenidate structurally resembles cocaine, a narcotic, and it is expected to have a preventive effect on immune system (Rofael et al., 2003).

Immunosuppression could be done by a variety of mechanisms which, besides the decrease of leukocytes, it could be through increasing catecholamines (Schedlowski et al.,1996).

Our study indicated that methylphenidate could influence the adrenal gland inducing thickness of zona glumerolosa and zona fasciculata in the adrenal cortex. The significant increase in the thickness of zona fasciculata indicated increase in the corticosteroids and subsequently significant increase in the cortisol, and subsequent suppression of the immune system.

Moreover, the thickness of medulla of the adrenal gland, responsible for synthesis and secretion of catecholamines showed a significant increase compared to the control group, which it was in turn another factor in suppression of the immune system in the present study. The serum cortisol level in experimental groups showed a significant

increase which could be an indicator of suppression in the immune system due to its inhibitory effect on proliferation of lymphocytes. This was in agreement with another study that showed effects of cocaine, with a similar structure to methylphenidate, on the adrenal gland and increase in the cortisol that induced suppression of the immune system (Rofael et al., 2003).

In the present study a significant decrease in the number of splenic plasma cells with a pattern of greater decrease in higher doses was seen. On the other hand, a significant increase in the number of megakaryocytes in spleen was observed. This increase showed that hematopoiesis could take place outside the bone marrow.

From the results of this study, preventive effect of methylphenidate on immunity could be deduced by decrease in plasma cells and also decrease in lymphocytes in different lymphatic organs.

Also, a study on the effect of morphine on the adrenal gland with similar findings to methylphenidate has been reported (Salback et al., 2001; Vinson and Brennan., 2013).

Investigations have shown that the effects of different drugs, opioids and methylphenidate on the immune system could be induced through three mechanisms including: Direct effect of these substances on immune cells in peripheral blood, effect on hypothalamic pituitary adrenal axis which indirectly induces cortisol increase and 3 activating sympathetic nervous system which causes circulating levels of epinephrine from the adrenal medulla as well as norepinephrine from sympathetic nerve terminal leading to increase in the catecholamines (Wang et al., 2002).

In other studies increase in the catecholamines due to usage of amphetamines has been observed. Methylphenidate could also affect immune cells in different organs by preventing their proliferation.16 Therefore, the present study indicated that methylphenidate influenced the spleen by significant decrease in plasma cells. Considering the spleen as the largest lymphatic organ and the only responsible organ for blood filtration, and so providing defense against blood antigens and microorganisms, reduction of plasma cells might represent an immuno-suppression.

On the other hand, significant increase in megakaryocytes in spleen, indicating a pathologic condition, implies inhibitory role of methylphenidate on immune system function. Also, increased catecholamine release has been associated with suppression of natural killer cell function and altered lymphocyte function (Schedlowski et al., 1993).

An analysis of the effects of amphetamine on proenkephalin-derived peptides in brain areas and immune cells in rats showed that acute as well as a repeated amphetamine treatment decreased the concanavalin-A-induced lymphocyte proliferation, concomitantly with an increase of free metenkephalin in nucleus accumbens, prefrontal cortex, spleen, thymus and splenic macrophages (Assis et al., 2006).

The possibility that the adrenergic system may stimulate the NK cells activity in the peripheral blood was confirmed by the studies of Schedlowski et al. (1993) and Benshop et al. (1997). Moreover, treatment with β-adrenoreceptor antagonist inhibits an increase in both circulating NK cells and NKCC elicited by stress or cathecolamine infusion (Glac et al., 2006).

The present study showed that lymphoid tissue of the cortex in thymus was denser with fewer cellular portions than medulla. Besides, the thickness was increased in capsule while decreased in medullar region in the experimental groups due to effect of amphetamines on thymus. In lymph nodes also the thickness of capsule in experimental groups compared to the control group due to the effect of amphetamines was observed. In conclusion, it could be suggested that caution should be considered in prescription of amphetamines due to their effects on proliferation of immune cells in various organs, peripheral blood and also on the most defensive organ against blood pathogens i.e. spleen and possibly substitution with other medications.

Acknowledgments

We would like to thank Dr. Omid Zehtab-var for his contributions.

References

Assis, MA., Collino, C., Flguerola, ML., Sotomayor, C., Cancela, L.M. (2006) Amphetamine triggers an increase in met-enkephalin simultaneously in brain areas and immune cells. J Neuroimmunol. 178: 62-75.

Benshop, RJ., Schedlowski, M., wienecke, H., Jacobs, R., Schmidt, RE. (1997) Adrenergic control of natural killer cell circulation and adhesion. Brain Behav Immune. 11: 321-332.

Bredholt, T., Ersvær, E., Erikstein, BS., Sulen, A., Reikvam, H., Aarstad, HJ., Johannessen, AC., Vintermyr, OK., Bruserud, O., Gjertsen BT. (2013) Distinct single cell signal athinone, cathine or norephedrine. Pharmacol Toxicol. 14: 35.

Bryant, HU., Bernton, EW., Holadyj, W. (1987) Immunosuppressive effects of chronic morphine treatment in mice. Life Sci. 41: 1731-1738.

Connor, TJ. (2004) Methylenedioxymethamphetamine (MDMA), (Ecstasy): a stressor on the immune system. Immunology. 111: 357-367.

Fazelipour, S., Tootian, Z.,Ghahri, SZ. (2014) Evaluation of histopathologic and histomorphometric changes of testicular tissue and gonadotropin levels following consumption of methylphenidate in male mice. Turk J Med Sci. 44: 1301-1309.

Fleshner, M., Deak, T., Nguyen, KT., Watkins, LR., Maier, SF. (2001) Endogenous glucocorticoids play a positive regulatory role in the anti keyhole limpet hemocyanine in vivo antibody response. J Immunol. 166: 3813-3819.

Flores, LR., Wahl, SM., Bayer, BM. (1995) Mechanisms of morphine induced Immunosuppression: Effect of acute morphine administration on lymphocyte trafficking. J Pharmacol Exp Ther. 272: 1246-1251.

Freire-Garabal, M., Balboa, JL., Nunez, MJ., Castano, MT., llovo, JB., Fernandez-Rial, JC., Belmonte, A. (1991) Effect of amphetamine on T-cell immune response in mice. Life Sci. 49: 107- 112.

Friedman, EM., Irwin, MR. (1997) Modulation of immune cell function by the autonomic nervous system. Pharmacol Ther. 74: 27-28.

Gagnon, L., Lacroix, F., Chan, J., Buttar, HS. (1992) In vitro effects of designer amphetamines on human peripheral blood mononuclear leukocytes proliferation and on natural killer cell activity. Toxicol Lett. 63: 313-319.

Glac, W., Borman, A., Badtke, P., Stojek, W., Orlikowska, A., Tokarski, J. (2006) Amphetamine enhances natural killer cytotoxic activity via β-adrenergic mechanism. J Physiol Pharmacol. 57: 125-132.

Liang, X., Liu, R., Chen, C., Ji, F., Li, T (2016) Opioid System Modulates the Immune Function: A Review. Transl Perioper Pain Med. 1: 5-13.

McEwen, BS., Biron, CA., Brunson, KW., Bulloch, K., Chambers, WH., Dhabhar, FS., Goldfarb, RH., Kitson, RP., Miller, AH., Spencer, RL., Weiss, JM. (1997) The role of adrenocorticoids as modulators of immune function in health and disease: neural, endocrine and immune interactions. Brain Res Rev. 23: 79-133.

Nunez –Iglesias, MJ., Castro- Bolano, C., Losada, C., Pereiro-Raposo, MD., Riveiro, P., Sánchez-Sebio, P., Mayán-Santos, JM., Rey-Méndez M., Freire-Garabal, M. (1996) Effect of amphetamine on cell mediated immune response in mice. Life Sci. 58: 29-33.

Pacifici, R., Zuccaro, P., Farré, M., Pichini, S., Di Carlo, S., Roset, PN., Ortuño, J., Pujadas, M., Bacosi, A., Menoyo, E., Segura, J., de la Torre, R. (2001) Effect of repeated doses of MDMA (ecstasy) on cell- mediated immune response in humans. Life Sci. 69: 2931-2941.

Richards, JR., Farias, VF., Clingan, CS. (2014) Association of leukocytosis with amphetamine and cocaine use. Sci World J. 22: 1-7.

Rofael, HZ., Turkall, RM., Abdel-Rahman, MS., (2003) Effect of ketamine on cocaine –induce immunotoxicity in rats. Int J Toxicol. 22: 343-358.

Ruginsk, SG., Uchoa, ET., Elias, LL., Antunes-Rodrigues, J., Llewellyn-Smith, IJ. (2011) Hypothalamic cocaine- and amphetamine-regulated transcript and corticotrophin releasing factor neurons are stimulated by extracellular volume and osmotic changes. Neuroscience. 186: 57-64.

Salback, A., Celik, I., Karabulut, AK., Ozkan, Y., Uysal, II., Cicekcibasi, AE. (2001) Effects of morphine on the rat lymphoid organs and adrenal glands: results of enzyme histochemical and histometric investigations. Rev Med Vet. 152: 691-698.

Schedlowski, M., Falk, A., Rohne, A., Wagner,

TO., Jacobs, R., Tewes, U., Schmidt, RE. (1993) Catecholamines induce altrations of distribution and activity of human natural killer (NK) cells. J Clin Immunol. 13: 344-351.

Schedlowski, M., Hosch, W., Oberbeck, R., Benschop, RJ., Jacobs, R., Raab, HR., Schmidt, RE. (1996) Catecholamines modulate human NK cell circulation and function via spleen-independent β-2-adrenergic mechanism. J Immunol. 156: 93-99.

Schedlowski, M., Jacobs, R., stratmann, G., Richter, S., Hädicke, A., Tewes, U., Wagner, TO., Schmidt, RE. (1993) Changes of natural killer cells during acute psychological stress. J Clin Immunol. 13: 119-126.

Seiden, LS., Sabol, KE., Ricaurte, GA. (1993) Amphetamine: effect on catecholamine systems and behavior. Ann Rev Pharmacol Toxicol. 33: 639-677.

Suter, W., Martus, HJ., Elhajouji, A. (2006) Methylphenidate is not clastogenic in cultured human lymphocyte and in the mouse bone –marrow micronucleus test. Mutat Res. 607: 153-159.

Vinson, GP., Brennan, GH. (2013) Addiction and the adrenal cortex. Endocr Connect. 2: R1-R14.

Wang, J., charboneau, R., Balasubramanian, S., Barke, RA., Loh, HH., Roy, S. (2002) The immunosuppressive effects of chronic morphine treatment are partially dependent on corticostrone and mediated by the μ-opioid receptor. J Leukoc Biol. 71: 782-790.

Witt, KL., Shelby, MD., Itchon-Ramos, N., Faircloth, M., Kissling, GE., Chrisman, AK., Ravi, H., Murli, H., Mattison, DR., Kollins, SH. (2008) Methylphenidate and amphetamine do not induce cytogenetic damage in lymphocytes of children with ADHD. J Am Acad Child Adolesc Psychiatry. 47: 1375-83.

Wrona, D., Sukiennik, L., Jurkowski, MK., Jur-

kowlaniec, E., Glac, W., Tokarski, J. (2005) Effect of amphetamine on NK- related cytotoxicity in rats differing in locomotor reactivity and social position. Brain Behav Immun. 19: 69-77.

Zuloaga, DG., Jacobskind, JS., Raber, J. (2015) Methamphetamine and the hypothalamic-pituitary-adrenal axis. Front Neurosci. 9: 178.

Permissions

All chapters in this book were first published in IJVM, by Faculty of Veterinary Medicine of University of Tehran; hereby published with permission under the Creative Commons Attribution License or equivalent. Every chapter published in this book has been scrutinized by our experts. Their significance has been extensively debated. The topics covered herein carry significant findings which will fuel the growth of the discipline. They may even be implemented as practical applications or may be referred to as a beginning point for another development.

The contributors of this book come from diverse backgrounds, making this book a truly international effort. This book will bring forth new frontiers with its revolutionizing research information and detailed analysis of the nascent developments around the world.

We would like to thank all the contributing authors for lending their expertise to make the book truly unique. They have played a crucial role in the development of this book. Without their invaluable contributions this book wouldn't have been possible. They have made vital efforts to compile up to date information on the varied aspects of this subject to make this book a valuable addition to the collection of many professionals and students.

This book was conceptualized with the vision of imparting up-to-date information and advanced data in this field. To ensure the same, a matchless editorial board was set up. Every individual on the board went through rigorous rounds of assessment to prove their worth. After which they invested a large part of their time researching and compiling the most relevant data for our readers.

The editorial board has been involved in producing this book since its inception. They have spent rigorous hours researching and exploring the diverse topics which have resulted in the successful publishing of this book. They have passed on their knowledge of decades through this book. To expedite this challenging task, the publisher supported the team at every step. A small team of assistant editors was also appointed to further simplify the editing procedure and attain best results for the readers.

Apart from the editorial board, the designing team has also invested a significant amount of their time in understanding the subject and creating the most relevant covers. They scrutinized every image to scout for the most suitable representation of the subject and create an appropriate cover for the book.

The publishing team has been an ardent support to the editorial, designing and production team. Their endless efforts to recruit the best for this project, has resulted in the accomplishment of this book. They are a veteran in the field of academics and their pool of knowledge is as vast as their experience in printing. Their expertise and guidance has proved useful at every step. Their uncompromising quality standards have made this book an exceptional effort. Their encouragement from time to time has been an inspiration for everyone.

The publisher and the editorial board hope that this book will prove to be a valuable piece of knowledge for researchers, students, practitioners and scholars across the globe.

List of Contributors

Tavakoli, A. and Shafiee, B.
Department of Clinical Sciences, Faculty of Veterinary Medicine, Islamic Azad Univeristy, Garmsar Branch, Garmsar, Iran

Hejazy, M.
Department of Basic Sciences, Faculty of Veterinary Medicine, University of Tabriz, Tabriz, Iran

Koohi, M.K.
Department of Basic Sciences, Faculty of Veterinary Medicine, University of Tehran, Tehran, Iran

Yousefi, M.H.
Department of Anatomy, Faculty of Veterinary Medicine, Semnan University, Semnan, Iran

Norouzian, H.
Department of Clinical Sciences, School of Veterinary Medicine, Lorestan University, Khorramabad, Iran

Dezfoulian, O.
Department of Pathobiology, School of Veterinary Medicine, Lorestan University, Khorramabad, Iran

Hosseini, H.
Department of Clinical Sciences, School of Veterinary Medicine, Islamic Azad University, Karaj, Iran

Chalmeh, A., Pourjafar, M., Nazifi, S. and Zarei, M.R.
Department of Clinical Sciences, School of Veterinary Medicine, Shiraz University, Shiraz, Iran

Imani, H., Baniadam, A., Mosallanejad, B. and Shabani, Sh.
Department of Clinical Science, Faculty of Veterinary Medicine, Shahid Chamran University of Ahvaz, Ahvaz, Iran

Behmanesh, M.A. and Erfani Majd, N.
Department of Histology, Faculty of Veterinary Medicine, Shahid Chamran University, Ahvaz, Iran

Shahriari, A.
Department of Biochemistry, Faculty of Veterinary Medicine, Shahid Chamran University, Ahvaz, Iran

Najafzadeh, H.
Department of Pharmacology and Toxicology,Faculty of Veterinary Medicine, Shahid Chamran University, Ahvaz, Iran

Khanamani Falahatipour, S., Rassouli, A. and Kiani, K.
Department of Pharmacology, Faculty of Veterinary Medicine, University of Tehran, Tehran, Iran

Hosseinzadeh Ardakani Y. and Akbari Javar, H.
Department of Pharmaceutics, Faculty of Pharmacy, Tehran University of Medical Sciences, Tehran, Iran

Zaharei Salehi, T.
Department of Microbiology, Faculty of Veterinary Medicine, University of Tehran, Tehran, Iran

Misaghi, A., Akhondzadeh Basti, A. and Gandomi, H.
Department of Food Hygiene and Quality Control, Faculty of Veterinary Medicine, University of Tehran, Tehran, Iran

Parsaeimehr, M.
Department of Food Hygiene and Quality Control, Faculty of Veterinary Medicine, Semnan University, Semnan, Iran

Zahraee Salehi, T.
Department of Microbiology and Immunology, Faculty of Veterinary Medicine, University of Tehran, Tehran, Iran

Azizkhani, M.
Department of Food Hygiene, Faculty of Veterinary Medicine, Amol University of Special Modern Technologies, Amol, Iran

Taheri Mirghaed, A.
Department of Aquatic Animal Health, Faculty of Veterinary Medicine, University of Tehran, Tehran, Iran

Saberi Afshar, F.
Department of Surgery & Radiology, Faculty of Veterinary Medicine, University of Tehran, Tehran, Iran

Shekarian, M., Baniadam, A. and Avizeh, R.
Department of Clinical Sciences, Faculty of Veterinary Medicin, Shahid Chamran University of Ahvaz, Ahvaz, Iran

Najafzadeh, H.
Department of Basic Sciences, Faculty of Veterinary Medicin, Shahid Chamran University of Ahvaz, Ahvaz, Iran

Pourmehdi, M.
Department of Food Hygiene, Faculty of Veterinary Medicine, Shahid Chamran University of Ahvaz, Ahvaz, Iran

Alishahi, M., Tulaby Dezfuly, Z. and Mohammadian, T.
Department of Clinical Sciences, Faculty of Veterinary Medicine, Shahid Chamran University of Ahvaz, Ahvaz, Iran

Abazari, A.
Graduated from Department of Animal Sciences, University of Mohaghegh Ardabili, Ardabil, Iran

Navidshad, B., Mirzaei Aghjehgheshlagh, F. and Nikbin, S.
Department of Animal Sciences, University of Mohaghegh Ardabili, Ardabil, Iran

Khaki, Z. and Fathipour, V.
Department of Clinical Pathology, Faculty of Veterinary Medicine, University of Tehran, Tehran, Iran

Masoudifard, M.
Department of Radiology and Sonography, Faculty of Veterinary Medicine, University of Tehran, Tehran, Iran

Khadivar, F.
Graduated student, Faculty of Veterinary Medicine, University of Tehran, Tehran, Iran

Shirani, D.
Department of Small Animal Internal Medicine, Faculty of Veterinary Medicine, University of Tehran,Tehran, Iran

Taheri, M.
Dr. Rastegar Laboratories, Faculty of Veterinary Medicine, University of Tehran, Tehran, Iran

Morovvati, H., Adibmoradi, M., Kalantari Hesari, A. and Moradi, H.R.
Department of Basic Sciences, Faculty of Veterinary Medicine, University of Tehran, Tehran, Iran

Mazaheri Nezhad Fard, R.
Division of Food Microbiology, Department of Pathobiology, School of Public Health, Tehran University of Medical Sciences, Tehran, Iran

Nemati, Gh.
Department of Food Hygiene and Quality Control, Faculty of Veterinary Medicine University of Tehran, Tehran, Iran
Nestlé Iran, Agriculture Service Department, Tehran, Iran

Shayan, P.
Department of Parasitology, Faculty of Veterinary Medicine University of Tehran, Tehran, Iran
Research Institute of Molecular Biological System Transfer, Tehran, Iran

Kamkar, A., Akhondzadeh Basti, A. and Noori, N.
Department of Food Hygiene and Quality Control, Faculty of Veterinary Medicine University of Tehran, Tehran, Iran

Eckert, B.
Research Institute of Molecular Biological System Transfer, Tehran, Iran

Ashrafi Tamai, I.
Department of Microbiology, Faculty of Veterinary Medicine University of Tehran, Tehran, Iran

Alishahi, M., Tulaby Dezfuly, Z., Mesbah, M. and Mohammadian, T.
Department of Clinical Sciences, Faculty of Veterinary Medicine, Shahid Chamran University of Ahvaz, Ahvaz, Iran

Alizadeh, S. and Rezaei, M.
Department of Clinical Sciences, Faculty of Veterinary Medicine, Urmia Branch, Islamic Azad University, Urmia, Iran

Veshkini, A.
Department of Clinical Sciences, Faculty of Veterinary Medicine, Tehran Branch, Islamic Azad University, Tehran, Iran

Safaee Firouzabadi, M.S., Haji Hajikolaei, M.R., Baniadam, A. and Ghadrdan Mashhadi, A.R.
Department of Clinical Sciences, Faculty of Veterinary Medicine, Shahid Chamran University of Ahvaz, Ahvaz, Iran

Ghorbanpoor, M.
Department of Pathobiology, Faculty of Veterinary Medicine, Shahid Chamran University of Ahvaz, Ahvaz, Iran

Hassankhani, M. and Aldavood, S.J.
Department of Small Animal Internal Medicine, Faculty of Veterinary Medicine, University of Tehran, Tehran, Iran

Khosravi, A.
Department of Microbiology, Faculty of Veterinary Medicine, University of Tehran, Tehran, Iran

Sasani, F.
Department of Pathology, Faculty of Veterinary Medicine, University of Tehran, Tehran, Iran

Masoudifard, M.
Department of Surgery and Radiology, Faculty of Veterinary Medicine, University of Tehran, Tehran, Iran

Ansari, F.
Iranian Evidence-based Center of Excellence, Tabriz University of Medical Sciences, Tabriz, Iran

Taheri, M.
Dr. Rastegar Research Laboratory, Faculty of Veterinary Medicine, University of Tehran, Tehran, Iran

Fazelipour, S.
Department of Anatomy, Islamic Azad University, Tehran Medical Sciences Branch, Tehran, Iran

Kiaei, M.
Pharmacist, Islamic Azad University, Tehran, Iran

Adhami Moghadam, F.
Department of Ophthalmology, Islamic Azad University, Tehran Medical Sciences Branch, Tehran, Iran

Tootian, Z. and Sheibani, M.T.
Department of Basic Sciences, Faculty of Veterinary Medicine, University of Tehran, Tehran, Iran

Gharahjeh, M.R.
Medical Student, Islamic Azad University, Tehran Medical Sciences Branch, Tehran, Iran

Index